Children and Families in Health and Illness

Marion E. Broome
Kathleen Knafl
Karen Pridham
Suzanne Feetham
Editors

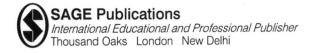

SAGE Publications
International Educational and Professional Publisher
Thousand Oaks   London   New Delhi

For information:

SAGE Publications, Inc.
2455 Teller Road
Thousand Oaks, California 91320
E-mail: order@sagepub.com

SAGE Publications Ltd.
6 Bonhill Street
London EC2A 4PU
United Kingdom

SAGE Publications India Pvt. Ltd.
M-32 Market
Greater Kailash I
New Delhi 110 048 India

Printed in the United States of America

Library of Congress Cataloging-in-Publication Data

Children and families in health and illness / edited by Marion E.
Broome ... [et al.].
    p. cm.
  Includes bibliographical references (p.) and index.
  ISBN 0-8039-5902-8 (cloth : acid-free paper).—
  ISBN 0-8039-5903-6 (pbk. : acid-free paper)
  1. Pediatric nursing. 2. Family nursing. 3. Pediatric nursing—
  Research. 4. Family nursing—Research. I. Broome, Marion.
  RJ245.C477 1998
  610.73'62—dc21   97-45403

98 99 00 01 02 03 10 9 8 7 6 5 4 3 2 1

Acquiring Editor:	Dan Ruth
Editorial Assistant:	Anna Howland
Production Editor:	Sanford Robinson
Copy Editor:	Joyce Kuhn
Production Assistant:	Denise Santoyo
Typesetter:	Danielle Dillahunt
Cover:	Ravi Balasuriya
Indexer:	Teri Greenberg
Print Buyer:	Anna Chin

CONTENTS

Preface   ix

PART I: HEALTH PROMOTION OF CHILDREN AND FAMILIES   1
Karen F. Pridham, Editor

1. Historical Overview of Health Promotion for Children
   and Families in Late 19th- and 20th-Century America   3

   Barbara Brodie

2. Integrative Review of Assessment Models for
   Health Promotion of Children and Their Families   15

   Margaret Grey

3. Integrative Review of Intervention Models for Health
   Promotion for Children and Families   56

   Laura L. Hayman

4. Implications for Practice, Education, and Research in
   Health Promotion of Children and Their Families   80

   Karen F. Pridham

PART II: RESPONSES OF CHILDREN AND FAMILIES TO ACUTE ILLNESS   97

Marion E. Broome, Editor

5. Historical Overview of Responses of Children and
   Their Families to Acute Illness   99

   Judith A. Vessey

6. Integrative Review of Assessment Models for Examining
   Children's and Families' Responses to Acute Illness   115

   JoAnne M. Youngblut

7. Integrative Review of Nursing Intervention Research on
   Acutely Ill Children and Their Families   142

   Janice Denehy, Martha Craft-Rosenberg, and Mary Jo Gagan

8. Acutely Ill Children and Their Families:
   Implications for Research, Practice, and Education   163

   Marion E. Broome

PART III: RESPONSES OF CHILDREN AND FAMILIES TO CHRONIC ILLNESS   177

Kathleen A. Knafl, Editor

9. Historical Overview of Responses of Children and
   Their Families to Chronic Illness   179

   Sandra A. Faux

10. Integrative Review of Assessment Models for Examining
    Children's and Families' Responses to Chronic Illness   196

    Joan K. Austin and Sharon L. Sims

11. Integrative Review of Intervention Research With Children
    Who Have Chronic Conditions and Their Families   221

    Janet A. Deatrick

12. Meeting the Challenges of Chronic Illness for Children
    and Families: Research Implications and Future Directions   236
    Kathleen A. Knafl

PART IV: CHILDREN AND FAMILIES AND
THE HEALTH CARE SYSTEM   247
Suzanne L. Feetham, Editor

13. Historical Overview of Health Care Delivery Models
    for Children and Their Families   251
    Doris J. Biester and Barbara Velsor-Friedrich

14. Community Infrastructures: Principles and Strategies
    for Improving Child Health Services   268
    Susan B. Meister

15. Issues in Health Services Research:
    Children and Families and the Health Care System   280
    Suzanne L. Feetham and Barbara B. Frink

    References   299

    Name Index   339

    Subject Index   351

    About the Contributors   359

PREFACE

The publication of this book culminates several years of planning, dreaming, and hard work on the part of many scholars in nursing of children and their families. The body of knowledge relevant to this area of research had grown steadily over the past few decades and it was time to systematically assess what we know, what it all means, and chart a productive future course for scholarly productivity. With the maturing of the subspecialty there was a critical need to synthesize and analyze where we've been, where we are, and where we need to go.

The book is organized into four parts that we believe best organizes the diversity of research related to the experience of health and illness of children and their families. In each part is a chapter that provides a historical overview, so that readers have a sense of the context within which our investigations with children and their families have evolved. In the first three parts (health promotion, acute illness, and chronic conditions), the historical chapter is followed by two chapters that examine the research related to the nursing of children and their families, with an emphasis on research conducted in the past decade. In the second chapter (assessment models), the methods used to measure the responses of children and their

families to health and illness are described. In the third chapter in each section, findings from studies examining the effectiveness of interventions are synthesized. Review of the second and third chapters makes clear the primary focus of nurse researchers on description of responses. There is yet much work to be done with interventions. Each of these three parts is then closed with a chapter by one of the editors, who reflect on the body of work in the area and share insights about where researchers need to focus in the future. The fourth and final section, health services research, reviews health policy and health and community systems for children and their families and analyzes areas and topics rarely addressed in the nursing literature of children and families.

We believe this book will be of use to a variety of audiences including students, clinicians, nurse scientists, and those in other disciplines. Traditionally, investigators in other fields have informed much of nursing research. It is our hope that by providing a critical synthesis of research done in nursing by such an outstanding cadre of nurse scientists, this book will inform those in other disciplines as well.

Dreams are never fulfilled without the hard work and contributions of many individuals. It was only through the efforts and patience of many scholars in pediatric and family nursing that this book became a reality. Authors applied their creativity and research expertise to the challenging task of examining existing literature and succeeded in making sense of it. Each of these chapters took the author(s) on an adventure. The task of synthesizing the body of knowledge in these various areas was quite new to most of us and we had little direction from our past.

We dedicate this book to all our colleagues in pediatric nursing, including researchers, clinicians, educators, administrators, and students of nursing—tomorrow's scholars! And we owe a debt of gratitude to those children and families who so generously allowed nurse researchers to understand an important (and often very private) part of their world. Finally,

we extend our deep appreciation to one individual in particular, Camille Kolotylo, MS, RN, who spent countless hours editing the final document. Without her dedication, publication of this book would have not been possible.

All extant forces point to a strong mandate and opportunity for nurses to develop, extend, and test their investigations of assessment and intervention models and to construct research-based models that will serve the complexities and challenges of tomorrow's health care systems. Nowhere is this opportunity greater, or the need more compelling, than in the areas of pediatric and family nursing. It is our intent that the ideas expressed in this book will afford nurse scholars and clinicians points of departure, directions, and new domains for future investigations.

PART I

HEALTH PROMOTION OF CHILDREN AND FAMILIES

■ *Karen F. Pridham, Editor*

1

■

HISTORICAL OVERVIEW OF HEALTH PROMOTION FOR CHILDREN AND FAMILIES IN LATE 19TH- AND 20TH-CENTURY AMERICA

■ *Barbara Brodie*

The management of infancy and childhood has an immense influence upon the health, vigor, and continuance of life; and the concurrent testimony of all intelligent men, who have examined the subject, is, that a great portion of debility, disease, premature deaths . . . is attributable to ignorance of physical laws and inattention to the physical wants, in the early years—the formative periods of life.

—Lemuel Shattuck, founder of America's sanitary movement
(1850/1976, p. 102)

Child and family health promotion involves a social movement to preserve, protect, and nourish the lives of American children. The movement found its historical origins in the last quarter of the 19th century, when the plight of immigrants in the nation's overcrowded cities struck a chord among concerned citizens, health professionals, and educators seeking ways to ameliorate social conditions that threatened the life and welfare of children and their families.

In response to the country's high infant mortality rates, the movement began in cities as a campaign to save babies' lives. Through the concerted efforts of health professionals and child welfare advocates, the movement spread beyond the cities and embraced the health needs of mothers and children of all ages. The emergence of health promotion as a social and intellectual field occurred with the contributions of child developmentalists who offered theoretical models to explain the dynamic transformation of infants into mature adults and the crucial role the family played in this process. Throughout the many societal changes of the past 100 years, the field of health promotion has remained steadfastly focused on the special needs of children and their families, thereby contributing to the preservation of children's lives and exerting an immense influence on the health, vigor, and continuance of American life.

■ *Role of Children in Society*

The health of their children has always been of concern to parents, but until the late 19th century, society had little or no interest in the subject. Philip Van Ingren, in his 1921 chronology of the development of infant hygiene in the United States, noted that, as a distinct entity, "the child had hardly been discovered before 1872" (p. 290). Prior to this time, pioneer physicians and educators wrote health advice books offering suggestions on ways to raise children and keep them healthy. In 1836, Ackerley's *Management of Children in Sickness and in Health* offered parents commonsense ways to keep their children well. Such advice as recommending that babies be fed a simple gruel and milk rather than sharing the family breakfast of "fish, perhaps salted and dried, sausages, hot bread or buckwheat cakes and hot coffee" (p. 76) was needed in an era when gastrointestinal disease was a leading cause of infant death.

The abandonment of infants on city streets did stimulate some public response in the early 1800s, leading to the establishment of several foundling homes and orphan asylums. These institutions, however, failed to save children because overcrowding and poor hygiene often led to shockingly high foundling mortality rates (Duffy, 1974). A woeful lack of medical knowledge about children's diseases contrib-

uted to the situation, and it was not until 1855 that the country's first children's specialty hospital was built in Philadelphia (Faber & McIntosh, 1966).

Society's concern for the health of children had changed drastically by the 1880s due to such social changes as industrialization, urbanization, and massive immigration. Cities grew quickly as their populations swelled with immigrants and rural Americans seeking employment and housing. Crowded into filthy and airless tenements, urban poor children, particularly infants, experienced exceedingly high levels of morbidity and mortality. Contagious and infectious diseases accounted for the suffering and deaths of most children. It would be this group of high-risk infants that would spark the birth of the modern child health movement (Smillie, 1955).

"Save the Babies" Campaign

In Chicago and New York City during the 1880s and 1890s, half of the children under 2 years of age and living in tenements did not survive. This exceedingly high mortality rate was due primarily to a severe form of gastroenteritis identified as cholera infantum. Appearing in epidemic proportions during the summer months, it struck quickly, afflicting its young victims with severe vomiting, diarrhea, and generalized weakness. Although its etiology was unknown, physicians suspected that it was a milk-borne disease because breast-fed babies were less susceptible to it than bottle-fed infants (Brodie, 1991).

The need of immigrant women to be employed and the then recent availability of rubber nipples encouraged a shift from breast to bottle feeding among mothers. The inability of city officials to provide clean, safe milk and water to their residents, however, led to the sale of raw, contaminated milk for infant consumption. To stem the resulting high infant mortality rate, concerned health professionals and child welfare advocates initiated a baby-saving movement, focusing first on providing children with clean milk. The campaign for clean milk was based both on the newly discovered scientific germ theory and its implications for the processing of milk and on the reformers' belief that mothers, especially immigrant mothers, were woefully ignorant of how to keep their infants healthy in an urban environment. These beliefs were translated into a public health movement to certify, pasteurize, and distribute safe milk to consumers and a health education movement to educate mothers in ways to feed their children safely (Shaftel, 1978).

The opening in 1893 of a milk depot in New York City where pasteurized milk was sold at cost or given free to indigent children marked a significant milestone in the milk campaign. Nathan Straus (1917), department store owner and humanitarian, subsidized the operation of milk plants and depots and became a national advocate in persuading local and state government officials to assume the responsibility of providing pasteurized milk to their youngest citizens. So successful were his depots that other philanthropic groups opened similar facilities in other cities.

Nurses were added to these milk depot staffs when it was recognized that many immigrant mothers lacked even a rudimentary understanding of how to prepare or store milk safely in their homes and that nurses were effective health teachers. Visiting nursing services, pioneered by Lillian Wald's Henry Street Visiting Nurses Service, had demonstrated that by educating mothers in ways to keep their infants healthy the infant mortality rate could be decreased. Nurses, experts in assessing and providing nursing care to the sick, offered mothers practical suggestions on ways to care for their children when ill and keep them healthy. As milk depot staff nurses, they visited the homes of families who had received pasteurized milk

and instructed the mothers on how to keep the milk cool in ice containers, how to prepare formulas and feed their infants, and about the necessity of domestic and personal hygiene (Barton, 1911). The scope of their health teaching also involved helping mothers adjust to the strangeness of American culture, its language, and city life (Melvin, 1983).

The slow realization that infant and maternal mortality rates could be reduced if mothers received prenatal supervision and were taught how to care for their infants led to the transformation of milk depots into prenatal and well-baby stations. Starting in 1910, physicians were employed by stations to provide infant and pregnant women medical screening and therapy. By 1920, municipal-supported public health departments offered similar maternal and child services in most American cities (Meckel, 1990).

Important to the development of the public health field and the baby-saving movement was the shift in emphasis from a single sanitary concern for clean milk to the education of mothers to be effective caretakers. Through the abilities of nurses to teach new health habits to mothers, the public health field expanded beyond its original goal of improving the sanitation of cities into a new phase of development: health promotion. While infant nutrition would remain fundamental to health promotional activities, the shift also acknowledged that "in the education of the mother in the care of herself and her baby, lies the strongest weapon for fighting infant mortality" (Report of the Executive Secretary, 1912, p. 19).

Infant mortality was thus redefined as a problem of uneducated mothers. Accepting this belief, health workers in infant dispensaries, public health agencies, and fresh air retreats for sick children diligently worked to bring scientific hygiene, nutrition, and health care advice into the lives of American children through their mothers (Meckel, 1990).

School Health Promotion

A second force in shaping the field of health promotion in the early 1900s was the budding school health education movement. Capitalizing on the recent passage of compulsory school attendance laws in most states, education and lay leaders began to explore ways to introduce health concepts into school programs and to address the special needs of poor children.

The involvement of school children in the maintenance of their own health was not a totally new concept. Since the 1870s, influenced by proponents of the European gymnasium movement, outdoor exercise and activities had been included in many school programs in the belief that the sedentary nature of school was detrimental to the development of healthy bodies. Proponents of the new health agenda believed that the value of personal hygiene, dental health, nutritious food, and proper sleep habits should be taught to school children to prepare them to become productive adults. By 1915, some of the more progressive schools included information on sexual hygiene in their health classes for adolescents (Lindsay, 1943).

The needs of immigrant school children, many of whom were malnourished and sick, drew the attention of school reformers who believed that crime, addiction, and violence grew from neglect of children's health problems. As part of the era's social reform efforts, physicians and dentists volunteered their services, and women's groups provided free breakfasts and lunches. Teachers welcomed this help because they knew that the state of the children's health affected their ability to learn (Cohen, 1964).

The introduction of automobiles to city streets in the 1910s saw an alarming increase in childhood accidents. City streets, particularly in tenement districts, doubled as roads for travel and commerce and as children's playgrounds. To prevent the accidental death and injury of children, local parks and school playgrounds were built, and street safety classes were added to the health promotional activities of school programs. Children learned the rules of the road, including understanding traffic lights and looking both ways before crossing a street, so that they might travel safely on the city streets (Zelizer, 1985).

The employment of school nurses in 1902 significantly aided the evolution of the health education movement. Beginning with an experiment devised by Lillian Wald to reduce the high levels of student absenteeism, school nurses demonstrated their effectiveness by detecting and treating children with minor illnesses and by making home visits to help families secure needed medical services (Hawkins, Hayes, & Corliss, 1994). Plagued with similar student health problems, other school systems in the country soon added nurses to their staffs. The addition of nurses to school districts not only helped children receive needed health care but also offered teachers, unprepared to teach health courses, the opportunity to work with nurses in developing health promotional activities. One of the most innovative of these activities was the initiation of "little mothers" clubs for school girls whose families depended on them for the care of their younger siblings. The clubs, which combined health classes and social activities, not only prepared girls to safely care and feed their younger siblings but also provided the girls with parenting skills to care for their own future children (Struthers, 1917).

Sally Lucas Jean, one of the early school nurses in Baltimore, became a national leader in developing the school health movement. Selected in 1914 by the Metropolitan Life Insurance Company to be the consultant for their new School Health Division, Jean contributed to the preparation of the company's child health pamphlets. She traveled throughout the country to work with teachers on using these pamphlets in their daily teaching plans and helped them develop creative health activities. Pageants, games, and local parades, all designed to

instruct children about
dental health, and ways
teaching methods used to
velop new health habits.
Jean served as the first d
Health Organization. This
posed of community lead
public health nurses and
headed a nationwide drive t
teachers keep the country's
and strong (Jean, 1949).

The school health moven
significantly to the advanceme
motional activities in several
added health education to the mi
can schools and enlisted the talent
the task of educating children t
sponsible for their own health ha
its research activities, which focu
to teach children of different age
responsibility for their own health,
mation was added to the body of hea
tion knowledge. The school health
also facilitated a productive relationsl
teachers, public health nurses, and p
that would lead to improvements in t
and welfare of children.

Many national organizations formed in the
first two decades of the 20th century reflect the
growing interest of society in the needs of children, among them the National Association for
the Study of Epilepsy and Care of Epileptics
(1901), the National Congress of Parents and
Teachers (1906), the Society of Mental Health
(1908), the American Home Economics Association (1908), the International Health Board
(1910), the Safety Institute of America (1911),
the National Organization for Public Health
Nursing (1912), the National Child Welfare
Association (1912), and the American Social
Hygiene Association (1914). All of these groups
worked with health personnel, child development experts, and government officials to initiate health surveys and preliminary research
projects and to institute special health promo-

; that would enhance the health of
ans, 1962).
f these organizations, under differ-
re still strong advocates for the
elfare needs of children—for ex-
National Congress of Parents and
now the Parent Teacher Associa-
National Organization for Public
ng is now the Public Health Nurs-
f the American Public Health As-

ic Medicine
ild Development

s awakening awareness that chil-
tuted a distinct group within the
that was worthy of saving also
e rise of pediatric medicine and
lopment experts. Both pediatric
nd the field of child development
rses a broadened base for health
activities. Advances in the field of
gy in the 1870s allowed physi-
he first time, to understand the etiology of children's infectious diseases. Abraham Jacobi, considered the father of pediatrics,
initiated pediatric hospital services in New
York City in 1860 and championed many
welfare campaigns that promoted the health
of children. It would be Dr. Luther Emmett
Holt, however, who would become the most
notable medical child health expert of the
time. Holt, Professor of Pediatrics at the College of Physicians and Surgeons of Columbia
University, published a child care manual in
1894 that became a best-seller. His book, *The
Care and Feeding of Children: A Catechism
for the Use of Mothers and Children's Nurses*
(Holt, 1894/1922), distilled knowledge from
scientific medicine and the field of child development to answer the most commonly
voiced questions of those who raised the na-

tion's children. Revised and expanded numerous times over the next 30 years, his baby book provided basic information on the physical and emotional needs of the developing infant, advice on how to manage common illnesses, and methods that could be used to keep children healthy. To promote infant health, Holt endorsed the prevailing medical belief of the era: that the feeding of the infant must follow a rigid time schedule. Failure to adhere to a feeding schedule was thought to compromise the child's physical maturation and threaten the proper formation of moral character. Echoing society's view that parents were responsible for the proper moral upbringing of their children, Holt advised parents to be loving disciplinarians. Such bad habits as thumb sucking, nail biting, dirt eating, bed wetting, lying, and masturbation were to be quickly prevented if the child was to grow into a mature, productive adult (Holt, 1894/1922).

Holt's belief that the pediatrician should be an active guardian of children's health and a highly skilled medical practitioner was transmitted to colleagues and medical students through his numerous professional publications. His pediatric textbook, *Diseases of Infancy and Childhood,* first published in 1897, incorporated in each of its nine revisions the newest information available in medical science, infant development, and the field of health promotion (Holt, 1897/1933).

The search for knowledge underlying human development captured the intellectual interest of psychologists, who in the 1890s began studying the process by which children are transformed into adults. Employing philosophical and scientific modes of inquiry, child psychologists and, later, psychiatrists generated innovative models to explain the unfolding of children's physical, intellectual, emotional, and social behaviors (Cravens, 1985). One of the first child developmentalists to appear was G. Stanley Hall. After years of study, he postulated that childhood was composed of a series of sequential stages from which the adult emerged. His landmark 1905 publication on the study of adolescents extended the length of childhood to include a turbulent adolescent period. This insightful work, which included several of the social factors that led some adolescents into delinquent behavior, aided school, health, and legal professionals in developing new strategies to promote the emotional and social adjustment of youths (Hall, 1905). His work also led to the establishment of juvenile courts and homes where adolescents in conflict with the law might be rehabilitated.

Arnold Gesell of the Yale Clinic of Child Development began his longitudinal studies on the developmental patterns of thousands of children in 1911. Gesell, both a developmentalist and a physician, refined and elaborated Hall's stage theory of development to include significant sequences or milestones that children achieved at different ages on their way to maturity. Gesell's extensive maturational studies identified behavioral characteristics and developmental tasks of children at various ages (Gesell & Ilg, 1943). For example, children between the ages of 24 and 36 months demonstrate characteristics of stubbornness and negativism. Labeled the "terrible twos" stage of development, the child's behavior in this phase reflects the desire for beginning independence from one's parents. Through his books, movies, teaching, and public lectures, Gesell offered professionals and the public a new appreciation and understanding of the changing nature of the child's personality (Gesell & Ilg, 1943).

■ Initiation of Government Child Health Services

The flow of immigrants into New York, Boston, and Philadelphia in the 1870s overwhelmed the limited sources of health care available to the ill poor. The inability of these cities' almshouses, hospitals, and medical dispensaries to meet the needs of the poor stimulated a number of church and women's groups to employ nurses to provide bedside nursing care to families residing in the tenement districts (Ewen, 1985). The growing numbers of indigent persons, however, especially infants and children soon outstripped these charitable efforts. At this point, concerned citizens, frightened at the alarmingly high infant mortality rates (288 per 1,000 live-born infants died in New York City in 1880), called on city officials to add health services to their public health departments (Bolduan, 1942).

Physicians and nurses, employed on a part-time basis, were sent to schools and tenements to find and care for ill children, but even these efforts proved inadequate to the task. One of the part-time physicians employed in 1901, Dr. Josephine Baker, proved to be a superb children's advocate and an excellent public health administrator. Rising quickly through the ranks of the health department, Baker demonstrated that the employment of full-time nurses to teach mothers how to keep their infants healthy was an effective strategy in reducing the city's infant death rate. By 1908, Baker gained the support of city officials to establish the country's first Bureau of Child Hygiene. This bureau, devoted to the study and preservation of the health of children, would lead the country in inventing, perfecting, and adapting methods of saving children's lives. The success of its program would lead other city health departments to initiate similar programs (Baker, 1939).

Staffed by dedicated physicians and nurses and supported by child welfare activists, the bureau organized a vital statistics department and developed a network of health care facilities needed to keep children alive and well. The network included infant and prenatal health stations, day nurseries for working mothers, children's dispensaries, and a public health nurse service that placed nurses in the homes of children. Each of these services used health promotional materials, written in the different languages of the immigrants served, to educate and encourage mothers to become better caretakers. Crucial to the success of the network was the ability of nurses to identify and gain the cooperation of mothers in the community. To earn mothers' trust, nurses learned to listen carefully to their concerns about their children prior to offering advice. Recognizing that the adoption of their advice was not always possible within the constraining conditions of tenement life, nurses quickly learned to respect a mother's decision to accept or not accept their recommendations. Assured that their decisions and opinions were respected, the mothers adopted many of the new health methods and learned to use the network's resources to solve family problems.

The Children's Bureau

The establishment in 1912 of the federal government's Children's Bureau was a direct outcome of the success rate of health professionals and welfare activists in the cities. Specifically, the idea originated in the experiences of two prominent social reformers of the era, Lillian Wald and Florence Kelley. Wald, a nurse and the director of the Henry Street Settlement House, and Kelly, a lawyer dedicated to improving employment conditions for women and children, believed that the health problems of mothers and children could be resolved only if the federal government become involved. They helped lead a coalition of social activists in convincing the government that the health of children and mothers was crucial to the vitality and social order of the country (Covotsos, 1976). Operating under its legal mandate to investigate and report on all matters pertaining to the welfare of children and child life, the bureau initiated a series of studies that focused on many dimensions of child life. Its innovative studies on infant and maternal mortality and morbidity, juvenile courts, orphanages, and child employment provided the country its first view of the health status of the nation's children.

Infant mortality, its causes and rates, was selected by the bureau as the subject of its first full-scale investigation. Data from official birth and death records and house-to-house canvassing revealed that 75% of neonatal deaths in the 10 communities studied resulted from three major causes: lack of prenatal care, gastrointestinal disorders, and respiratory diseases. The studies also verified what city health officials had learned: by educating mothers in self-care and in infant feeding and care that substantial decreases in infant mortality could be realized (U.S. Department of Labor, 1923).

To spread the gospel of health to rural mothers, the Children's Bureau distributed educational health pamphlets, posters, charts, and flyers. One of its most successful publications was its advice manual, *Infant Care,* published in 1914, that provided mothers basic advice on bathing, clothing, and choice of bedding and on how to lift an infant and care for its eyes, mouth, and ears. Detailed instructions on breast and bottle feeding, on the symptoms of common infant diseases, and when to see a physician added to the usefulness of the manual. It was so popular that from 1914 through 1921 nearly 1.5 million copies were distributed, many of them sent by congressmen to their constituents (Abbot, 1923).

Along with infant information, the Children's Bureau distributed information on prenatal care and the care of preschool- and school-aged children. The advice in the health materials covered child development, nutrition, and nursing care of ill children and the importance of physician guidance and care (Bradbury, 1962).

The popularity of the bureau's educational materials and the number of child care articles and health advice columns appearing in women's magazines of the era indicated American mothers' quest for guidance, which fueled the growth of the health promotion movement for decades.

Studies on the health status of rural mothers and babies from 1913 to 1917 revealed how inaccessible obstetrical and infant medical services were for families. Armed with this information and with the knowledge that over 50% of the nation's population and almost 60% of all children lived in rural areas, the Children's Bureau recommended in 1917 that the federal government help states provide maternal and infant health services to their rural communities (Covotsos, 1976). Public support for the idea grew when it was found that almost 30% of the young men drafted for World War I military services in 1918 were judged physically unfit to serve. A careful study of these unfit draftees emphasized the extent to which diseases during childhood were responsible for the men's damaging defects that, in the opinion of child experts, easily could have been prevented (Baker, 1918). Child advocates used this information to petition Congress to pass the Sheppard-Towner Act, designed to aid states in providing care for needy mothers and children. Although opposition to the legislation from the American Medical Association and powerful states rights advocates slowed its passage through Congress, the Federal Act for the Promotion of the Welfare and Hygiene of Maternity and Infancy (the Act's formal title) became law in 1921 (Mulligan, 1976).

States quickly took advantage of the nation's first grant in-aid health funds and established child hygiene bureaus to develop new health initiatives. State health department public health nurses and physicians, traveling to the most remote regions of their states, initiated infant/preschool and prenatal health clinics and health demonstrations, referred children with problems to physicians, made health visits, and distributed millions of health promotional leaflets. To deal with the rural communities' dependence on midwives, states established midwife educational programs on safe birthing techniques and mailed prenatal information directly to expectant mothers (Kalisch & Kalisch, 1978).

The public's response to this maternal and child health education was enthusiastic. The Children's Bureau reported that many families traveled long distances so that mothers and children could be examined and taught health care. For many mothers and children, these examinations and instructions were the first they had received (U.S. Department of Labor, 1923). Mothers wrote to state health departments thanking them for the health clinics and free pamphlets, noting that they had grown more confident and competent in their parenting skills and less isolated in raising their children (Ladd-Taylor, 1986).

The Sheppard-Towner Act was terminated in 1929, the result of powerful opposition from the American Medical Association, but during its 7-year existence the Act touched the lives of millions of American families. The educational dimensions of the states' programs raised public awareness of the needs of mothers and children for health promotional activities. Practicing physicians and nurses in rural communities, most educated prior to the development of the field of preventive medicine, also used the Children's Bureau's educational materials and consultants to update their knowledge in the new field of health promotion.

For the child welfare activists who dreamed of having the nation commit the necessary resources to provide mothers and children comprehensive health services, the loss of the Sheppard-Towner Act was a setback. The activists, however, did take pride in the nation's decreasing infant mortality rate and in the initiation of health conservation work among preschool rural children. During the Great Depression of the 1930s, the activists again supported the Children's Bureau's successful efforts in persuading Congress to reinstate funds devoted to maternal and child health services through Title V of the 1935 Social Security Act.

The Children's Bureau remained one of the nation's strongest advocates for the health of children for over 50 years. The restructuring of government agencies over the years, however, gradually divested the bureau of responsibility for researching children's health issues and of administering maternal and child health programs. Although no longer an independent bureau, it continues as part of the Department of Health and Human Services.

■ Advances in Preventive Medicine

The recognition that the vitality and economic growth of cities depended on their adoption of public health measures led to the establishment in the 1870s of municipal public health departments. Cities enacted sanitation laws that set the health standards for the quality of their food, milk, and water and established legal codes that governed the disposal of cities' sewage and garbage. Building codes were also enacted to improve cities' housing units. As the public health department came to be viewed as the official guardian of the city's health, the request that it provide health services to indigent infants and mothers appeared to child advocates a logical way to reduce the infant death rate (Duffy, 1992). In fact, the municipal public health departments' interventions effectively lowered cities' infant mortality rates. For example, New York City's infant mortality dropped from 144.4 per 1,000 births in 1906 to 94.6 by 1912—the lowest of any major American city (Larson, 1915).

New knowledge in the recently established field of immunology also contributed significantly to decreasing infant mortality and morbidity rates. In the 1910s, advances in immunology resulted in improvements in the smallpox vaccination and the development of a diphtheria immunization. The promise that the common communicable diseases that plagued and occasionally killed children could be controlled enticed researchers to intensify their efforts to find safe vaccines. By the 1940s, tuberculosis testing and immunizations for diphtheria, pertussis, and tetanus on a recommended age schedule were part of the preventive health care provided all children (Cone, 1979b).

Research in biochemistry beginning in the 1910s uncovered the role of vitamins in human nutrition and led to effective therapeutic and preventive measures for such common children's problems as rickets (vitamin D deficiency) and scurvy (vitamin C deficiency). In the 1920s, nutritional studies revealed children's need for a balanced diet of proteins, fats, carbohydrates, minerals (particularly iron and calcium), and such vitamins as A and the B complexes. The availability of height and weight charts, standardized in the 1930s, provided an effective tool to closely monitor the healthy development of children (Halpern, 1988). The new nutritional knowledge enabled health professionals to teach mothers the importance of providing a healthy diet for their children and preventing such diseases as rickets and obesity.

By the 1940s, vision and hearing screening tests were also part of the preventive health care provided children in physicians' offices and health clinics. These tests helped identify those children who required corrective devices before any developmental delays occurred.

■ *Child Development at Mid-Century*

A wealth of psychological, behavioral, and cognitive development theories and concepts appeared in the 1950s, 1960s, and 1970s. Sigmund Freud's theoretical formulations on the child's early psychological development, with its emphasis on the powerful role that parents, particularly mothers, played in shaping the child's personality, led to new insights into the psychological life of the individual (Hall, 1954). Freud's five-stage psychosexual development theory attempted to explain human development and to uncover reasons for mental illness. Erik Erikson, a follower of Freud, expanded and broadened Freud's theory to incorporate three additional stages that occurred in adult life. His theory also acknowledged the dynamic interactive effects of the family and society on the shaping of the individual. These theories aided parents and professionals in understanding children and in being able to anticipate potential emotional behavior of children at different ages. Erikson's theory also helped professionals respond to parents' questions with answers that were sensitive to each parent's stage of development (Erikson, 1963).

Behavioral theorists viewed the outside world as exerting the most powerful influence on the developing personality. From a behaviorist view, parents' and society's use of rewards or punishments in response to a child's behavior shaped the emerging personality of the child. This theory, although it ignores the inner life of children, including emotions, motivations, and mental prowess, provides additional insight into the shaping of human behavior (Skinner, 1974).

Jean Piaget, a cognitive developmentalist, made another significant contribution to understanding the maturation of the inner mental life of the child. Piaget viewed children as active participants in creating and interpreting the experiences of life. Building on their innate mental reflexes, children, through the processes of assimilation and accommodation, created an intellectual schema that allowed them to develop and process simple ideas into more complex mental thoughts and that contributed to understanding both the self and the outside world. Piaget's theory shed light on the importance of a child's experiences in developing this mental schema (Piaget & Inhelder, 1969).

To some degree, these conceptual views of human development served as a blueprint or map to the child's progression to adulthood. Health professionals incorporated concepts from the theories into their discussions with parents on how to handle their children's acts of disobedience, temper tantrums, and sibling fighting, among other behaviors. This new knowledge also aided professionals in helping parents anticipate and develop methods to avert health problems. For example, accidents, including poisoning, falls, and electrical burns, were now discussed with parents before their children reached the age when their curiosity and ability to ambulate made them prone to such accidents (Dixon & Stein, 1987).

The public's interest in learning more about the development of children was spurred by the post-World War II "baby boom." Between 1946 and 1964, 78 million American infants were born, and society sought new ways to protect their health and meet their educational needs. Parents, particularly mothers, found comfort and security in learning parenting skills from Dr. Benjamin Spock. Following in the popular, simple, and reassuring style of Dr. Holt's advice books, Spock's *Baby and Child,* first published in 1954, incorporated the new psychological developmental theories in his advice on parenting. A later book, *Dr. Spock Talks With Mothers* (Spock, 1964), in keeping with society's new permissive attitude toward children, encouraged parents not to be strict disciplinarians but, rather, to enjoy their children and be comfortable in doing what they thought best for them.

■ Children and Hospitals

The belief that health promotional activities fell outside the scope of clinical practice

of hospital nurses was drastically revised in the mid-1950s. Results of studies done in England on the effects of hospitalization on children radically altered the practice of hospital nurses and physicians. Research findings that documented that children under 4 years of age experienced emotional problems from maternal deprivation stimulated nurses to reexamine the hospital experience for children in their care (Robertson, 1958).

The first change was removal of restrictions on the time when parents could visit their hospitalized children. As nurses became more knowledgeable about child development and about the special need of hospitalized children for their mothers, they encouraged parents to remain with their children. In time, overnight accommodations for parents were made available in hospitals. The introduction of penicillin in the treatment of infections further supported the open visiting policy because the feared chance of cross infection was no longer a danger (Blake & Wright, 1963).

The increased time that parents and nurses spent together fostered a sense of cooperation and alliance in the care of the children. Nurses found opportunities in their interactions with parents to teach diverse health measures such as healthy nutrition, child safety, and ways to deal with siblings' anxiety and fears during the hospitalization period.

Advances in science and technology in the 1970s improved the survival rates of critically ill patients, especially premature infants. To keep pace with the health needs of the growing premature infant, nurses became highly proficient in working with parents to design discharge plans that assured continuity in the infants' care at home. Comprehensive health planning was essential to aid parents in coping with the special needs of the infant, especially the adaptations that had to be made in the family's daily life.

The availability of advanced technology also allowed many chronically ill children to return home to resume their lives. To successfully cope with the technology and special needs of these children, parents, but especially mothers, needed hospital and home health nurses to support them during the transition from hospital to home. Nurses provided crucial advice on how to deal with school issues and with the child's developmental needs (Marlow, 1969).

■ *A New Health Mandate*

Political and social events of the 1960s reawakened the country's interest in the needs of the poor for health, education, and related social services. Stimulated by the civil rights movement, federal initiatives were developed that targeted disadvantaged populations, especially the poor and minority families in urban and rural communities. As opposed to previous government policies that supported maternal and child health programs, the new initiatives focused on the health needs of families and communities. Basic to many of the programs was the belief that economic and social factors had seriously eroded the functioning of poor families. New community health centers worked closely with community schools to offer families comprehensive health services, including Head Start, nutritional and job training programs, and employment opportunities for the poor (Sedlak & Church, 1982).

Nurses, in a variety of roles, including their new role as pediatric nurse practitioners, developed health services and programs for families. Immunization programs, teen clinics, and mobile health units staffed by nurses provided needed services to disadvantaged children and their families. Characteristic of these new services was the focus on health promotion and on

disease and accident prevention (Bomar, McNeeley, & Palmer, 1989).

■ *Conclusion*

Many of the health problems of children at the turn of the century have been resolved. The communicable and infectious diseases that destroyed the lives of children in the past were conquered through the efforts of sanitation reform, the health promotion movement, improvements in the economic status of families, and advances in medical sciences. Nurses have played a significant role in society's battle to preserve the health and welfare of its children. The ability of nurses to translate scientifically based health knowledge into practical education for mothers, families, school children, adolescents, and teachers improved the children's chances of living and becoming productive citizens.

In place of yesterday's health problems, new challenges face today's families and child health professionals. Problems such as violence, homelessness, substance abuse, sexually transmitted diseases, adolescent pregnancies, the effects of environmental toxins, and developmental disorders define the health issues of today's children. The lesson learned from the past is that simple solutions to these problems do not exist. The progress made during the past century was the result of a comprehensive effort of citizens, health and educational professionals, and the government to meet the multiple needs of children and their families. Almost 150 years after the nation first embarked on a systematic effort to reduce mortality among its youngest citizens, Lemuel Shattuck's admonition that the successful "management of infancy and childhood has an immense influence upon the health, vigor, and continuance of life" (Shattuck, 1850/1976, p. 102) is still a valid claim.

2

∎

INTEGRATIVE REVIEW OF ASSESSMENT MODELS FOR HEALTH PROMOTION OF CHILDREN AND THEIR FAMILIES

∎ *Margaret Grey*

This chapter reviews the recent nursing literature on assessment of children and families for health promotion and presents the state of the art in literature on health promotion. Literature in MEDLINE and CINHAL from 1989 through June 1996 was searched using the following key words: health promotion, primary care, children, adolescents, models of care, nursing, and assessment. To be sure that no relevant studies were omitted from the review, a hand search of prominent nursing journals was also conducted, among them *Advances in Nursing Science, Image, Issues in Comprehensive Pediatric Nursing, Journal of Pediatric Health Care, Journal of Pediatric Nursing, Journal of School Health, Nursing Research, Pediatric Nursing,* and *Research in Nursing and Health.* Because the concepts of health promotion and disease prevention are used by multiple disciplines, relevant literature in public health and medicine was also

searched, especially studies by nurse authors. Studies dealing with ill children, ill premature infants, or interventions were eliminated.

Three questions were addressed in this review:

- What paradigms/models have guided nursing research dealing with assessment of children and families for health promotion and disease prevention?
- What methods have been used to study assessment for health promotion and disease prevention in children and families?
- What conclusions can be drawn about assessment of children and families for health promotion and disease prevention?

∎ Review of the Literature

Tables 2.1 through 2.13 show the studies that were reviewed, with information provided on each study's sample composition, design, measures, and major findings. Studies are grouped by content area within each table. The psychometric data presented are specific to the sample studied. The review identified 13 different models; in some cases, the model was inferred by the problem studied and the methods used.

Medical or Physiologic Model

The most commonly used model for health promotion assessment is the medical or physiologic model, distinguished by its emphasis on physiologic measurement and medical risk factors. Descriptions of normal variations in children's vital signs, especially blood pressure and temperature, and examinations of (a) risk factors for cardiovascular disease and how these change as children develop and (b) parents' and children's knowledge of risk factors for disease or health, such as breast feeding, alcohol and drug use, and skin cancer risk were the focus of 16 nursing research studies identified as using the medical or physiologic model (see Table 2.1).

Four of the 16 studies addressed questions regarding assessments of vital signs. Grossman (1991) and Grossman, Jorda, and Farr (1993) sought to determine the presence of circadian rhythms in school-age children's blood pressure using Dinamap monitors (Model 1846 SX-P, Critikon) and found that about one third demonstrated these rhythms. Pontius, Kennedy, Shelley, and Mittrucker (1994b) used experimental methods to examine the relative validity and reliability of various measures of temperature and found that TempaDot (PyMaH Corporation) was the most accurate method, with the oral site being the best site. Similarly, Haddock, Merrow, and Swanson (1996) examined the accuracy of axillary temperature in discriminating febrile and nonfebrile children, aged 7 days to 16 years, and found that axillary

temperatures had a sensitivity of only 27.8% in the ability to detect fever in febrile children.

Several groups of researchers—Berg, Swanson, and Juhl (1992), Cowell, Montgomery, and Talashek (1992), Davidson et al. (1991), Gilmer, Speck, Bradley, Harrell, and Belyea (1996), and Howard et al. (1991)—examined risk factors related to coronary artery disease in children and adolescents. Along with the physiologic measures of blood lipids, these studies used questionnaire measures of dietary intake and health behaviors, such as the Bloomsday Cardiovascular Fitness Questionnaire developed by Howard et al. (1991). Gilmer et al. (1996) published data on the psychometric properties of the instrument that they developed to measure cardiovascular risk factors in preadolescents. Cardiovascular risk factors were found to increase over time and to be associated with poorer diets, female gender, and oral contraceptive use but not family history.

Other researchers studied factors associated with knowledge of health risk by using descriptive designs and questionnaires they developed. Foltz (1993) studied skin cancer knowledge and practices and found that (a) there was substantial misinformation about risk, and (b) knowledge correlated highly with behavior. Sarvela and Ford (1992) found that about 25% of pregnant adolescents used cigarettes and alcohol and that these behaviors were associated with peer and parental substance abuse and history of previous mental health treatment. Francis, Williams, and Yarandi (1993) found a high prevalence of low hematocrit in young African American children in Head Start, and Feroli and Hobson (1995) found that 16.5% of preadolescent males and 13.7% of preadolescent females had anemia in two school-based health centers. Gilhooly and Hellings (1992) found that nurse practitioners spent about 9.5 hours per month dealing with breastfeeding concerns. Hill and Aldag (1996) found that among mothers of both term and low-birth-weight infants, those who smoked were more likely to stop breastfeeding earlier and that smoking was associated with insufficient milk supply. Most of the findings indicate that there are multiple areas of misinformation among parents and children, including skin cancer risk, risk behaviors in pregnant adolescents, and breastfeeding practices.

Studies using the medical or physiologic model were mainly descriptive. Many of the measures used were developed by the authors and had limited reliability and validity information reported. In addition, the convenience samples were often small. Thus, much work needs to be done to determine the risk factors associated with various health behaviors.

Developmental Models

Another model frequently used by researchers was the developmental model. The focus of developmental studies was on attainment of a specific developmental task or on testing a particular developmental theory, such as temperament. Nine such studies (7 descriptive and 2 psychometric analyses) were found. Sleep behaviors, temperament, toilet training, colic, health concerns, sex, and contraception were considered in clinical studies. In psychometric studies, the properties of the Nursing Child Assessment Teaching Scale (NCATS; Barnard, 1978) and stability of children's responses to questionnaires were evaluated (see Table 2.2).

Two studies examined sleep behaviors among infants and toddlers. Becker, Chang, Kameshima, and Bloch (1991) used a combination of established instruments, such as the Bates Infant Temperament Questionnaire (Bates, Freeland, & Lounsbury, 1979) and the Home Observation for Measurement of the Environment (HOME; Bradley & Caldwell, 1984), and semistructured interviews to determine that infants of adolescent mothers were more likely than those of older mothers to waken at night.

Using similar data collection methods, Jimmerson (1991) found that sleep problems in toddlers were associated with sleeping in a twin bed, spending less time in day care, and having a more difficult temperament, as measured by the Toddler Temperament Scale (Fullard, McDevitt, & Carey, 1984). Simons, Ritchie, and Mullett (1992) found that high-risk and low-risk infants did not differ in parental ratings of temperament as determined by the Revised Infant Temperament Questionnaire (Carey & McDevitt, 1978). Infant health risk was determined by medical record review.

Several other developmental issues were addressed through descriptive designs. Hauck (1991) used phenomenologic analysis to describe parents' decision making regarding toilet training. Covington, Cronenwett, and Loveland-Cherry (1991) assessed parental characteristics and behaviors associated with colic using multiple methods of assessment, including the Brazelton Neonatal Behavioral Assessment Scale (Brazelton, 1984). Similarly, Jacobson and Melvin (1995) used the Revised Infant Temperament Questionnaire (Carey & McDevitt, 1978) and other established instruments to determine that mothers of infants with colic were more likely than mothers of infants without colic to rate their infants as difficult and more bothersome. Family patterns of knowledge about sex and contraception were assessed with a questionnaire developed by Tucker (1990). Tucker found that grandmothers, mothers, and adolescent daughters have highly correlated amounts of information. McKay and Diem (1995) used an anonymous questionnaire to determine the health concerns of 1,416 adolescent girls and found that there were four categories of concerns—risk-taking behaviors, appearance, health promotion/future orientation, and psychological functioning. Of these, only concerns about appearance increased with age. In a study of early initiation of sexual intercourse, Porter, Oakley, Ronis, and Neal (1996), using an instrument developed by Bauman

text continued on p. 23

TABLE 2.1 Health Promotion Studies Using the Medical or Physiologic Model

Author(s) and Source	Sample	Design	Measure(s)	Major Findings
Pontius, S., Kennedy, A. H., Shelley, S., & Mittrucker, C. (1994b). Accuracy and reliability of temperature measurement by instrument and site. *Journal of Pediatric Nursing, 9*, 114–123	502 randomly selected children, ages 3 months–18 years, 56.2% male	Quasi-experiment	Temperature: TempaDot, IVAC, and glass thermometer; site: axillary, oral, and rectal	TempaDot provided the most clinically valid temperature measurement. Oral site was the most accurate, but in the axillary site both IVAC and TempaDot were off by 0.3° F. Inservice education did not change nurses' accuracy.
Haddock, B. J., Merrow, D. L., & Swanson, M. S. (1996). The falling grace of axillary temperatures. *Pediatric Nursing, 22*, 121–125	173 infants and young children, ages birth–16 years, 94 males	Quasi-experiment	Filac F1010 electronic thermometer	Axillary temperatures indicated sensitivity of only 27.8% in ability to detect fever in the febrile groups determined by oral or rectal temperatures. 58% of afebrile rectal-axillary differences and 77% of febrile rectal-axillary differences exceeded 2° F.
Grossman, D. G. S. (1991). Circadian rhythms in blood pressure in school-age children of normotensive and hypertensive parents. *Nursing Research, 40*, 28–34	Convenience 40 children, ages 8–10 years, 55% male 20 with parental history of hypertension 35% Caucasian, 10% Hispanic, 20% Asian, 35% African American	Descriptive Correlational	Blood pressure (BP): Dinamap monitor	Circadian rhythms present in 12 of 40; low phase occurred between 1200 and 1800 hours. No differences in circadian mesors (rhythm-adjusted mean) and amplitudes between children of normotensive parents and hypertensive parents.
Grossman, D. G. S., Jorda, M. L., & Farr, L. A. (1993). Blood pressure rhythms in early school-age children of normotensive and hypertensive parents: A replication study. *Nursing Research, 43*, 232–237	Convenience 60 healthy children, ages 7–9 years, 45% male 30 with parental history of hypertension 42% Caucasian, 37% African American, 22% Other	Descriptive Correlational	Blood pressure: Dinamap monitor	37 children had significant ultradian rhythms, with 3-hour cycles. These children differed from the others in height and weight but not age, race, gender, or parental BP status.

Citation	Design	Sample	Variables/Instruments	Findings
Howard, J. K. H., Bindler, R. M., Dimico, G. S., Norwood, S. L., Nottingham, J. P., Synoground, G., Trilling, J. A., Van Gemert, F. C., Kirk, M. C., Newkirk, G. R., Leaf, D. A., & Cleveland, P. D. (1991). Cardiovascular risk factors in children: A Bloomsday report. *Journal of Pediatric Nursing, 6,* 222–229	Descriptive	Convenience 78 healthy children, ages 7–18 years, 64.1% male 99% Caucasian, 1% Native American	New instruments for this study: Bloomsday Cardiovascular Fitness Questionnaire— health habits, medical history Coronary Risk Profile— family history about cardiovascular disease (CVD) Diet Habit Survey Total cholesterol High-density lipids (HDL–C) Weight Blood pressure	Children with higher cholesterol, lower HDL–C, and regular weight and height had significantly poorer diets, higher blood pressure, less exercise, and more stress.
Cowell, J. M., Montgomery, A. C., & Talashek, M. (1992). Cardiovascular risk stability: From grade school to high school. *Journal of Pediatric Health Care, 6,* 349–354	Retrospective Cohort, repeated measures	Convenience 195 high school students who participated in a 6th-grade risk-reduction program, 44.1% female Ethnicity not reported	Height Weight Blood pressure Heart rate Recovery Index Cholesterol	Risks for obesity and high cholesterol were stable. Heart rate recovery and blood pressure did not track. Females had higher cholesterol.
Berg, C. L., Swanson, D. J., & Juhl, N. (1992). Total blood cholesterol and contributory risk factors in an adolescent population. *Journal of School Health, 62,* 64-66	Descriptive	Convenience 452 students in the 10th grade, ages 13–19 years, 52% male 92% Caucasian, 7% Other	Cholesterol Age Gender Ethnicity Smoking history Blood pressure history Familial history of cholesterol Oral contraceptive use	Females had higher total cholesterol than males. Females who used oral contraceptives had higher cholesterol than nonusers.

TABLE 2.1. *Continued*

Author(s) and Source	*Sample*	*Design*	*Measure(s)*	*Major Findings*
Gilmer, M. J., Speck, B. J., Bradley, C., Harrell, J. S., & Belyea, M. (1996). The Youth Health Survey: Reliability and validity of an instrument for assessing cardiovascular health habits in adolescents. *Journal of School Health, 66,* 106–111	School-based convenience One suburban and one urban school, student mean age = 12.3 years, 47.5% male 82.3% Caucasian, 10.3% African American	Cross-Sectional Psychometric	Youth Health Survey Physical Activity Checklist, *alpha* = .70 Dietary Checklist, *alpha* = .84 Smoking Behaviors Scale, KR20 = .88 Attitudes Toward Exercise–Self, *alpha* = .80 Attitudes Toward Exercise–Others, *alpha* = .82 Peer's Health Behavior Scale, no *alpha* available Role Model Scale, KR20 = .89	Most scales had moderate to good psychometric properties. Physical Activity Checklist and Peer's Health Behavior Scale did not factor-analyze into meaningful factors. Most had good test-retest reliability, except for Attitudes Toward Exercise–Others.
Davidson, D. M., Van Camp, J., Iftner, C. A., Landry, S.M., Bradley, B. J., & Wong, N. D. (1991). Family history fails to detect the majority of children with high capillary blood total cholesterol. *Journal of School Health, 61,* 75–80	Convenience 1,118 children, ages 9–10 years, 48.6% male 18.2% Vietnamese, 16.3% Hispanic	Correlational	Parental CVD history Grandparental CVD history Total cholesterol	Of 157 children with cholesterol ≥ 200 mg low-density lipoprotein, only 0.9% had positive family history, varied by ethnic group. American Academy of Pediatrics (AAP) Guidelines would miss many.
Foltz, A. T. (1993). Parental knowledge and practices of skin cancer prevention: A pilot study. *Journal of Pediatric Health Care, 7,* 220–225	Convenience 60 parents, ages 23–49 years, attending pediatric offices of one health maintenance organization (HMO) 60% Caucasian	Descriptive Survey	Sociodemographics Skin cancer knowledge and practice survey created for the study, *alpha* for knowledge = .65 and for practice = .88	The most common areas of misinformation were risk phenotype, proper application of sunscreen, and translation of SPF (Sun Protection Factor) into safe time. Correlation of knowledge with practice was 0.64%.

Citation	Sample	Design	Measures	Findings
Sarvela, P. D., & Ford, T. D. (1992). Indicators of substance abuse among pregnant adolescents in the Mississippi Delta. *Journal of School Health, 62*, 175–179	Convenience 293 pregnant adolescents in two primary care clinics, mean age = 18 years, 29.2% married 72.6% Caucasian, 26.4% African American	Cross-Sectional Survey	Created for the study: behaviors of drug use, alcohol, cigarettes, caffeine, and over-the-counter (OTC) medications, *alpha* for knowledge = .11 and for attitudes = .70	24% smoked cigarettes, 20.4% used alcohol, and 5.2% used marijuana. Behaviors were predicted by peer and personal substance use behavior, parental substance use, and history of previous mental health treatment.
Francis, E. E., Williams, D., & Yarandi, H. (1993). Anemia as an indicator of nutrition in children enrolled in a Head Start program. *Journal of Pediatric Health Care, 7*, 156–160	Records of 467 children in Head Start, mean age = 55 months, equal number of males and females 75% African American	Retrospective Chart review	Hematocrit in health records	African American males had the lowest average value. Rural Caucasian females had the highest mean value. Caucasians > African Americans; males = females. 21.4% anemic; 81% of African Americans anemic.
Feroli, K., & Hobson, S. (1995). Defining anemia in a preadolescent African American population. *Journal of Pediatric Health Care, 9*, 199–204	School based 455 African American preadolescents, ages 11–15 years, 206 males	Medical Record review	Record review sheets Hematocrit factors—eating breakfast, Tanner stage, exercise, height, weight	Mean hematocrit was 40%, with the range 33%–52%. Anemia was found in 16.5% of the males and 13.7% of the females. Males at early puberty were more likely to have anemia than more mature males. Eating breakfast did not affect anemia status. Females who exercised fewer than 2 days a week were more likely to be anemic than those who exercised more. Weight and height did not affect anemia.
Gilhooly, J., & Hellings, P. (1992). Breast feeding problems and telephone consultation. *Journal of Pediatric Health Care, 6*, 343–340	Calls from 387 individuals, mostly mothers	Retrospective Chart review	Records of telephone consultation for breastfeeding concerns	9.5 hours/month to manage breastfeeding concerns: 31% requested general information; 24% requested referral; 25% led to consultation with service clinicians

TABLE 2.1 *Continued*

Author(s) and Source	*Sample*	*Design*	*Measure(s)*	*Major Findings*
Hill, P. D., & Aldag, J. C. (1996). Smoking and breastfeeding status. *Research in Nursing and Health, 19,* 125–132	400 lactating mothers and their healthy infants, ages 8–14 weeks 110 lactating mothers and their low-birth-weight (LBW) infants	Cross-Sectional Descriptive	Investigator-designed questionnaire on demographic, obstetric, and biobehavioral factors influencing breastfeeding duration	In both samples, women who smoked were more likely to stop breastfeeding early. Older and married mothers of term infants breast-fed longer than younger, nonmarried women. In the LBW sample, those who were employed breast-fed a shorter time. Smokers reported insufficient milk as a cause of decline in breastfeeding than did nonsmokers.
Purcell, A. C., O'Brien, E., & Parks, P. L. (1996). Cholesterol levels in children: To screen or not to screen. *Journal of Pediatric Nursing, 11,* 40–44	Convenience Private, suburban practice 415 children, age 2 years 86% Caucasian, 13% African American	Cross-Sectional Descriptive	Total cholesterol (TC)	7% had TC 200 mg/dl or higher. There was no relationship of TC < 200 mg/dl with family history of cardiac risk. Logistic regression showed that only gestational age (higher) was associated with high TC.

and Udry (1981) and Smith and Udry (1985), found that early initiation of sexual intercourse was common and that influences on such early initiation were complex.

Two studies dealt with psychometric issues related to instruments created for the assessment of developmental issues. Gross, Conrad, Fogg, Willis, and Garvey (1993) examined the correlates of the Nursing Child Assessment Teaching Scale (NCATS; Barnard, 1978) instrument to determine validity and found that NCATS scores correlated with maternal knowledge and education but not with depression or self-efficacy. Holaday, Turner-Henson, and Swan (1991) studied the stability of school-age children's survey responses and found that children's responses to subjective opinion questions about friends and activities had low stability, whereas immutable characteristics such as age, gender, and grade in school had acceptable to good stability.

These descriptive developmental studies relevant to health promotion and disease prevention further our knowledge of how children grow and develop and how their parents understand these phenomena. However, these studies again often relied on untested measures and convenience samples.

Community-Oriented Primary Care Model

Community-oriented primary care, as defined by Nutting (1987), deals with primary care services based on an epidemiologic framework, such that the researcher or provider focuses on issues of concern in a particular community. Given the community base of much health promotion practice in child health, it is not surprising that a number of studies using a community model were identified. The focus of these studies was on Acquired Immune Deficiency Syndrome (AIDS), adolescent pregnancy, injuries, violence, and health care needs

of children in communities. All the studies were descriptive in nature and, for the most part, dealt with prevalence of health problems (e.g., injuries), health needs in communities, and community-based knowledge (e.g., teenagers, teachers) about AIDS.

The nursing profession's interest in the prevention of AIDS and HIV transmission is reflected in the fact that several studies dealt with knowledge and attitudes of young people about AIDS. Glenister, Castiglia, Kanski, and Haughey (1990) used an established questionnaire (DiClemente, Zorn, & Temoshok, 1986) to survey primary grade teachers and students about AIDS knowledge and attitudes and found a substantial amount of misinformation. Using similar measures, Walker (1992) studied teenagers' knowledge of AIDS and associated behaviors and found that teenagers frequently participated in risky sexual behaviors.

SmithBattle (1996) used an interpretative, phenomenological approach to study the experience of adolescent mothers. She found that 16 mothers did not view their future as diminished by virtue of having a child. Anderson (1996) also used a qualitative approach to study substance use among adolescent females in detention and found that they had resolved to alter their substance use when released from detention.

Accidents are the leading cause of death in children from 1 year of age through age 15, and several studies dealt with injuries. Jones (1992) developed a questionnaire and surveyed pediatric nurse practitioners (PNPs) to determine their educational preparation and the clinical activities they routinely perform in injury prevention. Findings revealed that although most had preparation in injury prevention they did not routinely offer injury prevention advice. Lee and Bass (1990) studied accident report forms from a university-supported day care center and found that, although there were few serious injuries, the 3- to 5-year-old children were involved in accidents more than older or younger children were. Finally, Price, Desmond,

text continued on p. 27

TABLE 2.2 Health Promotion Studies Using the Developmental Model

Author(s) and Source	Sample	Design	Measure(s)	Major Findings
Becker, P. T., Chang, A., Kameshima, S., & Bloch, M. (1991). Correlates of diurnal sleep patterns in infants of adolescent and adult single mothers. *Research in Nursing and Health, 14*, 97–108	Convenience 46 first-time mothers: 23 adolescents, mean age = 16.8 years; 23 adults, mean age = 25.2 years 19 in each group at 12 months Low-middle socioeconomic status (SES) 45 Caucasians, 1 African American	Descriptive Correlational, with repeated measures	Sleep/Activity Record by mothers: percentage night sleep; variability of night sleep Bates Infant Temperament Questionnaire Home observation for Measurement of the Environment (HOME) Other established instruments No reliability data on current sample	Night sleep as percentage of total sleep was lower in the adolescent group than the adult group and increased significantly from 4 to 12 months. No differences were found in variability of night sleep. Adolescents scored lower on HOME but not temperament, stress, or support. Percentage night sleep correlated with parenting stress; variability of night sleep correlated with emotional support.
Jimmerson, K. R. (1991). Maternal, environmental, and temperamental characteristics of toddlers with and toddlers without sleep problems. *Journal of Pediatric Health Care, 5*, 71–77	Convenience 60 parents of toddlers, ages 12–36 months 30 with sleep problems, 30 without Suburban	Descriptive	Investigator-developed Sleep/Behavior Inventory Toddler Temperament Scale No reliability data on current sample	Nightwaking was present in 55% of the sleep-problem group. Toddlers with sleep problems were more likely to sleep in a twin bed instead of a crib, spent less time in day care, were less adaptable, and were more likely to have "difficult" temperaments.
Simons, C. J. R., Ritchie, S. K., & Mullett, M. D. (1992). Relationships between parental ratings of infant temperament, risk status, and delivery method. *Journal of Pediatric Health Care, 6*, 240–245	70 mother-father dyads and infants (39 low risk; 31 high risk), mean age of parents = 27.4 years, infants' ages 4–8 months Annual income = $15,000 Years of education mean = 14.3 years	Descriptive	Revised Infant Temperament Questionnaire Record review No reliability data on current sample	High-risk and low-risk infants were similar on easy-difficult profiles; high-risk infants were rated more adaptable and more positive in mood than low-risk infants. Low-risk infants delivered by cesarean section were less optimal in approach-withdrawal, adaptability, and mood.
Hauck, M. R. (1991). Mothers' descriptions of the toilet training process: A phenomenologic study. *Journal of Pediatric Nursing, 6*, 80–86	Convenience 10 Caucasian, middle-class mothers, ages 20–36 years, of toddlers, ages 13 months–4 years	Descriptive Phenomenologic	Interviews of individual mothers concerning the toilet-training process using interview guide	Five recurrent themes were identified: issues about timing, trajectory of success and failure, strategies used during the process, factors influencing the mother, and child skills and personality traits.

Reference	Sample	Design	Instruments	Findings
Covington, C., Cronenwett, L., & Loveland-Cherry, C. (1991). Newborn behavioral performance in colic and non-colic infants. *Nursing Research, 40,* 292–296	Convenience 119 married couples Fathers' ages 20–52 years, mothers' ages 19–41 years 117 Caucasian infants, 53% male, 32% with colic Enrolled prenatally; followed until age 4 months.	Descriptive	Investigator-developed questionnaire on colic Chart review Telephone interview for colic behaviors Brazelton Neonatal Behavioral Assessment Scale (BNBAS)	Colic and noncolic groups were not different on parent variables, except fathers were slightly more educated. Infants were not different, except for orientation cluster on the BNBAS.
Jacobson, D., & Melvin, D. (1995). A comparison of temperament and maternal bother in infants with and without colic. *Journal of Pediatric Nursing, 10,* 181–188	25 infants with colic, ages 4–8 months 30 infants without colic, ages 4–8 months	Descriptive Retrospective	Revised Infant Temperament Questionnaire Millor's Bother Scale No psychometric data on current sample	Mothers of infants with colic were more likely to rate their infant as difficult and were more bothered by their temperament dimension of mood than were mothers of infants without colic.
Tucker, S. K. (1990). Adolescent patterns of communication about the menstrual cycle, sex, and contraception. *Journal of Pediatric Nursing, 5,* 393–400	Snowball 179 African American women, ages 13–80 years, from 53 family units	Exploratory Descriptive	Investigator-developed survey about familial communication on menarche, sex, and contraception No psychometrics on current sample	Significant relationships were found within adolescent-mother-grandmother triads in amount of information received. Mothers were the major source of information. Significant negative relationship was found between amount of information received about sex and pregnancy before age 18 years. Communication about sex and contraception may not meet adolescent needs.
McKay, L., & Diem, E. (1995). Health concerns of adolescent girls. *Journal of Pediatric Nursing, 10,* 19–27	1,416 female students in Grades 7 through 10 from 38 schools in Ontario, Canada 90% Caucasian	Exploratory Descriptive	Investigator-developed 119-item questionnaire No psychometric information provided	Four factors of concerns were identified: risk-taking behavior, appearance, health promotion/future orientation, and psychological functioning. Health promotion and future concerns decreased with age, but concern about appearance worsened with age.

TABLE 2.2 Continued

Author(s) and Source	Sample	Design	Measure(s)	Major Findings
Porter, C. P., Oakley, D., Ronis, D. L., & Neal, R. W. (1996). Pathways of influence on fifth and eighth graders' reports about having had sexual intercourse. *Research in Nursing and Health, 19*, 193–204	Convenience 59 fifth graders 169 eighth graders; 50% male 38.9% and 66.1% Caucasian, respectively	Cross-Sectional Descriptive	Initiation of sexual intercourse (1 item) Demographic factors Costs and benefits of sexual intercourse—Bauman and Udry Scale, *alpha* = .87–89 Intimate behaviors—Smith and Udry Scale, *alpha* = .90 Personal norms (new items), *alpha* = .57	46% of fifth graders and 55% of eighth graders reported having initiated sexual intercourse. Influences on early sexual intercourse were complex, such that gender, use of alcohol, costs, and personal norms did not influence initiation directly but did indirectly through the frequency of other intimate behaviors.
Gross, D., Conrad, B., Fogg, L., Willis, L., & Garvey, C. (1993). What does the NCATS measure? *Nursing Research, 42*, 260–265	Convenience 128 mothers, mean age = 32 years, mean education = college 128 toddlers, mean age = 29 months 48% African American, 12% Hispanic, 3% Asian, 37% Caucasian	Psychometric Validity of NCATS	Nursing Child Assessment Teaching Scale (NCATS), interrater reliability = 85–87%, *alpha* = .71–85 Depression Scale, *alpha* = .88 Toddler Temperament Scale, *alpha* = .81 Two investigator-developed scales: Toddler Care Questionnaire (TCQ), *alpha* = .94 Knowledge of Infant Development Inventory (KIDI), *alpha* = .81	NCATS Parent subscale scores were related to maternal knowledge and education but not to depression and self-efficacy. Child subscale scores were unrelated to all variables, but significant differences were found between African American, Hispanic, and Caucasian mothers. NCATS tapped cognitive factors more reliably than other factors.
Holaday, B., Turner-Henson, A., & Swan, J. (1991). Stability of school-age children's survey responses. *Image: Journal of Nursing Scholarship, 23*, 109–114	76 randomly selected (from a total sample of 365) children with chronic illness, ages 10–12 years	Psychometric analysis using 3-way panel survey	Immutable characteristics (age, grade) Objective facts about activities Subjective opinions about friends and activities	Immutable characteristics and facts had acceptable to good stability. Opinion questions had low stability not associated with sex, age, and gender.

26

and Smith (1991) developed a questionnaire to measure urban adolescents' perceptions of guns and found that adolescents commonly had pistols, which they believed made them feel safe.

Several teams of researchers used survey methods and medical record abstraction to study the health needs of children. Attala, Gresley, McSweeney, and Jobe (1993) used a questionnaire to determine that school-age children in two midwestern counties had high need for educational services about drugs, sex, and AIDS. Murata, Mace, Strehlow, and Shuler (1992) used medical records to compare the health problems of homeless children to those of a national sample. They found that homeless children had significantly more communicable diseases, less acute noncommunicable diseases, and more injuries than the national sample. Richardson, Selby-Harrington, Krowchuk, Cross, and Quade (1995) also used medical record review to determine the effectiveness of the Early and Periodic Screening, Diagnosis, and Treatment Program (EPSDT) on rural children's health care. Kornguth (1990) reanalyzed data collected by the National School Health Services Program to determine the profile of children with high absenteeism. She found that the frequently absent child is most likely a female, from an ethnic minority group, and on medical assistance. The influence of type of after-school care on children's self-perceptions, as measured by Harter's (1985) Self-Perception Profile, and school performance was studied by Cutler, Smith, and Kilmon (1995), who found that type of care did not influence perception, school performance, or absenteeism.

Consensus techniques were used by Lavin, Shapiro, and Weill (1992) with school health workers to determine an agenda for school-based health promotion. Zadinsky and Boettcher (1992) also used consensus techniques with state health workers to determine preventability of infant mortality in a rural community. Techniques used in these studies included Delphi survey and integrative review of the literature. Using surveys, Weathersby, Lobo, and Williamson (1995) found that children and parents agreed on the need for school-based health services and the types of services that should be provided.

These descriptive studies suggest that homeless children have different health care needs than other children and that such needs may not be being met by existing programs, such as EPSDT. Further, the educational needs for school children include information about drugs, sex, and AIDS. Again, many studies used investigator-developed questionnaires without reported reliability or validity. Further, few studies have population-based samples or are replications of previous results, so findings must be considered preliminary.

Stress-Adaptation Models

Models of stress and adaptation are common models for nursing research. For the most part, these models are based on work of Roy and Roberts (1981) and Lazarus and Folkman (1984). Stressors associated with adolescence, the transition to parenthood, and coping behaviors for stressful situations in general were themes in the 18 studies reviewed, 13 of which were descriptive surveys, with 4 others psychometric analyses and 1 a content analysis (see Table 2.4).

Coping with life stressors in adolescence was identified as the problem in 5 surveys and 2 psychometric analysis. Measures used in these studies were obtained using established instruments. DeMaio-Esteves (1990) studied mediators (Ways of Coping Checklist; Folkman & Lazarus, 1985; introspectiveness) of daily stress (Hassles Scale; Kanner, Coyne, Schaefer, & Lazarus, 1981) and perceived health status using a stress-adaptation model in adolescent girls. Results showed that problem-focused coping had a mediating effect on the relationship between stress and perceived health status.

text continued on p. 40

TABLE 2.3 Health Promotion Studies Using the Community-Oriented Primary Care Model

Author(s) and Source	Sample	Design	Measure(s)	Major Findings
Glenister, A. M., Castiglia, P., Kanski, G., & Haughey, B. (1990). AIDS knowledge and attitudes of primary grade teachers and students. *Journal of Pediatric Health Care, 4,* 77–85	Convenience 345 pupils in Grades 4–8, ages 9–16 years; equal numbers of males and females; race not provided 55 staff members (50 teachers); 73% female; 90% Caucasian	Descriptive Survey	Knowledge and attitudes about AIDS, developed by DiClemente, Zorn, and Temoshok (1986), *alpha* = .74 National Center for Health Statistics survey on knowledge and attitudes about AIDS, *alpha* = .76	Pupils' knowledge was correlated with age, with no differences by gender. 89% were afraid of getting AIDS. Teachers did not consistently know facts on AIDS transmission, blood tests, and prevention. Results were similar between teachers and pupils.
Walker, S. H. (1992). Teenagers' knowledge of Acquired Immunodeficiency Syndrome and associated behaviors. *Journal of Pediatric Nursing, 7,* 246–250	Convenience 152 teenagers, ages 13–18 years, 48% male 97% Caucasian	Descriptive Survey	Questionnaire on AIDS knowledge (from DiClemente et al., 1986), *alpha* = .64	Overall knowledge scores increased significantly with age; 75% had fewer than 5 wrong responses. Main sources of information were radio/TV and magazines. 45% were sexually experienced; only 60% of the males used condoms consistently.
SmithBattle, L. (1996). Teenage mothers' narratives of self: An examination of risking the future. *Advances in Nursing Science, 17,* 22–36	16 adolescent mothers, ages 14–18 years, with infants, ages 8–10 months 9 Caucasians, 7 African Americans	Interpretive Phenomenological	Interviews	Themes included inheriting a diminished future, inventing a future from an impoverished past, and pressing into an open future. Themes suggested that teen mothers do not share the view that mothering jeopardizes their future.
Anderson, N. L. R. (1996). Decisions about substance abuse among adolescents in juvenile detention. *Image: Journal of Nursing Scholarship, 28,* 65–70	20 females, ages 13–18 years, in one juvenile detention center 10 Latinas, 7 African Americans, 2 Caucasians	Descriptive Ethnographic	Observations and investigator-developed interviews	Detained teens resolved to be abstinent in drug and alcohol use when freed. They had reservations about their ability to maintain sobriety once home.

Citation	Design	Sample	Measures	Findings
Jones, N. E. (1992). Injury prevention: A survey of clinical practice. *Journal of Pediatric Health Care, 6,* 182–186	Descriptive Survey	Convenience 64 pediatric nurse practitioners (PNPs), 64% older than 35 years, 97% female 79% master's-degree prepared	Investigator-developed questionnaire on characteristics, training in injury prevention, and clinical activities in injury prevention No psychometric data for current sample	97% reported content on injuries in the PNP program; 54% had continuing education in injuries. Only 27% reported giving injury prevention advice and recording it. Routine counseling was not provided on safety seats, seat belts, smoke detectors, safe hot water temperatures, syrup of ipecac, bicycle helmets, pedestrian safety, drinking and driving, or guns at home.
Lee, E. J., & Bass, C. (1990). Survey of accidents in a university day care center. *Journal of Pediatric Health Care, 4,* 18–23	Descriptive Record review	103 accident reports from a large university day care center involving 57 children, ages 6 months–6 years	Accident reports; methods of abstraction not reported	14% of children in day care had an accident, with the highest number in the 3- to 5-year age range; 44% involved boys, and 56% involved girls. 50% had one or more accidents in the year. Most accidents were associated with running or horseplay and occurred in the afternoon and out-of-doors. July had the highest incidence. Two required medical attention (human bite; staple in finger).
Price, J. H., Desmond, S. M., & Smith, D. (1991). A preliminary investigation of inner city adolescents' perceptions of guns. *Journal of School Health, 61,* 255–259	Descriptive Survey	Convenience 571 high school students in urban, low-socioeconomic-status (SES) districts 377 African Americans, 201 Caucasians	Investigator-developed questionnaire on demographics, gun ownership, and gun perceptions, *alpha* = .79	African American males were more likely than Caucasian males to have a pistol at home, less likely to have a shotgun, more likely to know someone who took a gun to school, and more likely to know someone who had been shot. African American females were more likely than Caucasian females to know someone who had been shot and know someone who took a gun to school and less likely to have fired a gun or have a shotgun or rifle at home. African American teens believed that guns make them feel safe and would protect them from criminals and that schools should have gun detectors. All believed that guns are too easy to obtain and there should be more gun control measures.

TABLE 2.3 *Continued*

Author(s) and Source	*Sample*	*Design*	*Measure(s)*	*Major Findings*
Attala, J. M., Gresley, R. S., McSweeney, M., & Jobe, M. A. (1993). Health needs of school-age children in two midwestern counties. *Issues in Comprehensive Pediatric Nursing, 16,* 51–60	49 administrators, 26 nurses, and 38 "informed parents" (113 total) from 2 Midwest counties	Delphi survey	Questionnaire on perceived health needs of school-age children and barriers related to meeting needs	High priority needs were primarily educational (drugs, sex, health, AIDS). Service needs were for school nurses, free or low-cost care, and parental concerns. High-priority barriers included lack of funds, lack of resources, low SES, not enough nurses, and parenting deficits. Administrators, nurses, and parents agreed for the most part.
Murata, J. E., Mace, J. P., Strehlow, A., & Shuler, P. (1992). Disease patterns in homeless children: A comparison with national data. *Journal of Pediatric Nursing, 7,* 196–204	Convenience 303 visits by clients, under age 18 years, to nurse-managed clinic at shelter 1985 data from National Ambulatory Medical Care Survey (NAMCS); 5,403 visits	Descriptive Comparative	Record review; NAMCS form	Homeless children were more likely to be non-Caucasian, older, and Hispanic. 17% lived on the street, and 8% were in shelters. 4.9% had no source of medical payment. Homeless children had more visits for communicable disease, prevention, and injuries and fewer visits for acute disease. Differences persisted when only Hispanics were examined.
Richardson, L. A., Selby-Harrington, M., Krowchuk, H. V., Cross, A. W., & Quade, D. (1995). Health outcomes of children receiving EPSDT checkups: A pilot study. *Journal of Pediatric Health Care, 9,* 242–250	76 children, ages birth–20 years, seen for Early and Periodic Screening, Diagnosis, and Treatment Program (EPSDT) visits during one 6-month period; 78% ethnic minority	Descriptive Medical record review	Closed and open items to abstract information from the medical record	43% of children had health problems identified, 22% received treatment, and 18% were referred for specialty care. Almost 1/3 of those referred for specialty care did not receive it.
Kornguth, M. L. (1990). School illnesses: Who's absent and why? *Pediatric Nursing, 16,* 95–99	3,000 children examined by the National School Health Services Program	Descriptive Secondary data analysis	Not reported	Children with the highest number of absences were female, ethnic minority, used public health clinic or services, and received medication. If the main source of health care was a school clinic, there were fewer absences due to illness.

Citation	Sample	Design	Instruments/Variables	Findings
Cutler, B. A., Smith, K. E., & Kilmon, C. (1995). Characteristics of fifth-grade children in relation to the type of after-school care. *Journal of Pediatric Health Care, 9,* 167–171	Convenience 154 fifth-grade children, mean age = 10.5 years, 46% male, in 3 types of after-school care: self ($n = 28$), sibling ($n = 20$), and adult ($n = 106$) 44% Caucasian, 33% African American, 23% Hispanic	Descriptive Correlational	Parents' responses to 3 items on after-school care form Harter's Self-Perception Profile for Children, $alpha = 0.71–0.82$ Substance use Academic performance and absenteeism	No differences were found between after-school care groups on self-perception, academic performance, or attendance. 10% to 12% of each group reported substance use, but more children in self-care used cocaine or marijuana than did those in the other two groups.
Lavin, A. T., Shapiro, G. R., & Weill, K. S. (1992). Creating an agenda for school-based health promotion: A review of 25 selected reports. *Journal of School Health, 62,* 212–228	25 reports on school-based health promotion published between 1989 and 1991	Integrative review	Not reported	Growing consensus about critical issues, urgency of concerns, and potential strategies. Five themes were identified: Education and health are interrelated; biggest threats to health are "social morbidities"; a more comprehensive, integrated approach is needed; health promotion and education efforts should be centered in and around schools; and prevention efforts are cost-effective and the social and economic costs of inaction too high and still escalating.
Zadinsky, J. K., & Boettcher, J. H. (1992). Preventability of infant mortality in a rural community. *Nursing Research, 41,* 223–227	5 physicians and 16 registered nurses from rural Georgia with expertise in maternal-infant care	Delphi survey	Case summaries of 26 infant deaths	First 2 rounds were used to develop a consensus of panelists' opinions about problems leading to high infant mortality rate. This created a decision tree that was used in Rounds 3 and 4 to evaluate case summaries. Significant differences were found between physicians and nurses on preventability, with nurses rating more cases as preventable.
Weathersby, A. M., Lobo, M. L., & Williamson, D. (1995). Parent and student preferences for services in a school-based clinic. *Journal of School Health, 65,* 14–17	Probability 199 students, ages 13–19 years, 49% male, 73% Caucasian 196 parents, 82% mothers, 83% having private physician	Descriptive Survey	Questionnaires developed from Center for Population Option's School Board Health Clinics Model	Students were less interested than parents. Both were interested in the availability of comprehensive services, including general health, reproductive, and counseling services.

TABLE 2.4 Health Promotion Studies Using Stress-Adaptation Models

Author(s) and Source	Sample	Design	Measure(s)	Major Findings
DeMaio-Esteves, M. (1990). Mediators of daily stress and perceived health status in adolescent girls. *Nursing Research, 39,* 360–364	Convenience 159 female adolescents, ages 14–16 years 86.2% Caucasian	Correlational Survey	Perceived health status, *alpha* = .85 Ways of Coping Checklist–Revised, *alpha* = .75–.79 Hassles Scale = daily stress, test-retest = .79 Introspectiveness, *alpha* = 89	Daily stress had a direct positive effect on perceived health status and on introspection. Introspection had a direct effect on health status. Introspection had a mediating effect on the relationship between daily stress and health status. Problem-focused coping had a mediating effect on the relationship between stress and health status; emotion-focused coping did not.
Gröer, M. W., Thomas, S. P., & Shoffner, D. (1992). Adolescent stress and coping: A longitudinal study. *Research in Nursing and Health, 15,* 209–217	Convenience 167 teenagers tested in 9th and 12th grade, 92 females 94% Caucasian	Longitudinal panel survey	Adolescent Life Change Event Scale Open-ended items on ways of coping with stress	Life events increased with age; females had more events. For them, siblings, relationships, and acne were the most problematic. Both females and males reported coping with stress mostly through active distraction techniques. In females, passive distraction increased with age, as did their self-destructive and aggressive coping behaviors. Stressful events were not related to coping.
Mahon, N. E., Yarcheski, A., & Yarcheski, T. J. (1993). Health consequences of loneliness in adolescents. *Research in Nursing and Health, 16,* 23–31	Convenience 325 adolescents, ages 12–21 years, 134 males 77% Caucasian	Correlational Survey	Revised UCLA Loneliness Scale, *alpha* = .89 Introspectiveness Scale for Adolescents, *alpha* = .87 Manifestations of psychological distress, *alpha* = .84 Perceived health status, *alpha* = .89	Loneliness contributes to introspectiveness, and both loneliness and introspectiveness contribute to reporting of symptom patterns. All of these contribute positively to perceived health status.

Study	Sample	Design	Instruments (alpha)	Findings
Grossman, M., & Rowat, K. M. (1995). Parental relationships, coping strategies, received support, and well-being in adolescents of separated or divorced and married parents. *Research in Nursing and Health, 18,* 249–261	244 matched adolescents from divorced/separated or married households, ages 13–20 years, mean = 16.6 years. Median time since divorce = 6.1 years. School based	Descriptive Cross-sectional Case-Control	Life satisfaction, *alpha* = .82–.83. Expectancy for success, *alpha* = .88–.91. Trait anxiety, *alpha* = .91–.92. Mental adjustment, *alpha* = .93–.94. Social support, *alpha* = .73–.90. Revised Ways of Coping Questionnaire, *alpha* = .84–.92. Life Events Checklist, no *alpha*	Perceived poor parental relationship, not family status, was associated with lower life satisfaction and sense of future and high anxiety in adolescents. Coping strategies and received support did not mediate the association between a perceived poor parental relationship and low levels of well-being.
Kelly, L. E. (1995). Adolescent mothers: What factors relate to level of preventive health care sought for their infants? *Journal of Pediatric Nursing, 10,* 105–113	49 adolescent mothers, ages 14–17 years. Urban well-child clinic setting. 39 African Americans, 8 Hispanics	Descriptive Correlational	Health beliefs, *alpha* = .72. Parenting stress, *alpha* = .93. Social support, *alpha* = .92. Investigator-developed scale of level of preventive health care	Mothers who maintained relationship with the child's father, scored high on "powerful others" and low on locus of control were more likely to practice better preventive health care.
Ferketich, S. L., & Mercer, R. T. (1995a). Paternal-infant attachment of experiences and inexperienced fathers during infancy. *Nursing Research, 44,* 31–37	Convenience. 79 experienced fathers and 93 first-time fathers, all over age 18 years. 70% Caucasian	Descriptive Longitudinal	Infant attachment, *alpha* = .66–.81. Parenting competence, *alpha* = .84–87. Self-esteem, *alpha* = .82–.87. Mastery, *alpha* = .66–.86. Marital adjustment, *alpha* = .76–.85. Family functioning, *alpha* = .77–.84. Depression, *alpha* = .83–.89. State anxiety, *alpha* = .92–.95. Social support, *alpha* = .93–.96. Life Experiences Fetal Attachment Scale, *alpha* = .85–.88	Infant attachment scores were not different for new versus experienced fathers. Fetal attachment was a major predictor of infant attachment for experienced fathers. For inexperienced fathers, fetal attachment and depression predicted attachment. Social support and stress had no influence on attachment.

TABLE 2.4 *Continued*

Ferketich, S. L., & Mercer, R. T. (1995b). Predictors of role competence for experienced and inexperienced fathers. *Nursing Research, 44,* 89–95	Convenience 79 experienced fathers and 93 Inexperienced fathers, all over age 18 years 70% Caucasian	Descriptive Longitudinal	Infant attachment, *alpha* = .66–.81 Parenting competence, *alpha* = .84–.87 Self-esteem, *alpha* = .82–.87 Mastery, *alpha* = .66–.86 Marital adjustment, *alpha* = .76–.85 Family functioning, *alpha* = .77–.84 Depression, *alpha* = .83–.89 State anxiety, *alpha* = .92–.95 Social support, *alpha* = .93–.96 Life Experiences Fetal Attachment Scale, *alpha* = .85–.88	Parental competence was similar by experience as were trajectories of change, increasing with time. Depression and partner relationships were predictive of competence for experienced fathers. Sense of mastery, family functioning, anxiety, and depression were predictors of competence for inexperienced fathers.
Mercer, R. T., & Ferketich, S. L. (1995). Experienced -and inexperienced mothers' maternal competence during infancy. *Research in Nursing and Health, 18,* 333–343	Convenience 136 experienced mothers and 166 inexperienced mothers, all over age 18 years 74% Caucasian	Descriptive Longitudinal	Infant attachment, *alpha* = .66–.81 Parenting competence, *alpha* = .84–.87 Self-esteem, *alpha* = .82–.87 Mastery, *alpha* = .66–.86 Marital adjustment, *alpha* = .76–.85 Family functioning, *alpha* = .77–.84 Depression, *alpha* = .83–.89 State anxiety, *alpha* = .92–.95 Social support, *alpha* = .93–.96 Life Experiences Fetal Attachment Scale, *alpha* = .85–.88	Maternal role competence was similar between experienced and inexperienced mothers. Inexperienced mothers became more competent over time. Self-esteem was a consistent, major predictor of maternal competence. For experienced mothers, maternal fetal attachment, readiness for pregnancy, and risk variables were also explanatory. Sense of control was also explanatory for inexperienced mothers.
Ryan-Wenger, N. M. (1990). Development and psychometric properties of the Schoolagers' Coping Strategies Inventory. *Nursing Research, 39,* 344–349	250 Caucasian children, ages 8–12 years, 54.4% male	Psychometric Analysis	Schoolagers' Coping Strategies Inventory (SCSI) Coping Inventory—teacher's observation of coping style Self-esteem Academic self-esteem stressors by self-report	SCSI has adequate internal consistency (.79) and moderate test-retest reliability (.73–.82). Construct validity was supported by lower coping scores among children with stress-related conditions. Divergent validity was demonstrated.

Citation	Sampling/Sample	Design	Measures	Findings
Ryan-Wenger, N. M., & Copeland, S. G. (1994). Coping strategies used by Black school-age children from low-income families. *Journal of Pediatric Nursing, 9,* 33–48	Convenience 59 African American children, ages 8–11 years Low socioeconomic status	Descriptive	Open-ended questionnaire on stress-related symptoms reported by teachers and children Schoolagers' Coping Strategies Inventory, *alpha* = .73–.80	Distraction and social support were most commonly used. Boys used relaxation more than girls. Girls used avoidance, aggressive motor activities, accepting responsibility, and spiritual activities.
Sharrer, V. W., & Ryan-Wenger, N. M. (1995). A longitudinal study of age and gender differences of stressors and coping strategies in school-age children. *Journal of Pediatric Health Care, 9,* 123–130	Convenience 101 children in parochial schools, ages 8–12 years school Majority Caucasian	Descriptive Longitudinal	Feel Bad Scale Schoolagers' Coping Strategies Inventory No psychometric data on current sample	Severity of stressors decreased significantly with age over 2 years, but frequency did not change. Boys used "watch television" or "yell or scream" more frequently than girls did. Girls used "cry" or "cuddle my pet" more often.
Meininger, J. C., Stashinko, E. E., & Hayman, L. L. (1991). Type A behavior in children: Psychometric properties of the Matthews Youth Test for Health. *Nursing Research, 40,* 221–227	Convenience 216 twins, ages 6–11 years, 53% female Mostly middle class	Psychometric Analysis	Matthews Youth Test for Health (MYTH) = Type A behavior Self-perceived competence and teachers ratings of competence	Two factors—Impatience-Aggression and Competitive Achievement-Striving—were derived and cross-validated, *alpha* = .82–.85. Construct validity was partially supported by the relationship between Type A components and teacher ratings. Children's ratings and global self-competence were not related to MYTH scores.
Sorenson, E. S. (1990). Children's coping responses. *Journal of Pediatric Nursing, 5,* 259–267	Convenience 32 children, ages 8–11 years 100% Caucasian	Descriptive Qualitative content analysis	Written health history from medical record Sentence completion list and response to potential daily stress-provoking situations Semistructured daily journals dealing with daily stressors, coping responses, and coping resources	21 categories among 4 themes of coping responses emerged. Themes were cognitive, cognitive-behavioral, behavioral, and interpersonal.

TABLE 2.4 *Continued*

Author(s) and Source	Sample	Design	Measure(s)	Major Findings
Yarcheski, A., Mahon, N. E., & Yarcheski, T. J. (1992). Validation of the PRQ85 social support measure for adolescents. *Nursing Research, 41,* 332–337	Convenience 325 adolescents, ages 12–21 years, 191 females 77% Caucasian	Psychometric Analysis/construct validity of PRQ85	Health, *alpha* = .88–.90 Symptoms, *alpha* = .78–.84 Social support, *alpha* = .84–.89	A four-factor solution, which was theoretically sound, was found, but *alphas* were low. Correlations suggested that these four factors were related, so the 17-item scale can be used as a total scale. Correlations were as expected, supporting construct validity.
Mahon, N. E., Yarcheski, T. J., & Yarcheski, A. (1995). Validation of the revised UCLA Loneliness Scale for adolescents. *Research in Nursing and Health, 18,* 263–270	Convenience 333 adolescents, ages 12–21 years, mean = 16.75 years 75% Caucasian	Psychometric Analysis	UCLA Loneliness Scale, *alpha* = .89 Time perspective, *alpha* = .87 Interpersonal solidarity, *alpha* = .89 Social self-confidence, *alpha* = .78	Factor analysis confirmed two factors—intimate–others loneliness and social–others loneliness. Construct validity was supported by significant associations between loneliness, future time perspective, close friend solidarity, and dependency. Slow tempo was not related to loneliness.
Gottlieb, L. N., & Baillies, J. (1995). Firstborn's behaviors during a mother's second pregnancy. *Nursing Research, 44,* 356–362	Convenience 80 preschool children, ages 18–60 months, 50% male, of expectant mothers: 20 only children 20 children of mothers in early pregnancy 20 children of mothers in mid-pregnancy 20 children of mothers in late pregnancy	Descriptive Comparative longitudinal	Preschool Behavioral Rating Scale, *alpha* = .58–.82 Administered monthly for 3 months	Young firstborn girls were more dependent than boys or older girls. Firstborns in the middle pregnancy group were more dependent at 20 weeks than at 24 and 28 weeks. Boys expressed more anger at separation than girls did. Older firstborns were more autonomous than younger firstborns.

Citation	Sample	Design	Measures	Results
Coffman, S., Levitt, M. J., & Guacci-Franco, N. (1995). Infant-mother attachment: Relationships to maternal responsiveness and infant temperament. *Journal of Pediatric Nursing, 10*, 9–18	Convenience 43 mothers, ages 20–40 years, of infants 98% Caucasian	Descriptive Longitudinal	2 investigator-developed scales: Close Person Satisfaction Scale = mother's perception of satisfaction with a close relationship, *alpha* = .95 Relationship Closeness Scale–Hassles Scale, *alpha* = .91 Infant Health Status Scale, no *alpha* available	Most women selected their husband or mother as their closest relation. Nine had a different significant other at 13 months following birth. Infant hospitalization, not infant risk status or major infant illness, was related to maternal stress and relationship change.
Friedemann, M. L., & Andrews, M. (1990). Family support and child adjustment in single parent families. *Issues in Comprehensive Pediatric Nursing, 13,* 289–301	103 single-parent and 271 two-parent families 56% Caucasian, 37% African American	Secondary analysis	Survey items concerning family support and adjustment	Single parents experienced stressors differently from those experienced by two-parent families. There were no differences in child behavior scores.

TABLE 2.5 Health Promotion Studies Using the Maternal Responsiveness Model

Author(s) and Source	Sample	Design	Measure(s)	Major Findings
Bloom, K. C. (1995). The development of attachment behaviors in pregnant adolescents. *Nursing Research, 44,* 284–289	Convenience 79 low-income, pregnant adolescents, ages 12–19 years, 86% single 60% African American, 38% Caucasian	Descriptive Longitudinal	Maternal-Fetal Attachment Scale Attachment assessment, interrater reliability = .93	Maternal attachment in adolescents began in pregnancy and increased over time, especially after quickening. Giving of self was less likely in younger adolescents. There was a positive relationship between attachment in the third trimester and affectionate behaviors following the birth.
Coffman, S., Levitt, M. J., & Guacci-Franco, N. (1993). Mothers' stress and close relationships: Correlates with infant status. *Pediatric Nursing, 19,* 135–140	Convenience 49 healthy mother-infant pairs 98% Caucasian Age of mothers: 22–41 years, mean = 31 Age of infants: 12–15 months, mean = 13 months; 29 males	Descriptive Correlational	Laboratory observation, interrater reliability = .50–.99	Infant temperament was more strongly related to attachment than to maternal responsiveness. Infants rated as anxious-avoidant in attachment were perceived by mothers as easier in temperament.
Karl, D. (1995). Maternal responsiveness of socially high-risk mothers to the elicitation cues of their 7-month old infants. *Journal of Pediatric Nursing, 10,* 254–263	Convenience 19 socially high-risk mother-infant dyads 42% single parents 80% Caucasian	Descriptive Naturalistic inquiry	Naturalistic videotapes of caretaking behaviors Investigator-developed scales to measure responsiveness and interaction No psychometric data on current sample	Mothers were generally emotionally depressed and unresponsive to infant cues. Adequate mothers more often responded appropriately to infant cues, were never physically unavailable, showed no anxiety, and were more positively responsive to infants' smiles and cries. Angry maternal mood was related to underresponse.
Beck, C. T. (1995). The effects of postpartum depression on maternal-infant interaction: A meta-analysis. *Nursing Research, 44,* 298–304	19 studies	Meta-analysis	Maternal interactive behaviors Infant interactive behaviors Dyadic interactive behaviors	Postpartum depression has a moderate to large effect on maternal-infant interaction.

Citation	Sample	Design	Instrument	Findings
Beck, C. T. (1996). Postpartum depressed mothers' experiences interacting with their children. *Nursing Research, 45,* 98–104	Purposive 19 married mothers who experienced depression after birth	Phenomenologic inquiry	Investigator-developed interview	Participants were overwhelmed by the responsibilities of caring for their children. Guilt, irrational thinking, loss, and anger filled their day-to-day interactions with their children. Sometimes, they "walled" themselves off and failed to respond to cues, leading to detrimental relationships with older children.
Gross, D., Conrad, B., Fogg, L., Willis, L., & Garvey, C. (1995). A longitudinal study of maternal depression and preschool children's mental health. *Nursing Research, 44,* 96–101	Community type 97 mothers with children, ages 2–3 years, and 97 mothers with children, ages 3–4 years 29% Caucasian, 50% African American	Longitudinal cohort	Social Competence Scale, *alpha* = .90–.92 Symptoms, *alpha* = .84–.92 Depression, *alpha* = .85–.88	Maternal depression was significantly related to competence and more behavior problems as reported by preschool teachers. Boys of depressed mothers were more likely than girls to have poorer social competence and more behavior problems.
Kristensen, K. L. (1995). The lived experience of childhood loneliness: A phenomenological study. *Issues in Comprehensive Pediatric Nursing, 18,* 125–137	Purposive 14 children, ages 8–10 years, 6 males 100% Caucasian	Phenomenologic inquiry	Investigator-developed interview	"Unhappily disconnected" emerged as the meaning of the complex and multideminsional experience of loneliness.

Gröer, Thomas, and Shoffner (1992) surveyed 167 teenagers using the Adolescent Life Change Event Scale (Mendez, Yeaworth, York, & Goodwin, 1980) and found that life events increased with age. Active distraction techniques, as determined by open-ended items about coping, were the most commonly used coping strategies. However, there were no relationships between amounts or types of life events, stressors, and ways of coping. The health consequences of loneliness in adolescents was the focus of a study by Mahon, Yarcheski, and Yarcheski (1993). Loneliness (as measured by the UCLA Loneliness Scale; Russell, Peplau, & Cutrona, 1980) and introspectiveness were found to contribute positively to perceived health status. In a study of adolescents from married and separated/divorced households, Grossman and Rowat (1995) found that the adolescents' perception of the parental relationship was associated more with life satisfaction than with family status. Further, Kelly (1995) found that adolescent mothers who maintained relationships with the child's father were more likely to practice better preventive health care for their children.

Gottlieb and Baillies (1995) examined distress and autonomy behaviors, as measured by the Preschool Behavioral Rating Scale (Gottlieb & Mendelson, 1990), in preschool children of pregnant mothers and nonexpectant mothers. They found that young, firstborn children of the pregnant mothers were more dependent and exhibited more anger and less autonomy than children of the nonexpectant mothers did.

Two studies on the experience of parenthood as a stressor were reported. Coffman, Levitt, and Guacci-Franco (1993) reported on a longitudinal descriptive study of 43 mothers of infants and found that the closest social support for the mothers was their mother or their husband, as measured by two instruments developed for the study: the Close Person Satisfaction Scale and the Relationship Closeness

Scale. Higher maternal stress was associated with the infant's hospitalization during the first year of life. Secondary analysis of family functioning data allowed Friedemann and Andrews (1990) to determine that single parents experienced different but not more stressors than two-parent families did.

In a series of studies of the impact of experience on parenting skills, Ferketich and Mercer (1995a, 1995b) and Mercer and Ferketich (1995) used a variety of established instruments to examine the competence of inexperienced and experienced mothers and fathers. They found that experience was not associated with attachment or competence but that the factors predicting attachment and competence varied for mothers and fathers and by experience.

Six studies dealt with coping strategies in school-age children and adolescents and the measurement used. Ryan-Wenger (1990) developed and validated the Schoolagers' Coping Strategies Inventory, and then in a separate study Ryan-Wenger and Copeland (1994) used it to describe the coping strategies chosen by African American school-age children from low-income families to deal with day-to-day events. They found that the instrument had acceptable reliability (*alpha* = .73 to .83) and that distraction and social support were the most commonly used strategies. They also found that (a) the severity of stressors assessed using the Feel Bad Scale (Lewis, Siegal, & Lewis, 1984) reported over time decreased but frequency did not decrease and (b) that boys and girls each used different coping strategies (Sharrer & Ryan-Wenger, 1995). Meininger, Stashinko, and Hayman (1991) reported on the psychometric properties of the Matthews Youth Test for Health (Matthews & Angulo, 1980), finding that two factors (Impatience-Aggression and Competitive Achievement Striving) were derived and cross-validated with acceptable reliability. Sorenson (1990) used content analysis of interviews to describe the coping behaviors of 32 well, school-age children and found four themes of coping responses—cognitive, cognitive-behavioral, behavioral, and interpersonal. Yarcheski, Mahon, and Yarcheski (1992) assessed the validity of the Personal Resource Questions (PRQ85) Social Support measure, developed by Brandt and Weinert (1981) for use with adolescents. Mahon, Yarcheski, and Yarcheski (1995) also reported on the validity of the UCLA Loneliness Scale. In both cases, the instruments were found to have acceptable reliability and validity for use with an adolescent population.

The consistency of the measures and methods used in these studies that emanated from a stress-adaptation model lends support to the conclusion that stressors are associated with alterations in health status and that certain coping behaviors may be helpful in dealing with stressors. Further, the measures used have been evaluated for reliability and validity.

Maternal Responsiveness Model

In 1995 and 1996, a number of studies were published that used maternal responsiveness as a framework (see Table 2.5). The majority of these studies focused on factors associated with maternal responsiveness, which has been found to be the single, most pervasive variable in infant attachment (Ainsworth, Blehar, Waters, & Wall, 1978). Bloom (1995) described the development of maternal attachment in a sample of 79 low-income pregnant adolescents and found that fetal attachment (Maternal-Fetal Attachment Scale; Cranley, 1981) increased beginning with quickening and that giving of self was less likely the younger the adolescent mother. Coffman, Levitt, and Guacci-Franco (1995) used laboratory observation of mothers and infants to describe the relationship of infant temperament to maternal attachment and responsiveness. Karl (1995) examined the effect of maternal depression on responsiveness to infant cues, Beck (1995, 1996) did the same

for maternal-infant interaction, as did Gross, Conrad, Fogg, Willis, and Garvey (1995) for social competence of preschool children. Finally, Kristensen (1995) used phenomenologic techniques to study children's experiences of loneliness.

Although these studies dealt with similar variables, the researchers used multiple types of designs, including phenomenologic and meta-analytic, to study attachment behavior. The richness of these methods and the consistency of findings, especially with regard to depression in mothers, suggest that maternal depression is a significant risk factor for attachment in young children.

Family Assessment/
Family Systems Models

Multiple studies used models based on the family as the focus. Two such models (McCubbin & Thompson, 1987; Wright & Leahey, 1994a) form the basis for a number of research studies dealing with health promotion in children. Five of the 9 studies included in this category were descriptive, 3 were psychometric analyses, and 1 was an ethnographic study (see Table 2.6). Topics dealt with the relationship of maternal symptoms of depression to childhood behavior and health status, psychometrics of family assessment tools, and child-rearing patterns.

Studies that use a family model most commonly examine the relationship of parental traits and states with child health status as an outcome. The studies reviewed here differed from those in the previous category because they did not describe an attachment model. For example, Hall, Gurley, Sachs, and Kryscio (1991) used the Center for Epidemiologic Studies-Depression Scale (CES-D; Radloff, 1977) and the Index of Parenting Attitudes (Hudson, 1982) to study the relationship of maternal depression and parenting attitudes with

text continued on p. 45

TABLE 2.6 Health Promotion Studies Using the Family Assessment/Family Systems Model

Author(s) and Source	Sample	Design	Measure(s)	Major Findings
Hall, L. A., Gurley, D. N., Sachs, B., & Kryscio, R. J. (1991). Psychosocial predictors of maternal depressive symptoms, parenting attitudes, and child behavior in single-parent families. *Nursing Research, 40,* 214–220	Convenience 225 mothers, ages 18–48 years 90% with annual income less than $10,000	Descriptive Correlational	Center for Epidemiological Studies–Depression Scale (CES-D), *alpha* = .86 Index of Parental Attitudes, *alpha* = .86 Preschool Behavior Questionnaire (PBQ), *alpha* = .84 Stressors, *alpha* = .80 Coping, *alpha* = .39–.66 Social support (FSSQ), *alpha* = .78 Family functioning, *alpha* = .96	5%–6% of the mothers had high depression symptoms, which were associated with greater everyday stressors, fewer social resources, and greater use of avoidance coping. Neither social resources nor coping strategies buffered the relationship between stressors and depressive symptoms. Maternal depressive symptoms predicted parenting attitudes. These attitudes predicted child behavior.
Hall, L. A., Sachs, B., Rayans, M. K., & Lutenbacher, M. (1993). Childhood physical and sexual abuse: Their relationship with depressive symptoms in adulthood. *Image: Journal of Nursing Scholarship, 25,* 317–323	Convenience 206 low-income mothers 59% African American	Descriptive	Violence, alpha not given CES-D, *alpha* = .89	36% of the mothers reported severe physical abuse during childhood. Prevalence of sexual abuse was 22%; more than half were violently abused. 51% reported depressive symptoms. Symptoms were associated with severe physical and sexual abuse. Women who experienced violent sexual abuse were 4-1/2 times more likely to report depressive symptoms.
Keltner, B. R. (1992). Family influences on child health status. *Pediatric Nursing, 18,* 128–131	Convenience 110 children, ages 3–5 years, in a Head Start program; 51% male 82% African American	Descriptive	Child's school health record Family Routines Inventory (FRI), test-retest = .79 Home environment, *alpha* = .80	51% of the children were healthy. Higher family routines and more stimulating home environments were positively correlated with child health status.

Citation	Sampling	Design	Instruments	Findings
Brown, P., Rustia, J., & Schappert, P. (1991). A comparison of fathers of high-risk newborns and fathers of healthy newborns. *Journal of Pediatric Nursing, 6,* 269–273	Convenience 18 fathers of healthy newborns and 18 fathers of newborns with health problems	Descriptive Comparison	Investigator-developed scales: Perception of Infant Scale Infant Care Activity Schedule Adjustment to Parenthood No psychometrics on current sample	Fathers of newborns with health problems performed significantly more infant care behaviors and had higher adjustment to parenthood scores 1 month following discharge from the hospital than did fathers of healthy newborns. There were no differences at 5 months after discharge.
Graham, M. V. (1993). Parental sensitivity to infant cues: Similarities and differences between mothers and fathers. *Journal of Pediatric Nursing, 8,* 376–384	Convenience 32 couples, ages 25–38 years, of 3-month-old infants	Descriptive Observation	Interpersonal reactivity, *alpha* = .84 Parental attitudes, *alpha* = .60 Marital adjustment, *alpha* = .89 Baby temperament, *alpha* = .56 Observation of parent response to infant cues	Interpersonal reactivity was associated with sensitivity to infant cues for mothers and fathers. Attitudes toward infant care were associated with sensitivity in mothers but not fathers. Nonverbal decoding ability, marital adjustment, baby temperament and gender were not related to sensitivity to cues. Mothers were significantly more empathic and had more positive attitude than fathers did.
Porter, C. (1994). As the twig is bent: Child rearing and working poor, older African American mothers. *The American Black Nursing Faculty Journal, 5*(3), 77-83	Convenience 3 mothers, ages 40–54 years, who participated in 4 weekly focus groups.	Ethnographic description	Focus group to elicit narratives tapping mothers' ideologies and practices for sex-role socialization	Child-rearing ideologies about and practices for differential sex-role socialization were influenced by environmentalist and behaviorist orientations. Ideologies and practices for the socialization of males into sex roles were contradictory.
Munet-Vilaro, F., & Egan, M. (1990). Reliability issues of the Family Environment Scale for cross-cultural research. *Nursing Research, 39,* 244–247	Convenience 57 Hispanics and 37 Vietnamese; no age range given	Psychometric Analysis	Family Environment Scale (FES)	*Alpha* ranged from .21 to .50, lower than reported by Moos and Moos (1986). Family concepts may be very different in different cultures.

TABLE 2.6 *Continued*

Author(s) and Source	Sample	Design	Measure(s)	Major Findings
Frankel, F. (1993). Sources of family annoyance (SOFA): Development, reliability, and validity. *Journal of Pediatric Nursing, 8,* 177–184	Convenience 235 parents of children, ages 2–12 years 65.5% Caucasian	Psychometric Analysis	Sources of Family Annoyance (SOFA)	Factor analysis revealed 2 subscales: Household Negatives and Child Negatives, *alpha* = .81–.91; test-retest = .93 and .71, respectively. SOFA discriminated between psychiatric clinic-referred parents. It also discriminated mothers on public assistance from mothers in a community sample.
Norwood, S. L. (1996). The Social Support APGAR: Instrument development and testing. *Research in Nursing and Health, 19,* 143–152	Convenience 220 postpartum patients, ages 14–38 years 98% Caucasian	Psychometric Analysis	Social Support APGAR, *alpha* = .88–.93	Social support scores were positively associated with favorable pregnancy outcomes and negatively associated with life stress.

child behavior as measured by the Preschool Behavior Questionnaire (Behar & Stringfield, 1974). In another study of maternal depression and abuse, Hall, Sachs, Rayans, and Lutenbacher (1993) found that 51% of women who were abused in childhood had depressive symptoms (CES-D). Keltner (1992) found that family routines, as measured by the Family Routines Inventory (Boyce, Jenson, James, & Peacock, 1983), and more stimulating environments were associated with better child health status as determined by school health records. Brown, Rustia, and Schappert (1991) compared fathers of high-risk newborns (now stable infants who had spent a minimum of 3 weeks in the Neonatal Intensive Care Unit or had a long-term health problem) with fathers of healthy newborns and found that the fathers of high-risk newborns were more involved in care and were better adjusted to parenthood at 1 month following discharge from the hospital. However, there were no differences at 5 months following discharge. Graham (1993) examined parental sensitivity to infant cues using observation and established scales and found that mothers were more empathic and had a more positive attitude toward their infants than fathers did. Porter (1994) used ethnographic methods to describe 3 working, poor African American mothers and concluded that models of sex-role socialization for males are different from those for females. Further, these socialization models provide contradictory ideologies and practices for males.

While there are multiple instruments available for family studies, using such instruments with various ethnic groups may create measurement problems. These problems were the topic of the psychometric study by Munet-Vilaro and Egan (1990), who examined reliability issues of the Family Environment Scale (FES; Moos & Moos, 1986) with different ethnic groups. Moos and Moos (1986) found serious problems in the concepts measured by the FES, with concepts varying by ethnic group.

The scale had low reliability (*alpha* = .20 to .50). Frankel (1993) developed the Sources of Family Annoyance (SOFA) Scale to measure the impact of potential stressors on mothers and fathers and reported its psychometric properties. Norwood (1996) evaluated the psychometric properties of the Social Support APGAR and found strong support for the reliability and validity of the instrument.

These studies for the most part used established instruments with acceptable reliability and validity. There appears to be some consistency in the finding that child health is associated with maternal characteristics, such as depressive symptoms or adjustment to parenthood.

Family Health Promotion Model

Pender (1982, 1987) developed the Health Promotion Model as an explanation of the determinants of health-promoting actions. A number of researchers based studies on this model, 4 of which dealt with assessment for health promotion in children and families. All these studies used descriptive designs and questionnaires to obtain data (see Table 2.7)

Houtrouw and Carlson (1993) studied the relationship between mothers' characteristics, beliefs about the vulnerability of their children to disease, and compliance with immunization schedules and found that mothers who perceived their children as vulnerable to disease were more likely to comply with immunization recommendations. Lenart, St. Clair, and Bell (1991) interviewed Cambodian refugee mothers about their child-rearing knowledge, beliefs, and practices. They found that these mothers used both traditional and clinic sources of information about child health. Logsdon (1991) studied the conceptions of health and health behaviors of preschool children by using a picture interview (Flaherty, 1986) with the children. The results indicated that young children view health as a positive

TABLE 2.7 Health Promotion Studies Using the Health Promotion Model

Author(s) and Source	Sample	Design	Measure(s)	Major Findings
Houtrouw, S. M., & Carlson, K. L. (1993). The relationship between maternal characteristics, maternal vulnerability beliefs, and immunization compliance. *Issues in Comprehensive Pediatric Nursing, 16*, 41–50	Convenience 40 mothers, ages 24–31 years, of children, ages 4–24 months 87.5% Caucasian 70% immunization compliant	Descriptive	Investigator-designed Communicable Disease Perceived Vulnerability, *alpha* = .91	No relationships were found between maternal characteristics, maternal vulnerability beliefs, and immunization compliance. Mothers who believe their infants had perceived vulnerability to disease had 60.6% compliance with immunizations.
Lenart, J. C., St. Clair, P. A., & Bell, M. A. (1991). Child-rearing knowledge, beliefs, and practices of Cambodian refugees. *Journal of Pediatric Health Care, 5*, 299–305	Convenience 40 Cambodian women, mean age = 37 years	Descriptive	Investigator-developed interview schedule to assess child-rearing knowledge, beliefs, practices, and information resources	Mothers used clinic and traditional sources for information. Mothers knew, for the most part, at what age children could perform specific developmental tasks. 50% reported that they would use clinics for 7 of 9 minor illnesses such as diarrhea, constipation, cough, and difficulty breathing.
Logsdon, D. A. (1991). Conceptions of health and health behaviors of preschool children. *Journal of Pediatric Nursing, 6*, 396–406	Convenience 30 children, ages 4–5 years, with no health problems, 26.7% male	Descriptive	Preschool Health Picture Interview	Health was conceptualized as a positive feeling state and the ability to participate in desired activities. Brushing teeth and eating were the highest-ranked health-promoting behaviors. Behaviors harmful to health were explained in terms of immediate physical consequences.

| Garcia, A. W., Norton-Broda, M. A., Frenn, M., Coviak, C., Pender, N. J., & Ronis, D. L. (1995). Gender and developmental differences in exercise beliefs among youth and prediction of their exercise behavior. *Journal of School Health, 65*, 213–219 | School based 286 children in 2 cohorts: 5th–6th grade and 8th grade; 48.3% male 63% Caucasian, 30% African American | Descriptive | Investigator-developed exercise log Self-esteem, *alpha* = .85 Health Perceptions Questionnaire, *alpha* = .85 Children's Self-Efficacy Survey, *alpha* = .77 Me Now and Future Scale: Children's Perceived Benefits/Barriers to Exercise Questionnaire, *alpha* = .77–.80 | Females reported less prior and current exercise, lower self-esteem, poorer health status, and lower exercise self-schema than males did. Eighth graders reported less social support for exercise and fewer role models than those in the lower grades did. In a path model, gender, differential of benefits/barriers, and access to exercise facilities directly predicted exercise. |

feeling state and that brushing one's teeth and eating the right foods were the most commonly performed health-promoting behaviors. Again, these studies used investigator-developed tools with limited psychometric evaluation presented, so the findings must be considered preliminary.

One study described an explicit attempt to test Pender's (1987) model on children's exercise behaviors. Garcia, Norton-Broda, Frenn, Coviak, Pender, and Ronis (1995) used a combination of investigator-developed and established tools to determine the factors associated with exercise behaviors in preadolescents and young adolescents. They found that females reported less exercise and that in addition to gender, the differential of benefits to barriers and access to exercise facilities predicted the children's exercise behavior. The results partially supported Pender's (1987) model.

Health Belief Model

The Health Belief Model was developed by Becker (1974) to help explain the likelihood of a person taking a particular health-related action. The model is based on the assumption that perceptions of one's subjective world predicts health behavior. The likelihood of taking such an action is presumed to be influenced by two major sets of variables—modifying factors (demographic, sociopsychological, and structural), which act on the likelihood of taking an action, and individual perceptions (psychological readiness, perceptions of barriers and benefits, perceived control, and health motivation). Three studies published in the 1995-1996 period explicitly tested the Health Belief Model with regard to children's health (see Table 2.8).

Hahn (1995) and Hahn, Simpson, and Kidd (1966) used it to explain the likelihood of parents of preschool children participating in programs related to alcohol, tobacco, and drug use prevention and found support for the model. Russell

and Champion (1996) found less support for the model in a study of hazards in the home with a sample of 140 low-income mothers of preschool children and hazards in the home. As with many of the studies of the Health Belief Model, the measures used in these studies are highly specific to the health behavior in question, so it is difficult to draw conclusions across them.

Bandura's Social Cognitive Theory

Bandura's (1986) social cognitive theory has two key components: perceived self-efficacy and outcome expectations. Perceived self-efficacy is the conviction that one can successfully execute the behavior required to produce desired outcomes and, as such, may be important to health-promoting behaviors. Four studies—3 descriptive, 1 quasi-experimental, and 1 psychometric analysis—that used a social cognitive framework were found (see Table 2.9). All dealt with adolescent risk-taking behaviors and were derived from Bandura's theory.

Descriptive studies using established instruments make up the majority of studies using Bandura's theory. Whatley (1991) found that health locus of control (measured by the Multidimensional Health Locus of Control Scale; Wallston, Wallston, & DeVillis, 1978), especially the influence of "powerful others," such as peers, explained more than 10% of the variance in risk-taking behaviors in adolescents, as measured by an instrument developed by the investigators. Mahon and Yarcheski (1992) described the characteristics of loneliness in adolescents as they relate to personality characteristics. DilOrio, Parsons, Lehr, Adame, and Carlone (1992) developed an instrument to measure safe-sex behavior in adolescents and young adults and reported initial validity and reliability analyses. Rozmus and Edgil (1993) reported rural adolescents' values, knowledge, and attitudes about AIDS. The investigators

TABLE 2.8 Health Promotion Studies Using the Health Belief Model

Author(s) and Source	Sample	Design	Measure(s)	Major Findings
Hahn, E. J. (1995). Predicting Head Start parent involvement in an alcohol and other drug prevention program. *Nursing Research, 44,* 45–51	Countywide convenience 300 parents, mean age = 29 years, of children in Head Start program 95% parents 90% female	Descriptive Correlational	Susceptibility Seriousness Barriers Beliefs Control, *alpha* = .79 Health motivation, *alpha* = .87 Stressors, *alpha* = .68 Role modeling, *alpha* = .87 Self-esteem, *alpha* = .85 Parental competence, *alpha* = .75 Parental alcohol and other drug use severity and knowledge, *alpha* = .70	Previous classroom involvement, barriers, county, and race predicted high attendance. Low attendance was associated with severity of alcohol and other drug use, benefits, and role modeling.
Hahn, E. J., Simpson, M. R., & Kidd, P. (1996). Cues to parent involvement in drug prevention and school activities. *Journal of School Health, 66,* 165–170	Focus groups 38 parents and preschool personnel	Descriptive	Focus group Investigator-developed instruments	Cues to action was the most frequently expressed construct of the Health Belief Model for promoting parent involvement with young children in an alcohol, tobacco, and drug prevention program. Enthusiasm for school activities was critical. Necessary incentives were transportation, child care, and other gifts.
Russell, K. M., & Champion, V. L. (1996). Health beliefs and social influence on home safety practices of mothers with preschool children. *Image: Journal of Nursing Scholarship, 28,* 59–64	Convenience 140 low-income mothers, ages 15–41 years (mean = 25.1 years), with preschool children, ages 1–3) years 97% African American	Descriptive Correlational	Susceptibility, *alpha* = .83 Seriousness, *alpha* = .94 Benefits, *alpha* = .81 Barriers, *alpha* = .72 Self-efficacy, *alpha* = .83 Social influence, *alpha* = .83 Knowledge, *alpha* = .75 Home accident prevention observation, interrater agreement = 90%–97%	Health beliefs, social influence, demographic, and experiential variables accounted for 51% of variance in hazard accessibility and 44% in hazard frequency. Home safety practices were predicted by high self-efficacy, previous injury experience, higher knowledge, older age, and child's birth position.

49

TABLE 2.9 Health Promotion Studies Using Social Cognitive Theory

Author(s) and Source	Sample	Design	Measure(s)	Major Findings
Whatley, J. H. (1991). Effects of health locus of control and social network on adolescent risk taking. *Pediatric Nursing, 17*, 145–148	Convenience 187 students, ags 14–19 years, 54% male	Descriptive Correlational	Multidimensional Health Locus of Control (MHLC), *alpha* = .51–64 Social support, *alpha* = .86 Risk taking, *alpha* = .91	Two MHLC subscales contributed to variance in risk-taking scores: Powerful Others (9.2%) and Internal Health (1.9%). Social support contributed 1.1%.
Mahon, N. E., & Yarcheski, A. (1992). Alternate explanations of loneliness in adolescents: A replication and extension study. *Nursing Research, 41*, 151–156	Convenience 113 early, 106 middle, and 106 late adolescents 72% Caucasian	Descriptive Correlational	Revised UCLA Loneliness Scale, *alpha* = .87–90 Maternal expressiveness, *alpha* = .88–93 Paternal expressiveness, *alpha* = .95–97 Interpersonal solidarity, *alpha* = .84–88 Personal resources, *alpha* = .89–91 Self-disclosure, *alpha* = .96–97 Shyness, *alpha* = .65–76 Self-esteem, *alpha* = .76–88 Emotional reliance, *alpha* = .74–.82	For early adolescents, the character set (self-disclosure, shyness, self-esteem, and emotional reliance) explained more variance in loneliness than the situational set (maternal and paternal expressiveness, close friend solidarity, and social support). For middle and late adolescents, the situational set explained more variance than the character set.
DiIorio, C., Parsons, M., Lehr, S., Adame, D., & Carlone, J. (1992). Measurement of safe sex behavior in adolescents and young adults. *Nursing Research, 41*, 203–208	Convenience Separate samples of 531 and 174 college freshmen; age range not given 80% Caucasian	Psychometric Analysis	Safe Sex Behavior Questionnaire (SSBQ) Self-expression, *alpha* = .91 Risk taking, *alpha* = .89	Content validity index = .98%, *alpha* = .82. Factor analysis of 5 factors. Construct validity of the SSBQ was supported by correlations with assertiveness and general risk taking.
Rozmus, C. L., & Edgil, A. E. (1993). Values, knowledge, and attitudes about Acquired Immunodeficiency Syndrome in rural adolescents. *Journal of Pediatric Health Care, 7*, 167–173	Probability 1,048 students in the 10th and 11th grades, 55% female	Descriptive	AIDS Knowledge and Belief Survey Value Survey Multidimensional Health Locus of Control, *alpha* = .55–62 Risk taking, *alpha* = 89	Students had more correct than incorrect knowledge about AIDS/HIV. Their personal values of an exciting life and pleasure were related to the likelihood of participating in risky behaviors. Attitudes were negatively related to the likelihood of participating in risky behaviors.

found that the adolescents had more correct than incorrect information.

The results suggest that Bandura's work may have relevance for the study of health-promoting behaviors in adolescents. Most of these studies used established instruments, with tested reliability and validity, thus creating more confidence in the findings.

Orem's Self-Care Model

Orem's (1971) conceptual framework of self-care forms the basis for much nursing research, but interestingly, little of this research deals with health promotion for children and families. Only one study—Moore and Gaffney's (1989)—was found that used Orem's framework for assessment concerning health promotion and disease prevention for children and families (see Table 2.10). This report of the psychometric analysis of the Dependent Care Agent questionnaire described the development and initial validation of an instrument to measure mothers' performance of self-care activities for children. Reliability was high at .91, and a 12-factor solution was isolated that supported Orem's model.

Comprehensive Assessment Model

C. Burns (1992) developed a new assessment model and tool concerning the health of children for pediatric nurse practitioners (PNPs). This tool integrates elements of the classical medical history, Gordon's (1982) functional health patterns, and development into one system. This model was tested by C. Burns (1993) in a study of the practice of three PNPs (see Table 2.11). Using a comprehensive taxonomy of diagnoses, C. Burns found that the PNPs used 3,000 diagnoses for 1,450 cases, and their scope of practice was variable. Although this is a new model, the application of

nursing diagnosis to health promotion and disease prevention for children and families has the potential to increase our knowledge.

Interaction Model of Client Health Behavior

Cox (1982) described the Interaction Model of Client Health Behavior to explain relationships between client characteristics, the client-provider relationship, and subsequent client behavior. Although many studies concerning adult clients use this model, only one study in the time period surveyed was found that dealt with children (see Table 2.12).

Farrand and Cox (1993) determined the contributions of sociodemographic variables, social influences (Family Environment Scale; Moos & Moos, 1986), intrinsic motivation (Health Self-Determinism Index for Children; Cox, Cowell, Marion, & Miller, 1990), and health perception (Child's Health Self-Concept Scale; Hester, 1984) to the health behaviors of preadolescent children (How Often Do You?; Stember, Swanson-Kaufman, Goodwin, Rogers, & Mathews, 1984). The results indicated that health behaviors are gender specific and that the models that predict them also vary by gender.

Problem-Proneness Behavior

The theory of problem-proneness behavior (Jessor & Jessor, 1977) suggests that adolescents who engage in one problem behavior are more likely to practice other problem behaviors, and that the dynamics between certain behaviors are dependent on the social ecology of the adolescent. One study used this model to examine the relationships of sexual risk taking to substance use and AIDS knowledge in pregnant and nonpregnant adolescents (see Table 2.13).

TABLE 2.10 Health Promotion Study Using the Self-Care Model

Authors and Source	Sample	Design	Measures	Major Findings
Moore, J. B., & Gaffney, K. F. (1989). Development of an instrument to measure mothers' performance of self-care activities for children. *Advances in Nursing Science, 12,* 76–84	Convenience 475 mothers of children, ages 1–16 year	Psychometric Analysis	Investigator-developed Dependent Care Agent Questionnaire	A 12-factor solution was isolated that supported Orem's (1971) requisition for self-care, *alpha* = .91.

TABLE 2.11 Health Promotion Study Using the Comprehensive Assessment Model

Author and Source	Sample	Design	Measure	Major Findings
Burns, C. (1993). Using a comprehensive taxonomy of diagnoses to describe the practice of pediatric nurse practitioners: Findings of a field study. *Journal of Pediatric Health Care, 7,* 115–121	Convenience 6 pediatric nurse practitioners	Descriptive	Record review using classification system	3,000 nursing diagnoses were recorded for 1,450 cases: 72% pediatric diseases, including 51% illnesses; 21% disease prevention and screening; 27% daily living problems; and 1% developmental problems.

TABLE 2.12 Health Promotion Study Using the Interaction Model of Client Health Behavior

Authors and Source	Sample	Design	Measures	Major Findings
Farrand, L. L., & Cox, C. L. (1993). Determinants of positive health behavior in middle childhood. *Nursing Research, 42,* 208–213	Convenience 260 children, ages 9–10 years, 54% female	Descriptive Correlational	Family Environment Scale, *alpha* = .71 Health Self- Determination Index for Children, *alpha* = .78 Child's Health Self-Concept Scale, *alpha* = .82 How Often Do You? (child health behavior), *alpha* = .84	Health behaviors were gender specific. Self-esteem, intrinsic motivation, and perceptions of health contributed to health behaviors. 53% variance in girls' behavior and 63% variance in the boys' behavior were explained.

Koniak-Griffin and Brecht (1995) used a new questionnaire with items from the Centers for Disease Control's Youth Risk Behavior Survey (Kolbe, 1990) together with the AIDS questionnaire developed by Flaskerud and Nyamathi (1990). The theory of problem proneness was supported, in that adolescents who used marijuana were more likely to engage in risky sexual behaviors.

■ Conclusions

The first question for this review asked what paradigms/models have guided nursing research dealing with assessment for health promotion/disease prevention. The preceding discussion demonstrates that in the period from 1989 to 1996, 13 models guided nursing research dealing with assessment for health promotion/disease prevention for children and families. These models ranged from a medical model to several nursing models, such as those developed by Orem (1971), Pender (1987), and C. Burns (1992).

Models developed in psychology and social psychology that have been used in assessing health behaviors and readiness for interventions in other fields or with adult populations were notably less prominent in the review of nursing literature on health promotion and disease prevention in children than might be expected. Neither Prochaska's Readiness for Change Model (Prochaska & DiClemente, 1983) nor Bruhn and Parcel's (1982) Model of Health Promotion was used to guide any of the nursing studies reviewed. Only the Health Belief Model (Becker, 1974) was used to develop studies, and it was used in only three studies, two of which were by the same author. It is possible that nurse researchers view the use of these models primarily for changing behavior in chronic illness, but the models also could provide potentially useful information for

health-promoting behaviors. It is possible too that these models have been used in studies with adults but not applied to problems in child health.

Although several studies used a physiologic or medical approach to assessment for health promotion for children and their families, none used the International Classification of Primary Care (Wood, 1992) to categorize patients or complaints. This omission may be due to the relative newness of this approach and the lag time in adapting its use in primary care research. Although these models provide information about assessment for health promotion, models developed in other disciplines may help provide a stronger basis for health promotion practice in nursing and across disciplines.

The second question addressed by this review asked what methods have been used to study assessment for health promotion and disease prevention in children and families. The designs, samples, and measures for each study are summarized in Tables 2.1 through 2.13.

The methods used in the studies reviewed are almost all descriptive. Most researchers used interviews or questionnaires to collect the data. In many instances, psychometric information about the tools used in the population studied was not provided. Many of the researchers used small samples, but a number of studies had adequate samples for statistical power. Only a few studies were qualitative; the majority were quantitative, descriptive studies, or psychometric analyses. Some of the concepts central to health promotion and disease prevention need to be further explicated using qualitative methods.

Many of the studies involved descriptions of single variables or bivariate relationships rather than full tests of the models under study. This finding suggests that, despite the centrality of assessment and health promotion to child health nursing, the study of this aspect of nursing science is in its infancy. More work on concept development and measurement of constructs in

TABLE 2.13 Health Promotion Study Using the Theory of Problem-Proneness Behavior

Authors and Source	Sample	Design	Measures	Major Findings
Koniak-Griffin, D., & Brecht, M. (1995). Linkages between sexual risk taking, substance use, and AIDS knowledge among pregnant adolescents and young mothers. *Nursing Research, 44,* 340–346	Convenience 58 pregnant adolescents and 93 nonpregnant adolescents, ages 12–20 years, mean = 16.6 years 64% Latina, 25% Caucasian, 11% African American	Descriptive Comparative	Sociodemographic and background information CDC Youth Risk Behavior Survey, *alpha* = .55–.87 AIDS Questionnaire, *alpha* = .90	Multiple high-risk behaviors were reported. Current pregnancy, history of marijuana use, and African American race were strong predictors of having had multiple sex partners. Pregnant adolescents were also more likely to have unprotected sex. AIDS knowledge was not a significant predictor of high-risk sexual behavior.

health promotion models and in model testing must occur before a prescriptive approach to health promotion and disease prevention, based on empirical research, can be obtained.

The majority of the studies reported relied on convenience samples. Because health promotion, disease prevention, and primary care are by definition community based, more population-based studies need to be conducted. Further, aside from studies of risk-taking behaviors, little work has been reported on health promotion knowledge and its correlates in non-Caucasian, non-middle-class populations. It is acknowledged that such populations may be more difficult to study, but because primary care services delivered by nurses are mostly to underserved populations, understanding these groups is important (Grey & Flint, 1989). It is also important to determine if the models studied in Caucasian populations will be valid for studies that include other population groups. Preliminary data suggest that the instruments available need work to establish reliability and validity in population subgroups.

Finally, this review attempted to draw conclusions about the assessment of children and families for health promotion. Unfortunately, the lack of more than one or two studies in any one area makes drawing conclusions difficult. A key finding of this review is the relative lack of sustained research in any one area. Only a few nurse researchers have published more than one study in the same area of inquiry. This finding may be a result of limiting the review to the past 7 years, but the reference lists of the studies reviewed support the view that few researchers have sustained productivity in any research area. This lack of research program development suggests that the field is ripe for future inquiry.

Although few topics were addressed by more than one or two studies, the topic of HIV/AIDS was dealt with in a number of studies, most of which dealt with risk behaviors and knowledge among adolescents. Information about this topic is important for providers of health promotion and disease prevention services because of the need to understand what clients understand before attempting to change behavior. The consistency of findings that children and adolescents have substantial correct knowledge about risky behavior but that their behavior does not reflect this knowledge suggests that assessing readiness to change behavior may be more important than knowledge per se. Clearly, more research that replicates findings and extends findings from one setting or population to another is needed in other areas of inquiry, such as injuries and violence.

An area in which there is some agreement concerns adolescent stress and coping. Stress and coping, especially problem-focused coping, were consistently associated with variations in health status. Such information is important for assessing the health-promoting behavior of teens and should be taken into account by providers working with teens.

It is clear from this review that researchers interested in health promotion and disease prevention in childhood must develop sustained programs of research that deal with the serious problems in health promotion and disease prevention. These problems include violence, immunization compliance, and accidents. For the most part, few studies in these important areas of assessment have been published in the recent past. For example, only one study of immunization status was found. Only by developing sustained programs of research in these topic areas will our knowledge of children's and families' health promotion needs be expanded. Further, new models of health promotion and disease prevention may emerge from such sustained programs of research.

3
■

INTEGRATIVE REVIEW OF INTERVENTION MODELS FOR HEALTH PROMOTION OF CHILDREN AND FAMILIES

■ *Laura L. Hayman*

Promoting the health of children and families has been a major goal of professional nursing practice. Throughout the past two decades, however, health promotion and disease prevention have captured increased attention in both the research and clinical agendas of numerous, diverse disciplines and have emerged as priority areas for nurse scholars and clinicians. This emphasis, as Grey (chap. 2 in this volume) observed, is reflected in the number of existing paradigms/conceptual models designed to guide research and clinical practice in health promotion and disease prevention. Documents including *Healthy People 2000: National Health Promotion and Disease Prevention Objectives for the Year 2000* (U.S. Department of Health and Human Services [USDHHS], 1990), *Health Promotion for Older Children and Adolescents* (Na-

tional Institute of Nursing Research [NINR], 1993), and *Bright Futures: Guidelines for Health Supervision of Infants, Children and Adolescents* (Green, 1994) provide further evidence of the multidisciplinary attention focused on health across the life span.

This chapter presents the state of the art and science in conceptually based, health-promoting interventions for children and families with the ultimate goal of informing clinical practice and future research. Three questions are addressed in this review:

- What paradigms/conceptual models have guided research focused on health promotion and disease prevention interventions with children and families?
- What dimensions of health promotion have been addressed?
- What conclusions can be drawn?

■ *Background*

The methods and content selected to address the questions raised in this review were based in part on principles developed by the World Health Organization (1984) to guide the direction of health promotion globally and by the health status objectives for the nation defined in *Healthy People 2000* (USDHHS, 1990). Consistent with principles advanced by the World Health Organization, health is viewed from a developmental-contextual lifespan perspective as a multidimensional phenomenon—a positive process of reaching one's potential in physical and nonphysical domains. As Millstein (1989) observed, this process is mediated by the interaction of systems within and outside the individual, including the biological, cognitive, and emotional systems as well as the social, economic, and political systems such as the family, neighborhood, community, race, culture, and country. Health promotion and disease prevention are viewed as distinguishable, complementary processes (Pender, 1987). Health-promoting interventions, the primary focus of this chapter, consist of activities designed to increase the level of well-being of children and families. In contrast, primary disease prevention consists of activities designed to decrease the probability of specific illnesses or dysfunctions in children and families (Pender, 1987). Because these processes/activities are complementary and implemented in tandem in clinical practice, research that focused on preventive interventions was not excluded from this review.

Although not intended as an exhaustive review, it does include research identified through a comprehensive literature search (emphasizing the time period 1989 through 1995) using MEDLINE and CINHAL with the following terms: health promotion, interventions, children, adolescents, families, models of care, and nursing. Terms added sequentially were derived from the health status goals/objectives for health promotion as defined categorically in *Healthy People 2000* (USDHHS, 1990). These included physical activity/fitness, nutrition, tobacco, alcohol and other drugs, family planning, mental health, violent and abusive behavior, and educational and community-based programs. Recent documents together with reports emanating from relevant multidisciplinary panels (Blumenthal, Matthews, & Weiss, 1994; Harlan, Kalberer, & Vogel, 1994; Lamberty & Barnard, 1994) were also reviewed.

Several assumptions about health guided the inclusion of content and the organization of this chapter:

- By definition, at both the individual and population level, health is a multidimensional construct necessitating multidisciplinary research and practice.
- Health and behavior are inextricably linked across the life span.
- Childhood and adolescence are critical periods for the development of health-promoting behaviors.
- Effective health promotion strategies must target the individual child and that child's contexts of development.

Collectively, the guiding principles, definitions, and assumptions point to the importance of paradigms/models of health promotion that provide for individual, family, and community-based interventions.

Numerous conceptual models have been developed to guide health promotion initiatives, but few have been applied in the design of health promotion interventions for pediatric populations. Together with highlighting their specific research applications, several conceptual models are discussed that have guided research in health promotion interventions for children and families. Emphasis is placed on the utility of the respective models for intervention-focused research designs and clinical practice with children and families across settings and contexts.

■ *Focus on Individuals: The Health Belief Model*

The Health Belief Model (HBM) was originally developed at the U.S. Public Health Service to explain why individuals did not participate in programs to prevent or detect disease (Hochbaum, 1958; Rosenstock, 1960, 1966). Throughout the past four decades, the model has been further developed and applied to adherence, sick role, and health promotion behaviors (Becker, 1974; Rosenstock, 1990) and, most recently, development of children's health beliefs and expectations (Bush & Iannotti, 1990). The original conception of the HBM is illustrated in Figure 3.1. In this model, the likelihood of health-related behaviors is a function of (a) the level of threat posed by the health problem as determined by both the individual's perception of the severity of the problem and perceived vulnerability/susceptibility to it; (b) the individual's perception of benefit to be derived from engaging in a behavior to reduce the threat versus perception of barriers to performing the behavior; and (c) an internal or external trigger or cue to action (Becker & Maiman, 1980). After considerable research with the HBM and in an attempt to increase its explanatory power, Rosenstock, Strecher, and Becker (1988) added Bandura's (1977) concept of self-efficacy, the belief or conviction that one could successfully execute the behavior required to produce the desired outcome. Other modifications to the original HBM were suggested by A. C. Burns (1992).

The Children's Health Belief Model (CHBM; Bush & Iannotti, 1990) incorporates the major elements of the HBM together with variables derived from three other conceptual systems: Social Learning Theory (SLT; Bandura, 1972), Cognitive Developmental Theory (CDT; Inhelder & Piaget, 1985), and Behavioral Intention Theory (BIT; Fishbein & Ajzen, 1975). With its emphasis on external social and physical influences on acquisition and maintenance of behaviors, SLT provides for inclusion of environmental variables (including familial influences) associated with children's health-related attitudes and behaviors (Bush & Iannotti, 1985; Lewis & Lewis, 1982). CDT emphasizes the role of developmental changes in cognitive processes that influence children's understanding of social and physical events (Bibace & Walsh, 1980; Mickalide, 1986; Natapoff, 1978). BIT, although not emphasized in the pediatric literature, is noteworthy for its inclusion of reference group norms, emphasis on specific behaviors as compared with abstractions and inferences for which children are not cognitively prepared, and indication that behavioral intentions are the best available predictors of behaviors (Bush & Iannotti, 1990). The resulting model, as applied to children's expected medicine use for five common health problems, is illustrated in Figure 3.2. Consistent with Gochman and Saucier (1982) and other recent recommendations for optimal health promotion and disease prevention with children and families (Green, 1994), the CHBM places children's health behavior within its personal and social context. As such, it recognizes the relationship of children's health behavior to their personal attributes (beliefs, expectations, motives, cognitive processes) and the influence of external social factors (families, peers, social groups) on these attributes (Bush & Iannotti, 1990).

The CHBM was evaluated in a study of children's expected medicine use for five common health problems (Bush & Iannotti, 1990). The

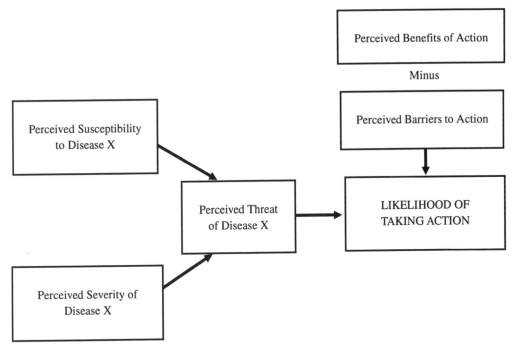

Figure 3.1. Health Belief Model

sample consisted of 270 urban preadolescents (stratified by socioeconomic status, grade level, and sex) and their primary caretakers (93% mothers). Of the study children, 56% were African American, 33% were Caucasian, and 11% were Hispanic or "other." Children and their caretakers were interviewed individually. Two major hypotheses, derived from prior results in this program of research (Bush & Iannotti, 1988), were tested: (a) CHBM variables predict children's expectations to take medicine, and (b) caretaker health beliefs and expectations increase the ability to explain children's states of readiness and expectations to take medicines. Regression analyses evaluated the influence of the child's primary caretaker on the child's expected medicine use. Individual differences in children's motivations, perceived benefits and threats, and expectations to take medicines were partially explained by caretakers' perceptions of their children. Path analysis evaluated hypothesized causal rela-

tionships in the CHBM, accounting for 63% of the adjusted variance in children's expected medicine use. Two readiness factors—perceived severity of illness and perceived benefit of taking medicines—had the highest path coefficients, with illness concerns and perceived vulnerability to illness accounting for a smaller but significant portion of the variance. Cognitive and affective variables, notably children's health locus of control, contributed to indirect paths between demographic and readiness factors.

The results of this study underscore the complexity and multiple sources of influence on children's health-related behaviors and suggest the CHBM as a viable explanatory model. As Tinsley (1992) observed, the CHBM is one of the most comprehensive models to date to focus on how familial, demographic, and attitudinal factors shape children's developing health beliefs and behaviors. As such, the model has potential for intervention-focused research with children and families. Requisite to such

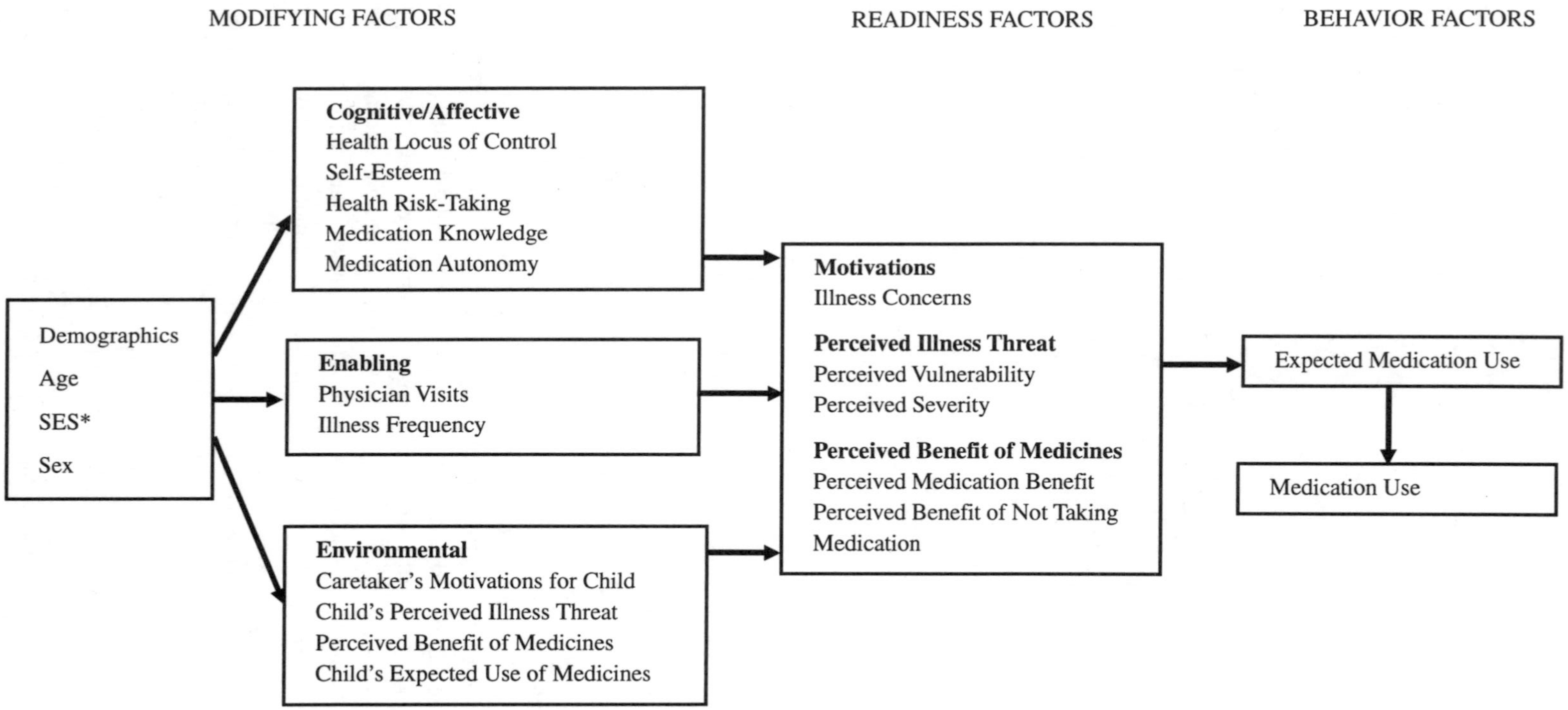

Figure 3.2. Children's Health Belief Model (CHBM)

*SES = socioeconomic status.
SOURCE: Bush and Iannotti (1990).

intervention studies is an examination of the utility of the CHBM in predicting the targeted health behavior in the population under study. Similar to the HBM, operationalizing and testing the full model requires a large sample. Additional directions for future research include testing the model with population-based multiethnic samples and delineating the relationships between self-esteem, health locus of control, and risk taking as they interact to influence health-related behaviors.

■ *Focus on Individuals:*
Theory of Reasoned Action
and Theory of Planned Behavior

The theory of reasoned action (TRA; Ajzen & Fishbein, 1980; Fishbein & Ajzen, 1975), also referred to as the BIT, was designed to predict an individual's intention to perform a behavior (under volitional control) in a specific, well-defined setting. A major assumption, as illustrated in Figure 3.3, is that behavioral intention is the immediate determinant of behavior; all other factors that influence behavior are mediated through this variable.

The strength of the intention to perform a behavior is a function of two factors: *personal attitude* toward the behavior and *social influence* of the environment or general subjective norms on the behavior. Attitude is determined by (a) the belief that a particular outcome will occur if the behavior is performed and (b) an evaluation of that outcome (Carter, 1990). Social norm is determined by an individual's (a) normative belief about what significant others think and (b) the motivation to comply with those expectations.

The theory of planned behavior (TPB; Ajzen, 1985, 1989) adds another intention-mediating factor, *perceived control* (ease or difficulty of achieving the outcome), and attempts to account for behaviors that are beyond volitional control. Perceived behavioral control reflects both past experience and anticipated obstacles, resources, and opportunities (Jemmott & Jemmott, 1994). It is noteworthy that perceived behavioral control and perceived self-efficacy, derived from Bandura's (1986) Social Cognitive Theory (SCT), are similar constructs.

The TRA was applied by Jemmott and Jemmott (1991) in a study of AIDS risk behavior in 103 sexually active, unmarried, collegiate African American women. This study, the first step in a program of research, was designed to determine the usefulness of the framework for targeting interventions to change AIDS risk behavior among women. Specifically, the study tested hypotheses regarding personal (attitudinal) and social (normative) influences on intentions to use condoms, a behavior that would reduce women's risk of sexually transmitted HIV infection. Consistent with the theory, women's anonymous responses to a mailed survey indicated stronger intentions to use condoms (in the next 3 months) among those with favorable attitudes toward condoms and among those who perceived subjective norms more supportive of condom use. Behavioral beliefs related to attitudes focused on the adverse effects of condom use on sexual enjoyment. Key normative influences were respondents' sexual partners and mothers. Personal factors (women's attitudes) were a stronger determinant of intentions to use condoms than were their perceptions of normative influences, particularly among women with above-average AIDS knowledge.

The results of this study provided direction for using the TRA in conjunction with SCT to guide a program of research focused on modifying perceptions of adverse effects of condom use on sexual enjoyment among adolescent women (Jemmott, Jemmott, Spears, Hewitt, & Cruz-Collins, 1992).

Research in progress, funded by the National Institute of Nursing Research (NINR),

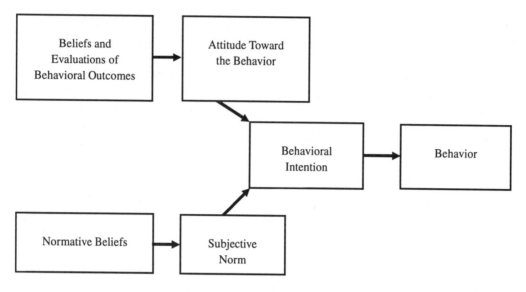

Figure 3.3. Theory of Reasoned Action
SOURCE: Ajzen and Fishbein (1980).

illustrates the application of Ajzen's (1985, 1989) TPB to health-promoting interventions among 356 African American adolescent mothers, ages 15–18 years (Schwarz & O'Sullivan, 1993). Even though this research is still in the data collection phase, it is noteworthy because it is a randomized controlled trial (RCT) of practice and community-based interventions stimulated by comprehensive longitudinal observations of health behaviors and outcomes of adolescent mothers and is modeled on an adaptation of the theory of planned behavior. The conceptual model includes operationalization of the major constructs, including personal (beliefs, attitudes, values) and social (perceived social norms) factors, and emphasizes mediators of perceived behavioral control (personality type, depression, stress) as they interact to influence behavioral intentions and outcomes. A major outcome targets sexual indicators of health status (regular use of condoms and effective hormonal contraception). The 356 adolescent mothers were enrolled during their postpartum hospitalization and randomized to intervention ($n = 178$) or control ($n = 178$)

groups. Measured at the nurse-managed, multidisciplinary, teen/well-baby practice site, assessments of both personal and social factors and behavioral intentions provide the baseline information necessary for the individualized interventions that target behavioral control and its study-specific mediators. Noteworthy is the emphasis on provider-patient collaboration/ negotiation in the development of this aspect of the intervention plan implemented at the practice site by nurse-health educators. The nurse-health educator intervenes to alter perceived social norms in the practice and home sites respectively. Between-group differences in outcomes together with model-specific personal and social factors are assessed at 18 months' postpartum in the home environment by blinded members of the research team.

Effective implementation of the TRA and the TPB in health promotion or disease prevention interventions requires a comprehensive survey of the target population (Carter, 1990). Specifically, as illustrated by Jemmott and Jemmott (1991) and Schwarz and O'Sullivan (1993), the foci of interventions and the outcomes perceived as most important must be identified (a priori) by the individuals targeted for behavior change. Consideration also must be given to developmental variables (not directly specified in these theories) known to influence children's and adolescents' understanding of health and illness (Bibace & Walsh, 1980; Mickalide, 1986). The complexity of these theoretical approaches (reasoned action and planned behavior) necessitates substantial resources for full and effective implementation in health promotion interventions. Thus, these theories are often used to identify the specific targets for interventions alone or in conjunction with other theoretical approaches, including SCT.

■ *Focus on Individuals and Environments: Social Learning Theory and Social Cognitive Theory*

Social Learning Theory (SLT) and Social Cognitive Theory (SCT) were articulated by Albert Bandura (1977, 1986) to address both the psychosocial dynamics underlying health behavior and the methods of promoting behavior change. The SCT also emphasizes the effects of cognitive processes on behavior. Central to both theories is the explanation of human behavior in terms of a triadic, dynamic, and reciprocal model in which behavior, personal factors (including cognitions), and environmental influences all interact (Perry, Baranowski, & Parcel, 1990). Among the crucial personal factors are the individual's capabilities to symbolize the meanings of behavior, foresee the outcomes of given behavior patterns, learn by observing others, self-determine or self-regulate behavior, and reflect and analyze experience (Bandura, 1986). Recently, Bandura (1995) emphasized self-efficacy as a major determinant of health-related behavior

across the life span. Collectively, these personal factors have been major influences in designing effective health education and promotion programs, including those focused on children, adolescents, and families. In the development of contemporary health promotion programs, however, emphasis has been placed on multicomponent interventions directed simultaneously at the individual and the environment (Flynn, Worden, Seckler-Walker, Badger, & Geller, 1995; Simons-Morton, Simons, Parcel, & Bunker, 1988; Stone, McGraw, Osganian, & Elder, 1994; Stone, Perry, & Luepker, 1989). Within this framework, environment reflects a range of factors (i.e., family, peers, school) that have the potential to influence behavior but are physically external to the individual. The inclusion and operational definitions of person, environment, and behavior have contributed to the application of these theories with diverse groups in a range of settings. Table 3.1 provides definitions of and implications for intervention for the major model constructs.

SCT was used in conjunction with other theories to guide a number of multicomponent intervention studies funded by the National Heart, Lung, and Blood Institute (NHLBI) focused on cardiovascular health promotion and disease prevention in childhood and adolescence. Stone et al. (1989) provided a synthesis of the school-based studies illustrating the versatility and effectiveness of SCT. Although the designs and methods differed among these studies, most of the SCT constructs listed in Table 3.1 were operationalized in each study.

Stone et al. (1994) also detailed the process evaluation of the recently completed Multicenter Child and Adolescent Trial for Cardiovascular Health (CATCH). The purpose of this NHLBI-funded project, grounded in SCT (Luepker et al., 1996), was to test the effectiveness of a multicomponent, school-based, cardiovascular health promotion program for public elementary school students. A random sample of 96 elementary schools at four sites

TABLE 3.1 Major Concepts in Social Learning Theory and Implications for Interventions

Concepts	Definitions	Implications
Environment	Factors that are physically external to the person	Provide opportunities and social support
Situation	Person's perception of the environment	Correct misperceptions and promote healthful norms
Behavioral capability	Knowledge and skill to perform a given behavior	Promote mastery learning through skills training
Expectations	Anticipatory outcomes of a behavior	Model positive outcomes of healthful behavior
Expectancies	The values that the person places on a given outcome, incentives	Present outcomes of change that have functional meaning
Self-control	Personal regulation of goal-directed behavior or performance	Provide opportunities for self-monitoring and contracting
Observational learning	Behavioral acquisition that occurs by watching the actions and outcomes of others' behavior	Include credible role models of the targeted behavior
Reinforcements	Responses to a person's behavior that increase or decrease the likelihood of reoccurrence	Promote self-initiated rewards and incentives
Self-efficacy	The person's confidence in performing a particular behavior	Approach behavior change in small steps; seek specificity about change sought
Emotional coping responses	Strategies or tactics that are used by a person to deal with emotional stimuli	Provide training in problem solving and stress management; include opportunites to practice skills in emotionally arousing situations
Reciprocal determinism	The dynamic interaction of the person, behavior, and the environment in which the behavior is performed	Consider multiple avenues to behavioral change including environmental, skill and personal change

NOTE: From "How Individuals, Environments, and Health Behavior Interact: Social Learning Theory" (Table 8.2, p. 166), by C. L. Perry, T. Baranowski, and G. S. Parcel, in *Health Behavior and Health Education,* edited by K. Glanz, F. M. Lewis, and B. K. Rimer, 1990, San Francisco: Jossey-Bass. Copyright 1990 by Jossey-Bass Inc., Publishers. Reprinted with permission.

in California, Louisiana, Minnesota, and Texas participated. CATCH objectives were designed to reduce dietary intake of fat and sodium, increase levels of moderate to vigorous physical activity, and promote abstention from tobacco use (Stone et al., 1994). Interventions focused on changing the school health and physical education curricula, school food service, policies for school tobacco use, and structured activities for families of CATCH students (Stone et al., 1994). In this regard, the CATCH exemplifies the integrated approach to school-based health promotion. Guided by SCT, the functions of process evaluation targeted program

implementation, quality control and monitoring, and an explanation of program effects (Stone et al., 1994). The process evaluation plan enabled understanding of how the program functions within the school organizational system as well as the extent and fidelity of program implementation. Such information is essential for replication and dissemination of intervention protocols across geographic sites and in the determination of the linkages between interventions and outcomes. For example, as illustrated in the CATCH, process evaluation data will be useful in examining outcome differences between schools within and across the four geographic sites, documenting the quality and minimum dose necessary to achieve desired outcomes, and the differential effects of the respective interventions on those cardiovascular risk outcomes. Preliminary results underscore the importance of process evaluation in multisite, multicomponent interventions and support the utility and effectiveness of SCT in guiding this comprehensive process (Elder et al., 1994).

The Heart Smart Cardiovascular School Health Promotion Program (Arbeit et al., 1992; Butcher et al., 1988) and the Family Health Promotion Program (Johnson et al., 1991) illustrate the application of SCT by a multidisciplinary team using multicomponent interventions in a school-based setting with extension to families at risk for cardiovascular disease. Heart Smart builds on and extends the Bogalusa Heart Study (Berenson, 1980), an observational investigation of cardiovascular risk factors in a well-defined pediatric population. The Heart Smart Program illustrates the application of a conceptual model in building the science base in both cardiovascular health promotion and risk reduction (disease prevention). The two components of the Heart Smart Program, family and school, illustrate respectively the differences between high-risk and population-based approaches to cardiovascular disease prevention. In epidemiologic terms, the goal of the individual high-risk approach is to identify individuals at risk and target interventions accordingly. Population-based approaches attempt to shift the distribution of risk factors by interventions designed to change the patterns of risk within that targeted population. As illustrated in this program and in the published literature, the population approach to disease prevention is often referred to as health promotion.

Within the SCT framework, both components of the Heart Smart Program targeted several of the health status objectives defined in *Healthy People 2000* (USDHHS, 1990). Spe-

cifically, objectives for the population-based school component were these:

- Adoption of dietary patterns consistent with American Heart Association Guidelines (Weidman, Kwiterovich, Jesse, & Nugent, 1983; reducing dietary fat intake to < 30% of total energy intake, reducing saturated fat intake to < 10% of total energy intake, reducing sodium chloride intake to < 5 grams per day, attainment and maintenance of ideal body weight)
- Adoption of physical activity patterns and behavioral skills conducive to lifetime physical fitness
- Deterred onset of cigarette smoking and other unhealthful behaviors through the promotion of self-esteem and cognitive and attitudinal awareness

To achieve the SCT-derived objectives of the Heart Smart Program, interventions targeted at both the individual and transformation of the school environment were implemented. A comprehensive health curriculum was focused on four areas: cardiovascular physiology, eating behavior, exercise behavior, and coping skills. Emphasis was placed on self-esteem, self-responsibility, decision making, and assertiveness. Modification of school lunch menus to reduce sodium and sugar by 50% and fat by 30% was recommended. Cardiovascular healthy food choices were provided to allow students to practice positive health decisions and to provide for program evaluation. A "Superkids–Superfit" physical education program, featuring aerobic conditioning and personalized fitness, was implemented as part of the comprehensive curriculum.

Also, in the intervention schools, comprehensive cardiovascular risk-factor screening was conducted in the fall, winter, and spring to operationalize the SCT construct of reciprocal determinism (the dynamic interaction of the person, behavior, and environment in which the behavior is performed). The results provided participants with periodic feedback regarding physiologic risk factors (serum lipids, blood pressure, indices of obesity/ponderosity), which were also viewed as outcome indicators (measurements at the spring data point).

Additional environmental support mechanisms, central to SCT, were the development of a school health advisory committee composed of teachers, administrators, parents, and representatives from the school lunch and physical education staffs. The committee devised and implemented adjunct health promotion strategies for the school and home environments (i.e., health fairs, fun runs). An extensive parent education and volunteer program provided additional support for behavior change. In both the school and home-based components of the Heart Smart Program, Bandura's (1986) four steps to self-efficacy, an important mediating variable in behavior change, were emphasized: modeling, positive past experiences, accurate knowledge and appropriate communication skills, and correct interpretation of physiologic reaction (feedback provided from the cardiovascular screenings).

The Heart Smart Program (Arbeit et al., 1992; Butcher et al., 1988) was initiated in four elementary schools in a suburb of New Orleans. The site was selected because of its racial and socioeconomic diversity: 55% Caucasian, 32% African American, 8% Vietnamese, and 2% Hispanic. The unit of randomization was the school; however, analyses were restricted to fourth and fifth grades in each school. Of 870 eligible fourth and fifth graders at the four schools, 530 (61%) received parental consent and were enrolled in the study. The design specified assessment and measurement of physiologic risk factors (fasting lipid profiles, blood pressure, and indices of obesity/ponderosity), dietary evaluation (self-reports of school lunch menu choices, nutrient analysis of school lunch recipes, and plate waste analysis), fitness evaluation (1-mile run/walk completion

times), and a cardiovascular health knowledge test at selected intervals throughout the school year.

Outcome indicators, used to evaluate the effectiveness of the interventions, were measured at the spring data point for the following: cardiovascular risk factors, content of school lunches, physical fitness, and cardiovascular health knowledge. Although the school was the unit of randomization, postintervention analyses were conducted, with individual students in participating schools as the units of analysis. Acknowledging this limitation, results provide support for SCT in guiding components of the Heart Smart Program and in transforming the school environment. Specifically, participating children in the two intervention schools demonstrated significant increases in high-density lipoprotein cholesterol (HDL-C), whereas their control counterparts demonstrated a consistent decrease. With students assigned to quartiles according to pre- and post-changes in risk factors (total cholesterol, ponderosity, systolic and diastolic blood pressure), children in the quartile showing the greatest cholesterol reduction also had the largest number of healthful food choices (61% selecting three or more healthful foods, compared with 42% in the quartile with the least lipid reduction). Likewise, among children in the quartile showing the greatest reduction in ponderosity ($n = 32$), 81% selected three or more healthful foods, compared with 47% in the quartile of children with the least reduction. For pre- and post-systolic or diastolic blood pressure changes, no similar trend was observed. Physical fitness, as gauged by 1-mile run/walk times, improved significantly on an age/sex-specific basis; those who improved their walk/run times manifested systolic blood pressure decreases an average of 1.6 mmHg. Subscapular and triceps skinfolds also decreased 4.4 mm and 2.8 mm, respectively. Finally, improvements in the walk/run performance were related in predicted directions to the entire cardiovascular risk profile. Collectively, the results emphasize the utility of SCT as applied in a multicomponent, short-term intervention in cardiovascular health promotion in a school-based setting. Observations also indicate a relationship between behavior change and physiologic changes (Arbeit et al., 1992).

The utility and versatility of SCT was also demonstrated in the family health component of the Heart Smart Program (Johnson et al., 1991), which targeted high-risk children and their families and was designed to accomplish the same objectives as the school-based Health Promotion Program described above. The multidisciplinary program was developed to serve as a model for family-based cardiovascular health promotion and risk reduction that could be applied in other settings. It was implemented with 19 fourth and fifth graders (and 23 parents), who were selected as probands based on results of cardiovascular risk-factor screening conducted in the school environment.

The 12-week intervention consisted of eight 90-minute sessions (presentations, activities, group aerobic exercise) and three nutrition, exercise, and counseling sessions. Interventions were provided to groups of families, except for the counseling sessions that were conducted for individual families. Developmental level was considered in the educational sessions; children and parents attended separate sessions held in the school during the evening and on Saturday morning. Guided by SCT, the nutrition module taught at each session consisted of a brief didactic presentation, group discussion, modeling, and hands-on activities. Cooking demonstrations, games, and a cardiovascular health picnic not only focused on illustrating health concepts but afforded interactive hands-on experiences. Similar to the nutrition module and consistent with SCT, the exercise module incorporated several teaching-learning approaches including didactic presentations on

energy expenditure, group exercise sessions that progressed from 10 to 30 minutes' duration over the 12-week intervention, and competitive aerobic games. Other didactic sessions focused on skill acquisition necessary for behavior change in these high-risk families: self-monitoring of eating and exercise; consumer-health-oriented grocery shopping and label reading; recipe modification; healthy snacking; and social support, self-efficacy, and self-management skills necessary for maintenance. Families were also counseled in eating and exercise behavior by a behavioral specialist and a nutritionist or physical educator. Contingency contracts were voluntarily negotiated with each family member and a choice of reward was offered for performance. Self-monitoring of eating and exercise behavior was accomplished with biweekly food records and exercise logs; extensive training in record keeping was provided. Attendance at 75% or more of the intervention sessions was rewarded with incentives.

Postintervention, both children and parents showed positive changes in eating habits and physical activity and significant changes in health knowledge and blood pressure levels. The results support SCT in guiding intensive, short-term interventions focused on a high-risk approach to disease prevention.

Even though both components of the Heart Smart Program illustrate optimal application of SCT, several limitations that restrict generalizability of results are noteworthy. The Heart Smart Program used a nonrandom, one-site sample with insufficient power to determine intervention effects. Methodologically, as the investigators acknowledge, the school was the unit of randomization; however, postintervention analyses focused on individual students in participating schools. Nevertheless, similar to CATCH and other effective school-based health promotion initiatives (Stone et al., 1989), the Heart Smart Program illustrates the human and fiscal resources necessary to transform the school to an environment conducive to health promotion and disease prevention. Time-limited granting mechanisms, unfortunately, do not allow for long-term, longitudinal interventions with concomitant process and outcome evaluations. Thus, it is not possible to determine if the results observed in the Heart Smart Program were sustained through childhood into adolescence and/or what specific SCT-derived interventions influenced the outcomes achieved. Although SCT was effective, it is not clear what aspects of the framework were most useful in either Heart Smart Program component. Finally, the family health promotion component, while effective in achieving short-term behavior change in high-risk individuals, was not effective as a family-based model. The challenges inherent in engaging the family as a unit of care for health promotion notwithstanding, Heart Smart captured high-risk members of selected families, not the family unit (Feetham, 1990; Ryan & Hayman, 1996).

The versatility of SCT allows for numerous applications in health promotion initiatives focused on children and adolescents in a range of settings. Effective implementation, as illustrated in the Heart Smart Program, requires comprehensive knowledge and awareness of the model constructs as demonstrated in the target population. For example, approaches to enhancing self-efficacy will necessarily vary as a function of developmental and sociodemographic factors. Operational definitions of environment, left to the discretion of the investigator or practitioner, may include family, peers, school, and/or other contextual variables. Within these categories, the specific targets for optimal intervention also must be identified. Taken together, these caveats point to the importance of comprehensive assessment and the benefits of conceptually based programs of research that progress from observation to intervention.

■ Focus on Individuals and Environments: Model of Health Promotion

Bruhn and Parcel (1982) elaborated the model presented in Figure 3.4 for the specific purpose of health promotion initiatives with children, adolescents, and families.

The model emerged from a 1979 multidisciplinary conference that focused on health behaviors in children. After reviewing existing models, conference participants recommended a conceptual framework consisting of family influences, developmental and psychological characteristics of the child, children's health behavior, and children's health status (Bruhn & Parcel, 1982). Bruhn and Parcel's Model of Health Promotion combines parental influences and the child's developmental and personality characteristics to influence health behaviors, which result in health outcomes or "health status indicators." The model allows for reciprocal influences (i.e., the health status of the child potentially influences the health of parents). Bruhn and Parcel (1982) incorporated the factors defined in the Predisposing, Reinforcing, and Enabling Courses in Educational Diagnosis and Evaluation (PRECEDE) community-planning model of Green, Kreuter, Deeds, and Partridge (1980) as potential influences on health behaviors in children. However, it was postulated that these factors—predisposing, reinforcing, and enabling—exhibit considerable intra- and interindividual variation. Thus, this part of the model lacks specificity and relies on the investigator or practitioner for operational definitions. However, as defined by Green et al. (1980), these factors are hypothesized to mediate prevention-related behavior change. Predisposing factors, derived from the HBM (Rosenstock, 1966), provide the motivation for behavioral intention. Enabling factors, derived from SLT (Bandura, 1977) are

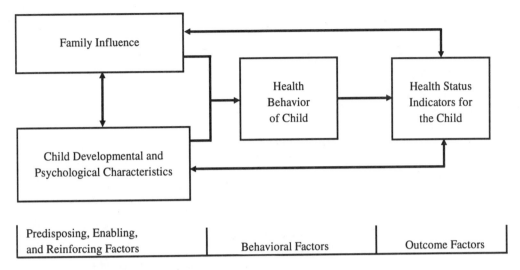

Figure 3.4. The Bruhn and Parcel Model of Health Promotion

hypothesized to provide behavioral capability, including the skills required for successful performance of the behavior. Reinforcing factors, derived from SLT (Bandura, 1977), provide behavioral reinforcement; they include societal, family, and peer support for performance of the behavior.

Application of this model is illustrated in Cardiovascular Health in Children (CHIC I; Harrell, McMurray, Frauman, Bangdiwala, & Levine, 1995; Harrell et al., 1995), a randomized, controlled field trial designed to determine the prevalence of cardiovascular risk factors in third- and fourth-grade children in rural and urban settings and to compare the effectiveness of two interventions designed to reduce these risk factors. Although CHIC I was completed recently and only the school-based intervention results are available (Harrell et al., 1995), it is noteworthy for its conceptualization, methodology, and multidisciplinary interventions focused on understudied children and youths. Funded in 1990 by the National Institute of Nursing Research, CHIC I emphasized Bruhn and Parcel's (1982) Model of Health Promotion (MHP) with selected variables from

Pender's (1987) Health Promotion Model (HPM). Its conceptualization and empirical indicators are presented in Table 3.2.

The school-based intervention· segment (Harrell et al., 1996) of CHIC I was conducted in 12 schools in North Carolina, stratified by geographic region and urban/rural setting. Two schools were randomly selected within each of six strata defined by the state's three geographic regions and by two (urban or rural) settings. Subjects were 1,274 third and fourth graders (48% male). The intervention, taught by regular classroom and physical education teachers, provided all children in the 6 intervention schools with an 8-week exercise program and 8 weeks of classes on nutrition and smoking. In implementing the intervention, teachers used the American Heart Association's (1989) Lower and Upper Elementary School Site Program Kits, which contained information about selecting heart healthy foods, the importance of regular physical exercise, the dangers of smoking, and ways to combat pressure to smoke.

Also used was the investigator-designed physical activity intervention (3 times per week

TABLE 3.2 CHIC I: Application of the Bruhn and Parcel Model

Variable	Measurement Used
[FAMILY INFLUENCE]	
Family history of CVD	Parental questionnaire
Parental risk factors	Parental questionnaire
Socioeconomic status	Hollingshead Four-Factor Index
[CHILD DEVELOPMENTAL AND PSYCHOLOGICAL CHARACTERISTICS]	
Age, gender, race, rural/urban	Child's questionnaire
Health knowledge	AHA Intermediate-level Heart Smart test
Health locus of control	Child's Health Locus of Control (Parcel & Meyer, 1978)
Behavioral factors **[HEALTH BEHAVIOR OF CHILD]**	
Activity habits	Know Your Body Health Habits Survey (Oaks, Warren, & Harsha, 1987) (modified by investigators)
Smoking habits	
Eating habits	
Outcome factors **[HEALTH STATUS INDICATORS FOR CHILD]**	
Blood pressure	Mercury manometer
Total serum cholesterol	Reflotron (BMD)
Obesity	
Height/weight index	Balance beam scales
Triceps skinfold	Lange caliper
Activity tolerance	Heart rate at rest and after 6 and 12
Physical work capacity (PWC-170)	minutes on bicycle ergometer

for 8 weeks) that focused on exercising large muscle groups through noncompetitive, aerobic activities. Children in the 6 control-group schools did not receive any specific intervention: however, they did participate in their usual health instruction and were assessed in the same manner as those in the 6 intervention-group schools. Specifically, cardiovascular risk factors (health behaviors, total cholesterol, blood pressure, aerobic power, and measures of adiposity) were assessed in all study participants at baseline and at 2 weeks' postintervention (posttest). As illustrated in Table 3.2, the cardiovascular risk factor variables were defined and operationalized within Bruhn and Parcel's (1982) Model of Health Promotion.

Data were analyzed at the school level with survey regression models and at the individual level with multiple analysis of variance (MANOVA) and analysis of covariance (ANCOVA) models. Because the school was the unit of randomization, primary analyses were conducted first at that level. In these analyses, compared with children in the control schools, children in the intervention schools had significantly greater health knowledge (7.9% more correct as measured by the Heart Smart test; see Bruhn & Parcel, 1982) and a significant increase in self-reported physical activity as measured by an adapted version of the Know Your Body Health Habits Survey (Oaks, Warren, & Harsha, 1987). No statistically significant differences in physiologic variables were observed in the school-based analyses. However, trends for those in the intervention groups were a reduction in total cholesterol (-5.27 mg/dl), an increase in aerobic power, a reduction in body fat, and a smaller rise in diastolic blood pressure than found in control-group children (Harrell et al., 1995). In individual-level analyses, significant differences (as measured by changes from baseline to posttest) were observed for total cholesterol, adiposity as measured by skinfolds, and aerobic power. The collective results of this segment of the CHIC I suggest that a classroom-based population approach can improve cardiovascular risk profiles in elementary school children.

Similar to other school-based initiatives (Luepker et al., 1996; Stone et al., 1989), CHIC I results support the efficacy of an integrated approach to health promotion and disease prevention executed in the school environment. Consistent with results generated in three major community-based health promotion initiatives (Minnesota's statewide Heart Project, Pawtucket [Rhode Island], and Stanford [California]) and those from a community-based nutrition intervention for school-age children (Shannon et al., 1994), the CHIC I results underscore the importance of long-term interventions (combined with periodic boosters) in maintaining treatment effects.

Collectively, these results suggest that Bruhn and Parcel's (1982) Model of Health Promotion (1982) provided a useful framework for selected aspects of CHIC I. As seen in Table 3.2, the model guided the selection of the major study variables, but because it provides minimal specificity with regard to interactions, reciprocal influences, and other process characteristics, how interventions could be derived is not clear. It is noteworthy that CHIC II, in progress, is guided by an investigator-developed framework (adapted from CHIC I) emphasizing developmental contextual interactions and influences on health behavior and health outcomes (Harrell et al., 1995). Because CHIC II is designed to follow this cohort through the adolescent transition and incorporates an environmental-level intervention, a framework emphasizing relevant contextual factors (i.e., peers) was considered more appropriate (Harrell et al., 1995).

As Grey observed (chap. 2 in this volume), Bruhn and Parcel's (1982) model has been underutilized in health promotion initiatives focused on children and adolescents. As CHIC I (Harrell et al., 1995) demonstrated, this model may be most useful in the initial conceptualization of a research design, particularly in descriptive studies with young children. Although family influences are instrumental, the family is not operationalized as a unit. Similar to SCT, operational definitions of model constructs, particularly the environment, are left to the investigator. Most important, for intervention-focused research or practice, the lack of specificity in process characteristics limits the utility of the Bruhn and Parcel (1982) Model of Health Promotion.

■ Focus on Families: Model of Family Influences on Health Behavior

Conceptually based family-unit studies, as reflected in the nursing literature, have increased substantially in the past decade (Feetham, Meister, Bell, & Gilliss, 1993; Whall & Loveland-Cherry, 1993). As Grey (chap. 2 in this volume) observed, several studies based on family system models (McCubbin & Thompson, 1987; Wright & Leahey, 1994a) and Pender's (1987) HPM focused on assessment for health promotion. Despite families being targeted for health-promoting interventions, studies have not included the family as a unit of analysis. In recent independent reviews of this literature, Whall and Loveland-Cherry (1993) and Riley-Lawless (1995) identified this area of inquiry as a priority for future family research. As no conceptually based family-unit intervention studies were found, this section focuses on a synthesis of available findings that provide direction for health promotion research and practice.

Current models and conceptualizations of optimal health point to the importance of biological, social, and environmental factors (Blumenthal et al., 1994; Millstein, 1989). Because families are a major component of children's social and environmental contexts, recent recommendations, including *Bright Futures* (Green, 1994), emphasize family involvement in health promotion. These recommendations for family-focused health promotion are based, in part, on results of several lines of inquiry, including familial aggregation studies and research on parental influences on health behaviors and health status during childhood and adolescence. Noteworthy, as Green (1994) acknowledges, is the need for additional empirical validation of the proposed guidelines.

Familial aggregation studies have been conducted primarily to determine the genetic and environmental influences on physiological and behavioral risk factors for chronic disease as well as indicators of health status. In one of the most comprehensive and cited reviews of family determinants of health behaviors, Sallis and Nader (1988) concluded that physiological risk factors for chronic disease, including hyperlipidemia, hypertension, and obesity, and behavioral factors, including patterns of smoking behavior, physical activity, and dietary intake, are aggregated within families. Recognizing that estimates of environmental influence on physiological and behavioral factors varied across studies, Sallis and Nader emphasized the need for further delineation of familial environmental influences on health behaviors over time. To that end, a conceptual framework, based on an integration of SCT (Bandura, 1977) and Skinnerian learning principles (Skinner, 1953) was articulated (Sallis & Nader, 1988).

Developed with the ultimate goal of influencing family-based, health-promoting interventions, the Model of Family Influences on Health Behavior (see Figure 3.5) emphasizes the role of intrafamilial processes (modeling influences) in the acquisition and maintenance of health-related behaviors. Particularly noteworthy is the emphasis on factors external to the family unit, such as the neighborhood, schools, peers, and the media (Sallis & Nader, 1988). Viewing family health behaviors and outcomes within these contexts is consistent with ecological models (Bronfenbrenner, 1979; Moos, 1980; Sallis & Owen, 1997).

Results of several recent studies support Sallis and Nader (1988) and point to the importance of examining both genetic and environmental sources of variation in future investigations (Hayman, Meininger, Coates, & Gallagher, 1995; Heller, DeFaire, Pedersen, Dahlen, & McClearn, 1993). Consistent with early, population-based, twin-family studies (Namboodiri et al., 1985), Hayman, Meininger, Gallagher, and Whalen (1994) observed familial aggregation of the lipid profile and obesity. Genetic analyses (Meininger, Hayman, Coates, & Gallagher, 1988, in press) and nongenetic analyses (Hayman et al., 1995) indicated that environmental factors contributed to the observed expression of both inter- and intraindividual differences in physiological risk factors for cardiovascular disease during the school-age and adolescent periods of development. Collectively, these results point to the importance of family-based, health-promoting interventions. To this end, using longitudinal data from this twin-family cohort (Hayman, Meininger, Stashinko, Gallagher, & Coates, 1988) and a synthesis of Pender's (1996) Revised Health Promotion Model (Revised HPM) and von Bertalanffy's (1968) General Systems Theory, analyses in progress are designed to examine familial aggregation of health behaviors with emphasis on implications for health-

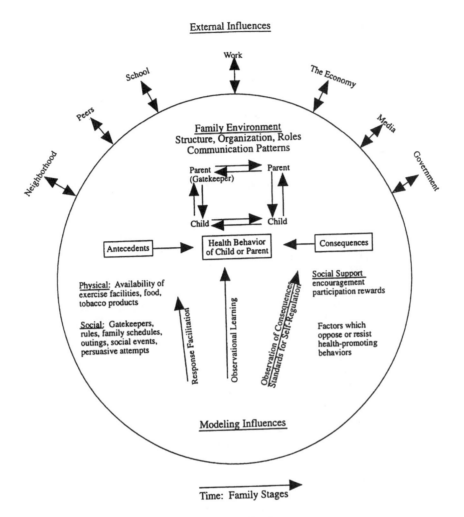

Figure 3.5. A Model of Family Influences on Health Behaviors

NOTE: From "Family Determinants of Health Behaviors" (chap. 6, p. 112) by J. S. Sallis and P. R. Nader, in *Health Behavior: Emerging Research Perspectives,* edited by D. S. Gochman, 1988, New York: Plenum Press. Copyright © 1988 by Plenum Publishing Corporation. Reprinted with permission.

promoting interventions (Whalen, 1996). Similarly, Sallis and Nader's (1988) model and the longitudinal, twin-family data combine to explicate the role and functions of the family unit in health promotion during the adolescent transition (Riley-Lawless, 1996).

Additional insights concerning genetic factors, parenting, and the family environment have evolved from twin-family and adoption studies (Plomin, 1994). In summarizing results from these investigations, Plomin (1994) em-phasized the usefulness of genetic research for the identification of specific environmental influences on developmental processes. For example, across disciplines, attention has focused on the influence of the nonshared family environment, the component that contributes to between-sibling variation in characteristics and behaviors.

Twin and twin-family studies have demonstrated that environmental effects on behavioral development are primarily attributable to nonshared processes and experiences (Plomin, 1995). Applied to health promotion of children and adolescents, this type of investigation would address why children in the same family differ in beliefs, attitudes, and behaviors as well as health outcomes. As Plomin (1995) suggested, the research implications point to the importance of studying more than one child per family, to assess environmental influences specific to each child, and to identify environmental processes that differ for two children growing up in the same family.

Parental influences on health behaviors in childhood and adolescence have been investigated from several different theoretical perspectives. Early work in this area emphasized maternal influences on children's health behaviors and health outcomes (Alpert, Kosa, & Haggerty, 1967; Morris, Hatch, & Chipman, 1966). Later, within a developmental-SCT paradigm, Baumrind (1991) investigated parenting influences on health-related risk behaviors. The cohort for this landmark study consisted of 139 parents and children, the latter assessed at 4, 9, and 15 years of age. The major purpose was to examine the effects on adolescent competence and substance use of the following parenting styles: authoritative, democratic; authoritarian-permissive, nondirective; and rejecting-neglecting, disengaged. An authoritative (democratic) parenting style was associated with healthy development, high competence and self-esteem, internal locus of control, and minimal maladaptive risk-taking behaviors, independent of developmental stage in both males and females. In contrast, authoritarian and disengaged parenting hindered healthy development as measured by these same outcome indicators. These results are consistent with several other studies that examined parental influences on risk-taking behaviors (Cohen, Richardson, & LaBree, 1994; Pulkininen, 1983; Shedler & Block, 1990).

Noteworthy among these studies is the longitudinal investigation of parenting behaviors and adolescent risk taking in a large ($n = 2,300$)

representative, multiethnic sample (Cohen et al., 1994). The purpose of this prospective cohort study was to identify which specific parenting behaviors were associated with the onset of alcohol and tobacco use among 1,034 fifth graders and 1,266 seventh graders surveyed annually for 4 and 3 years, respectively. Results underscore the importance of parenting behaviors in relationship to adolescent disruptive/risk-taking behaviors. Specifically, children who reported that parents spent more time with them and communicated more frequently had lower onset rates of using alcohol and tobacco as measured at the final data point. Parental monitoring and positive relationships were protective factors for risk-taking behavior and substance-using friends. Disruptive, risk-taking behavior increased the odds of adolescent drinking and smoking at the final data point (Cohen et al., 1994). Collectively, the results provide further evidence of the associations between parenting behaviors and adolescent health-related behaviors. Thus, Cohen and colleagues (1994), consistent with other recent recommendations (e.g., Green, 1994), suggested targeting this aspect of the family environment in primary prevention efforts.

Additional evidence for the role of the family in health-promoting interventions emanates from studies based on SCT (Epstein, Valoski, Wing, & McCurley, 1994; Nader et al., 1989; Perry et al., 1989). Although the family was not the unit of intervention, the results of these studies converge to suggest the feasibility and importance of parental involvement in initiating and maintaining health-related behaviors in childhood and adolescence.

The challenges inherent in intervention research focused on the family unit notwithstanding, the collective results of research cited in this section and that reviewed by Grey (chap. 2 in this volume) point to the importance of using conceptual models in building the cross-disciplinary science base in this aspect of health promotion.

■ *Focus on Contexts: Ecological Models*

As Sallis and Owen (1997) observed, ecological models consider the connections between individuals and their environments. Although several models of health promotion and health and behavior incorporate environment as an influencing factor, the distinguishing characteristic of ecological models is the definition of environment as the "space outside the person." Sallis and Owen (1997) provide a comprehensive review of ecological models and their relevance for future health promotion research and practice. In so doing, they elaborate critical components of ecological models/frameworks and articulate the defining feature of their (developing) model, which emphasizes the explicit treatment of relations between the person and the physical environment. In both research and practice initiatives, this ecological perspective focuses on factors in the natural physical environment (e.g., weather and geography) and the constructed physical environment (e.g., architecture, transportation, entertainment, and recreation infrastructures). Sallis and Owen (1996) also emphasize and explicate social and intrapersonal factors. For example, supportive behaviors of significant others, social climate, culture, and regulatory policies are defined as part of the social environmental factors. Intrapersonal factors, emphasized in other sections of this chapter, focus on demographics as well as biological, cognitive, affective, and behavioral characteristics. Applicable at the individual level, these intrapersonal factors interact with social and physical environmental factors as key determinants of health-promoting behaviors.

Although Sallis and Owen (1997) have not elaborated all the specific individual-environmental linkages as they interact to influence health behaviors, they emphasize the need to consider both social and physical environments within key behavior settings such as the home, school, and neighborhood. This explication of environment is particularly applicable to health promotion research and practice with children and families because it acknowledges, on several levels of analysis, specific contexts in which health behaviors develop and are maintained. For example, in designing health-promoting interventions for school-age children, this perspective would target the family home environment, including exposure to healthful foods, exercise equipment, and smoke-free air. Within the contexts of school and community, targets for intervention would include exposure to healthy school lunch programs, smoke-free buildings, space, equipment, and other resources designed to increase physical activity and accessible, affordable healthful food products. Implementation of such interventions would necessarily require attention to the regulatory policies that influence these environments in which health behaviors develop and are maintained.

In a comprehensive review of the impact of ecological theory on intervention research in maternal and child health, Black and Danesco (1994) offered several observations relevant to health promotion research and practice with children and families. First, they acknowledged the need for ecological studies that use experimental designs, particularly randomized clinical trials. Although Bronfenbrenner's (1979, 1993) ecological model has influenced the practice of maternal and child health, few studies were based on this framework. In applying the framework to developmental and behavioral issues, emphasis has been on the child and his or her proximal environment, such as relationships within the family unit. Distal, contextual influences, such as the impact of sociopolitical factors, have received minimal research attention (Black & Danesco, 1994). Particularly noteworthy was the absence of research focused on health-promoting interventions with children and families (Black & Danesco, 1994).

Research in progress illustrates the application of ecological theory in the conceptualization and design of a longitudinal, randomized clinical trial (RCT) focused on promoting the health and development of high-risk, extremely-low-birth-weight (ELBW) infants (Pridham, 1995). Specifically, the major purpose of this short-term RCT is to test the effectiveness of an intervention (guided participation) for aiding mothers and family members of ELBW infants at risk for chronic lung disease in developing competencies for infant feeding and for supporting each other in infant feeding practices. Guided participation, adapted from Rogoff (1990), is an arrangement for learning and development of a practice (i.e., caregiving) through the relationship of a less experienced person (i.e., a mother) with a more experienced, skilled, or resourceful person (i.e., a nurse; Pridham, 1993). Stated in other terms, guided participation is an apprenticeship in problem solving and graduated practice of skills and assumption of responsibility as expertise is acquired (Pridham, Limbo, Schroeder, Thoyre, & Van Riper, in press). As applied in this RCT with the 50 mother-infant dyads randomly assigned to the intervention group, guided participation begins in the neonatal intensive care unit (NICU) at 2 weeks postbirth and continues through the infant's first post-term 12 months in the home environment. Assessments of maternal and family member competencies in infant feeding and supporting each other in feeding practices are made just prior to the infant's NICU discharge (at approximately 35 weeks postconceptional age), at term age, and at 1, 4, 8, and 12 months postterm age.

Operationalization of the intervention in this RCT illustrates the application of ecological theory in extending beyond the proximal environment (i.e., the family unit) to dimensions of the distal environment, including the provider network (nurse, physician, social worker, dietitian, psychologist) and contextual influences (extrafamilial resources). For example, the nurse who is the intermediary of the guided participation intervention collaborates with a social worker who addresses family needs (housing, transportation, financial support), with a dietitian who oversees the infant's diet, and with a clinical psychologist who provides consultation about therapeutic interactions with family members (Pridham, 1995). Additional assessments, conducted at 1 and 12 months postterm age, focus on both the proximal (family functioning) and the distal (family relationships with health care providers) environment. Also examined are the costs of acute illness care for infants in both the intervention and usual care groups. Thus, relevant contextual influences on outcomes are incorporated.

Bronfenbrenner's (1993) model emphasized the need to examine the influence of contextual interactions in intervention research. As applied to future health promotion research, this emphasis suggests an intervention based on the interaction of familial and community factors as they relate to health and health outcomes. For example, the financial status of a family unit interacts with health care services available and accessible in the community to influence the health status of children and families. Investigations based on this approach would progress from observations of the target population to interventions designed to impact this interaction of family and community contexts.

As Stokols (1992) observed, a social-ecological view of health promotion has implications for theory development and basic research as well as public policy, community intervention, and program evaluation. Applications of this perspective, including the models defined by Bronfenbrenner (1979, 1993), Moos (1980), and Sallis and Owen (1997), point to the importance of programs of research that progress from observation to intervention and from main effects of singular contexts to contextual interactions. By definition, research and practice based on this perspective require multidisciplinary teams.

■ *Summary and Conclusions*

This chapter presented the state of the art and science in conceptually based, health-promoting interventions focused on children and families, with the ultimate goal that of informing clinical practice and future research. To that end, the research cited contributes to the cross-disciplinary science in this aspect of health promotion and highlights the operationalization of major model constructs as applied to the dimensions of health promotion outlined in *Healthy People 2000* (USDHHS, 1990).

This approach was selected over an exhaustive review focused primarily on nurse-initiated studies for several reasons. First, as illustrated in this chapter, health promotion is not a discipline-specific phenomenon. Building the knowledge base necessary to inform clinical practice requires a creative synthesis of cross-disciplinary science generated through systematic, longitudinal programs of research. Second, as Grey (chap. 2 in this volume) notes, existing programs of nursing research focus on assessment for health promotion/disease prevention. Because building the science base in a given area of inquiry normally progresses from assessment/observation to intervention, it follows logically that conceptually based intervention research is just beginning to emerge. Finally, although numerous studies cited in this chapter were not nurse initiated, nurses participated in various roles, including recruitment and retention of participants, implementation of the intervention, evaluation of the results, and publication of major findings. Taken together these observations point to the impor-

tance of defining optimal roles for nurses and nursing in health promotion research.

Several observations emerged from examining the utility of the respective paradigms/models for intervention-focused research designs and clinical practice with children and families across settings and contexts. Normally, as Harrell and colleagues (1995) and Jemmott and colleagues (1992) illustrated in their respective programs of research, building the science base in a specific area of inquiry requires more than one conceptual model. Independent of temporal trends across disciplines, paradigm shifts occur for several reasons. In research focused on children and families, developmental and contextual factors vary over time, necessitating models that capture and characterize change at both the individual and environmental levels of analysis.

Although several models presented herein address both individual and environmental/contextual factors, emphasis on the processes and mechanisms of change, the foci of interventions, and targeted outcomes vary from model to model. For example, as illustrated in the research cited, SCT can be operationalized to apply specifically to intraindividual variation in health-related behaviors and health outcomes over time. Ecological perspectives are required to conceptualize the interaction of multiple contexts such as the family, school, and community on both individual and aggregate-level health behaviors and outcomes. Taken together these observations support the adaptation and integration of conceptually consistent theories and models in the design and implementation of programs of research.

Pender's (1987) HPM and Revised HPM (Pender, 1996) illustrate the integration of conceptually consistent theories and models. Previously the HPM had been applied in health promotion research focused only on adults; however, initiatives in progress are adapting the HPM for research on children, adolescents, and families (Pender, 1996).

The uniqueness of both versions of the HPM allows for ease of adaptation to specific health behaviors across the life span. Specifically, the Revised HPM (Pender, 1996) emphasizes and integrates SCT (Bandura, 1986) and constructs from expectancy-value theory (Feather, 1982) within a nursing perspective of holistic human functioning. As such, the resulting model affords examination of the multidimensional nature of health-promoting behaviors and suggests critical points for preventive interventions. Included in the Revised HPM are factors known to influence health-promoting behaviors: individual characteristics and experiences, behavior-specific cognitions and affect, interpersonal influences (family, peers, providers), and situational influences. The inclusion of these factors within the well-defined conceptual framework allows examination of individual and environmental/contextual variables as they interact to influence health-promoting behavior. As Pender (1996) acknowledges, both versions of the HPM remain to be validated with pediatric populations. Funded by the NINR, research in progress at the University of Michigan Child/Adolescent Health Behavior Research Center is designed to address this goal (Pender, 1996).

The integration of developmental concepts, Bronfenbrenner's (1979) ecological model, and Milio's (1986, 1988) public health policy framework forms the organizing conceptual framework for the multidisciplinary Center for the Study of Health Behaviors in Vulnerable Youth located at the University of North Carolina School of Nursing at Chapel Hill. Funded by a trans-Institute NIH initiative (P20 NR, HD, MH 03003), the center focuses on the initiation and maintenance of health-promoting and health-compromising behaviors in vulnerable youths. Populations targeted are migrant and seasonal farmworker children, children with chronic conditions, and minority youths

and their respective families. Application of the integrated conceptual framework affords examination of the individual and environmental/contextual factors as they interact to influence targeted health outcomes (Miles & Harrell, 1991).

Across the paradigms/models and the research cited, several themes have emerged that provide direction for future health promotion initiatives. For example, on the individual level, both self-efficacy and empowerment are suggested as important influences on health and health behaviors across the life span. As demonstrated in the Heart Smart Program (Arbeit et al., 1992) and in the CATCH (Luepker et al., 1996; Stone et al., 1994), empowerment is an essential ingredient for consumer self-care. As Igoe (1991) observed, self-efficacy is enhanced by developmentally and contextually appropriate empowerment strategies. Similarly, in population-based approaches to health promotion, as demonstrated in the school-based component of the Heart Smart Program (Arbeit et al., 1992), empowerment emerges as an important outcome mediating variable.

The operational definitions as well as the emphasis placed on the role, structure, and functions of the environment in health promotion vary between and within models. As illustrated in the application of SCT to the research cited, environment may include such contexts as family, school, and/or community. Normally, the specific aims of the research provide direction for how these contexts are viewed and emphasized as part of the intervention. For example, in SCT-grounded, school-based studies (Stone et al., 1989), intensive efforts were focused on transformation of the school environments. Simultaneously, multidimensional interventions were targeted at changing individual health-related behaviors. Predetermined outcomes (end points) measured change at both the individual and environmental level. Disentangling the relative contributions of individual versus environmental interventions and linking interventions and outcomes, however, requires knowledge generated through ongoing process evaluations. Demonstrated uniquely in the CATCH (Stone et al., 1994), process evaluation provides insights on the intervention-outcome linkages, including dose-response relationships, as well as on the mechanisms through which interventions influence outcomes. This information is essential in intervention research because it enables more effective and efficient replication and dissemination.

As illustrated in this chapter, conceptually based intervention research has advanced the science base in the area of health promotion with children and families. Yet recent results from population-based health surveys (Willard & Schoenborn, 1995) indicate slow progress toward realization of the objectives stated in *Healthy People 2000* (USDHHS, 1990). A cursory glance at the health-status indicators of our nation's children shows patterns of physical activity, dietary intake, and smoking behaviors, observed in population-based surveys, that do not bode well for the health of the nation in the next millennium. Thus, with *Healthy People 2000* (USDHHS, 1990) objectives as outcome indicators and collective results of cross-disciplinary research as process/progress indicators, substantial work remains to be done. Because many questions regarding intervention-outcome linkages remain unanswered, it is clear that optimal approaches to health promotion, on both the individual and population level, will require cross-disciplinary collaboration. As Pridham (chap. 4 in this volume) emphasizes, the art and science of nursing could add substantively to the health of our nation's children and families in the next millennium.

4

■

IMPLICATIONS FOR PRACTICE, EDUCATION, AND RESEARCH IN HEALTH PROMOTION FOR CHILDREN AND THEIR FAMILIES

■ *Karen F. Pridham*

Health promotion is a major function of professional nursing (Laffrey, Loveland-Cherry, & Winkler, 1986; Pender, Barkauskas, Hayman, Rice, & Anderson, 1992; Smith, 1990), and has been from its beginning (Nightingale, 1860/1969). Nursing has a history of responding to socially defined needs for the promotion of children's health. Furthermore, nurses have often taken the lead in setting and implementing agendas to secure better health conditions and resources for children. Health promotion for children and their families is a substantial component of community health nursing practice and the basis of the responsibility nurses take for the social-emotional needs of hospitalized children (Brodie, chap. 1 in this volume).

Health promotion is health care directed toward growth, development, improved well-being, increased resiliency or adaptability in the face of stressors, and accomplishment of health-relevant tasks, including enhancing the environment in which children live (Brubaker, 1983; McLaughlin, 1982; Pridham & Schutz, 1985; Simeonsson, 1994; Walker, 1992). Although health promotion is different from disease prevention (Laffrey et al., 1986; Smith, 1990), the promotion of health presupposes the prevention of disease (Brubaker, 1983). The aim of preventive interventions may be not only to counteract risk factors but also to strengthen protective factors (Coie et al., 1993). Both of these aims operate to promote health.

The contemporary emphasis that policymakers give to achieving the best possible health outcomes for all sectors of the population while containing costs (Margolis, Carey,

Lannon, Earp, & Leininger, 1995) supports an even greater role in health promotion for nurses in all settings of care. Acceptance by nurses of an enlarged health promotion role and leadership in the advancement of effective health promotion programs and strategies means a commitment to research of issues that are significant to the public and to the development of cutting-edge theory and practice (Meleis, 1990).

Nurses have drawn substantially from social, psychological, educational, medical, and developmental sciences for their health promotion research. The diversity of ideas about health promotion that nurse scholars employ increases the possibilities of raising meaningful questions and developing health promotion knowledge (Meleis, 1990). The collaborative and family- and community-centered traditions of nursing practice for the health promotion of children (Brodie, chap. 1 in this volume; Pender et al., 1992) are consistent with a significant health promotion role for nurses and health promotion practice that is well attuned to societal needs. For nursing to capitalize on these strengths and to merit health promotion leadership, the nursing research addressed to health promotion must be carefully examined with the aim of determining what needs to be done and how.

This chapter examines what has been accomplished in the recent nursing assessment and intervention research for the health promotion of children (i.e., infants, young children, school-age children, and adolescents) and explores challenges for the future. The aims, theoretical models, and methods of this research are discussed from the perspective of the research reviewed in the assessment and intervention chapters and from the perspective of directions to be taken in the future. This discussion is followed by a review of directions that health promotion practice and scholarship indicate for nursing education.

■ The Aims, Theoretical Models, and Methods of Health Promotion Research

Examination of the aims, theoretical models, and methods of nursing health promotion assessment and intervention research concerns five major issues:

- The health problem, practice, or outcome that is the topical focus of the research, that is, the research agenda
- Nature of the research questions asked
- Assessment and intervention models used
- Research design and methods
- Programs of research

Each of these issues is discussed in relation to assessment and intervention strategies in tandem.

Research Agendas

Research agendas stem from investigators' research commitments, beliefs about the types of health promotion problems that need to be solved, and ideas concerning appropriate solutions. The research agendas expressed in assessment research are to determine the need for health promotion in a specific population of children, identify factors associated with health behaviors and health promotion activities, and develop instruments to measure needs, influencing factors, and health behaviors as outcomes of health promotion.

Specific health problems for assessment research reviewed by Grey (chap. 2 in this volume) are risks for cardiovascular disease, skin cancer, HIV infection, sexual behavior and pregnancy, substance use, and immunization status—all topics of concern in the 1990 health objectives for the nation (Mason, 1991; McGinnis, Richmond, Brandt, Windom, &

Mason, 1992; U.S. Department of Health and Human Services [USDHHS], 1990). Other assessment issues are activities of daily living (e.g., sleep, toilet training), child characteristics or behavior (e.g., temperament, colic), and how mothers teach their young children to accomplish tasks. Although questions concerning these daily living issues are not directly aimed at what has been defined as major child health problems, they are concerned with behavior and interactive patterns that may support or interfere with health and potentially provide a base for study of the processes that elicit and maintain or thwart health-promoting behaviors.

The intervention research that Hayman reviewed (chap. 3 in this volume), like the assessment research, concerns health problems addressed in *Healthy People 2000: National Health Promotion and Disease Prevention Objectives for the Year 2000* (USDHHS, 1990) and everyday activities and behaviors that have implications for health promotion or disease prevention. Risk factors for chronic disease and health-related behaviors predominate as the health problems targeted in the cross-disciplinary literature. Whereas assessment research has targeted children of all ages, the populations targeted by intervention research primarily have been school-age children and adolescents.

Research Questions

The types of questions addressed in both the assessment and intervention research reviewed reflect the level of the theory that nurse researchers have available to them and choose to use. In assessment studies, this level was in some cases a single factor—for example, a problem or condition. Although much of the factor-relating assessment research describes health indicators in a demographic context, some assessment research has addressed questions about implied predictive or explanatory

relationships between influencing factors and outcomes specified by multicomponent models. Questions concerning development or learning over time are not yet evident in the nursing health promotion literature.

Assessment studies derived from Stress Adaptation Models reflect several assumptions. First, times of life transition and life events that are commonly viewed as being stressful are associated with increased risks for health problems. Second, support of an individual's coping will promote health by reducing the risk associated with the transition or stressful event or condition. Some of the studies derived from this model were descriptions of coping behaviors or strategies, whereas other studies related variables within the model to each other, one of them longitudinally. Much theoretical and empirical work remains to be done to clearly link coping conditions and behaviors to health outcomes.

Health promotion research questions also reflect the unit of concern. Assessment and intervention research that focuses on social units such as the family and community rather than on individuals is limited. Several studies in both the assessment and intervention modes were concerned with the health behaviors and responses of family members other than those of the target child and of the health-promoting actions of clinicians or teachers. Hayman (chap. 3 in this volume) reviews family aggregation studies and research on parental influences on the health behaviors and health status of children in the context of the implications for family-based, health-promoting interventions. Although derived from family assessment, family systems, family health promotion, or interaction models, these studies, for the most part, concern individual members of a family rather than the family as a unit. However, the development of theoretical frameworks that include factors external to the family unit, such as the neighborhood, schools, peers, and the media (see Hayman's review in chap. 3 of Pender's Revised Health Promotion Model and the Sallis and Nader framework) and results of familial aggregation studies, also reviewed by Hayman, support the mounting of assessment and intervention research targeted at a family or community aggregate.

Several programs of health promotion research have targeted the school environment or community. The Heart Smart Cardiovascular School Health Promotion Program (Arbeit et al., 1992; Butcher et al., 1988), reviewed by Hayman (chap. 3 in this volume) was designed to transform the school environment in respect to a comprehensive health curriculum, cardiovascular healthy food choices in school lunches, and a physical education program that included aerobic conditioning and personalized fitness. The Cardiovascular Health in Children controlled field trial (Harrell et al., 1995) included a population-based approach in the form of a classroom-based intervention. This intervention included cardiovascular health information provided by teachers and an exercise program.

The Community-Oriented Primary Care Model (Nutting, 1987), applied in assessment research, has been used to frame epidemiological questions concerning the prevalence in communities of health problems (e.g., injuries), community health needs, and community conditions that support health knowledge and healthy behavior or that compromise health (e.g., homelessness; see Grey, chap. 2 in this volume). Although the intervention research often has a setting beyond the family (e.g., day care, school), little evidence of organizations, communities, and extant social policy as foremost research settings was apparent in the literature reviewed. Lavin, Shapiro, and Weill (1992) were singular in their reports of school-based health promotion programs. Multiple sources of health promotion strategies, including the efforts of individuals, community organizations, industry, and government, are likely to be needed to accomplish a complex, multifaceted task (Hurrelmann, 1990; Lawrence, Arbeit, Johnson, & Berenson, 1991).

Assessment and Intervention Models

Health promotion assessment and intervention research is oriented to specific target health behaviors and predictors by the investigator's beliefs and assumptions (i.e., theoretical frame) about what needs to be promoted for achievement of health. Nurse researchers have examined physical, physiologic, behavioral, cognitive, and social phenomena as health outcomes. In recent years, nurse researchers working in both the assessment and intervention modes have, to an increasing extent, been examining competencies either as factors assumed to influence outcomes or as outcomes of importance in themselves. Perceived self-efficacy, a component of Bandura's (1986) Social Cognitive Theory, may be viewed as a type of competency. The relationship of self-efficacy to adolescent health behaviors or outcomes such as risk taking, loneliness, sexual behavior, and pregnancy-prevention behavior is a prime example of the interest of nurse researchers in competencies that promote health (Jemmott & Jemmott, 1992). This type of interest shows increasing attention to the theoretical underpinnings or models of health promotion and to further the explanation and prediction of health outcomes.

Self-efficacy studies are conceptually related to life-skills training programs tested by investigators in other disciplines (Botvin & Tortu, 1988; Dusenbury & Botvin, 1992; Kelder & Perry, 1993; Rhodes & Englund, 1993). Life-skills training programs generally are comprehensive programs designed specifically to develop competencies for successful living and, consequently, to prevent such problems as substance abuse. Competence enhancement approaches included in these programs emphasize broadly applicable skills such as problem solving, decision making, resisting interpersonal and media influences, increasing self-control and self-esteem, asserting oneself, coping with stress, and relating to others. Dusenbury and Botvin (1992) cautioned that the effectiveness of competence enhancement approaches with youths who have limited life opportunities, due to disadvantage and poverty, requires concurrent provision of healthy and adaptive options for education, work, recreation, and community participation. This note of caution supports the need for interventions designed to empower individuals and aggregates. Millstein, Petersen, and Nightingale (1993) observed that programs addressed to individuals were most effective in the context of societal and community change, including elimination of poverty.

Nursing assessment and intervention research in which competencies are incorporated into the theoretic model appears to be developing strength and prominence. Moore and Gaffney's (1989) psychometric analysis of an instrument to assess dependent care agent behavior enhances nursing's resources for the study of competencies. Competency-focused research could be expanded beyond knowledge and self-efficacy to other competencies such as relating, communicating, problem solving, and decision making. Nurse researchers who are primarily concerned with the promotion of the health of healthy children, the subject of this book section, could find useful theoretical and empirical support in the study of Hollen and Hobbie (1993) concerning risk behaviors and decision making of adolescent long-term survivors of cancer.

The conceptual entities in models used for assessment and intervention also merit comment. The models generally include both child and parent characteristics, attributes, or resources (e.g., knowledge, attitudes, beliefs, and behavior) and aspects of the environment. Models, for the most part, have specified the environment in terms of social groups (e.g., family, school, and community). However, physical aspects of the environment (e.g., food, air, and water), geographical aspects, and living conditions that present risks to health are also relevant to health promotion (Beaver, 1995; Goldman, 1995; McLaughlin, 1982; Syme, 1986). Sallis and Owen (1997) have charted a direction for health promotion research and practice in the model they are developing to explicate relationships between persons and the physical environment.

The importance of including genetic factors in models of behavioral, physical, and physiologic health outcomes is certain to increase with the advent of the Human Genome Project and rapidly advancing knowledge (Lessick & Forsman, 1995; Williams & Lessick, 1996). Family history is the genetic factor in Hayman, Meininger, Stashinko, Gallagher, and Coates's (1988) model of genetic and environmental influences on cardiovascular risk in childhood. Specification of genetic and nongenetic (i.e., environmental) factors, as Hayman, Meininger, Coates, and Gallagher (1995) did in a recent study of the influences of obesity on risk factors for cardiovascular disease, will help determine the environmental and potentially modifiable components of behavioral or physiologic risk factors. Plomin (1995) observed, from accumulated research findings, that environmental effects on behavior are primarily experiences and processes not shared among the children in a family, making it imperative to examine the experiences and processes specific to an individual child.

McKinlay (1993) argued that social system factors (e.g., organizational priorities and practices, professional behaviors, and governmental policies) may offer more promise for promoting health than targeting individual risks (McGinnis, 1992). Examples of community-based prevention or health promotion programs originating in other disciplines are the Healthy Heart Program (Shea, Basch, Lantigua, & Wechsler, 1992) and the Heart Smart Cardiovascular School Health Promotion Program (Arbeit et al., 1992; Butcher et al., 1988). The time is ripe to build on the pioneering work that Milio (1970) did to improve the health of children and their families in a central-city health center.

The relationships between conceptual entities in models used for assessment and intervention research at this time are largely portrayed as links between entities rather than as specific types of relationships. How well the relationships are specified reflects the state of the art of theory and of research that advances the development of theory. For example, the social and physical environment may affect health by moderating the child's developmental pathways and biological vulnerabilities (Beaver, 1995; Crockett & Petersen, 1993). Accounting for these moderating effects in assessment and intervention models would strengthen their descriptive, explanatory, and predictive power. Lindley and Walker (1993) explained moderating and mediating effects and methods of analysis to test their presence. Interrelationships of all factors expected to contribute to health-promoting actions have had limited examination in the nursing literature, using such techniques as path analysis or structural equation modeling. An exception is the analysis of Pender's (1987) Health Promotion Model (Johnson, Ratner, Bottorff, & Hayduk, 1993). Illustrations of structural equation modeling to examine health promotion theory can be found in literature originating in other disciplines (Ellickson & Hays, 1991; Nowacek, O'Malley, Anderson, & Richards, 1990).

Hayman (chap. 3 in this volume) suggested that examination of multicomponent theoretical models using techniques to evaluate causal relationships was needed prior to mounting intervention studies. The study of children's medicine use, derived from the Child Health Belief Model that Hayman reviewed, exemplifies the type of questions about, and analysis

of, complex relationships that will aid the advancement of intervention research.

The models that nurses have used for assessment and intervention studies were constructed with an undifferentiated population-at-large in mind. How models must be formulated for specific populations and cultures is beginning to be addressed in the health promotion literature. Airhihenbuwa (1992) claimed that the health crises in African American communities were directly related to the failure to devise a health intervention model suited to the cultural practices and values of African Americans. A critical dimension of the framework (the PEN3 model; Airhihenbuwa, 1990-1991) for health promotion and disease prevention in African American communities that Airhihenbuwa developed is the cultural appropriateness of health beliefs.

Research Design and Methods

Issues of research design relevant to assessment and intervention studies are the following:

- Strategies for examination of complex relationships
- Investigation of processes through which an intervention affects outcomes
- Study of learning (i.e., development)
- Exploration of health promotion from the perspective of children and their families
- Examination of the accessibility and usefulness of health promotion activities for various populations of children and their families, including economically and socially disadvantaged children
- Methods for the study of health promotion at the level of organizations, communities, and social policy.

These issues are discussed in respect to both the nursing research and to other health promotion research.

Current theory of health promotion, for the most part, posits multiple predictors of health promotion actions or outcomes—for example, the Bush and Iannotti (1990) Children's Health Belief Model and the Bruhn and Parcel (1982) Model of Health Promotion. However, as Grey observed (chap. 2 in this volume), most of the relationships examined in assessment studies have been bivariate rather than multivariate. An exception is Bush and Iannotti's (1990) investigation of relationships within the Children's Health Belief Model using path analysis (Hayman, chap. 3 in this volume).

Delineation of the structure of relationships between variables in complex assessment models, including relationships between explanatory variables as well as between explanatory and outcome variables, requires research designs that support application of methods of structural analysis, such as structural equation modeling (Loehlin, 1992).

Structural analysis of relationships in complex, multidimensional and multicomponent models generally requires a relatively large number of study participants for power, that is, to reject the model if it is wrong (Loehlin, 1992). One consequence of this practical issue is that the entire model may not be testable in one research study. Depending on resources and the availability of persons in the population of interest, nurse researchers may need to plan investigations involving complex assessment models in stages, beginning with the variables for which the literature provides most evidence of importance or with variables that best represent a theoretically or clinically important concept.

Study of the process or mechanisms through which an intervention has an effect on outcomes is a variant of the issue concerning examination of complex relationships. For the most part, the intervention studies reviewed were designed to learn the effect on targeted health outcomes of multicomponent interven-

tions. These studies were not designed to examine the mechanisms and processes through which the intervention affected outcomes. Explanatory mechanisms include the context in which the intervention is offered. The context moderates the effect of the intervention on health outcomes. Explanatory mechanisms also include child, parental, familial, and community characteristics and attributes that mediate the effect of the intervention on outcomes. Theory of health-promoting behavior and health outcomes for children in respect to causal relationships, moderating and mediating variables, and relationships between the explanatory variables is yet to be developed and tested.

The development of health promotion behavior and participation in health promotion activities is a personal expression of learning and commitment or valuing. Nurses have not yet examined the process of learning health promotion behavior, whether through natural occurrence or through intervention. Assuming that nursing has the function of putting a person in the best condition to achieve, regain, and maintain health (Nightingale, 1860/1969) and that learning advances this condition, supporting and understanding the process of learning health promotion behavior, is central to nursing practice and research.

The examination of processes of learning behavior for health-promoting practices is thwarted by limitations in the theories nurses use. These theories primarily focus on the learning of tasks with deliberate instruction rather than on learning that occurs through interaction with a more expert person in a socially valued activity (Rogoff, 1990). This type of learning, in the context of everyday activities, is more likely to characterize the development of health-promoting practices than participation in formal instruction.

Investigation of learning for health promotion activities could be advanced by specification of entities proximal to the desired behavior or practice (e.g., using condoms to protect oneself from AIDS or getting one's child immunized). These entities include personal competencies and environmental supports that a person, family, or organization could marshal. Several investigators included knowledge, which accrues from competencies, as a variable in their studies (Glenister, Castiglia, Kanski, & Haughey, 1990; Jemmott & Jemmott, 1992; Lenart, St. Clair, & Bell, 1991; Sarvela & Ford, 1992). Competencies include such skills as valuing, seeking information, observing and reflecting, performing, problem solving, and communicating with others (Pridham & Schutz, 1985). Competencies are best examined in the context of the social structures that support them (Fisher, Bullock, Rotenberg, & Raya, 1993).

How children and their families gain competence for health-related tasks is a question for longitudinal study. Longitudinal research designs, which are needed for study of learning processes, were not prominent in the assessment and intervention literature reviewed. Gröer, Thomas, and Shoffner (1992) used a longitudinal design to survey adolescents in the 9th grade and later in the 12th grade about increase or decrease in life-change events and in specific ways of coping with stress with increasing age. Coffman, Levitt, and Guacci-Franco (1993) used a longitudinal design to examine change in mothers' close relationships between the birth of an infant and 13 months later. Hayman and her colleagues (1995) examined cardiovascular disease risk factors that were associated with change in obesity from the school-age years to adolescence. With advancement of theory of processes that undergird the development of health-promoting behavior and practices and research programs concerning this development, an increase in the number of longitudinal studies could be expected. The importance of research design is

the support or constraint it presents to the pursuit of specific types of questions. For the most part, both assessment and intervention questions have been posed from the perspective of an external observer rather than from the perspective of the person or persons experiencing health promotion activities or the absence of such activities. Exceptions to the external perspective are the assessment studies of Hauck (1991), who interviewed mothers concerning the process they used to toilet train their toddler; Porter (1994), who used a focus group to elicit mothers' narratives concerning their beliefs and practices for sex-role socialization; and Lenart and colleagues (1991), who interviewed Cambodian women about child-rearing knowledge, beliefs, practices, and information resources.

Questions about what things are like or the nature of the situation, if asked from the perspective of the persons whose health promotion behavior and activities are of interest, could help investigators better understand health and what promotes or hinders it from the perspective of experience. Discourse about how health promotion activities are experienced could help explain why interventions fail or succeed. Furthermore, discourse about what a person expects to happen and intends to do and the criteria used to determine if aims are successfully accomplished could advance understanding of the meanings that health promotion activities have in a person's life and actions taken (Hampshire, 1959; Miller, Galanter, & Pridham, 1960). Exploration of these meanings and actions would include what conditions or supports are needed for health-promoting practices. This type of exploration could provide a framework for culturally astute health promotion activities on the part of nurses.

A person's expectations, intentions, and evaluations are units of experience that are built into internal working models of self in relation to others and to the physical world (Bowlby,

1988; Pridham, 1993). These internal working models operate dynamically in goal-corrected activity (Bowlby, 1982), whether deliberately or only indirectly aimed at health promotion. Research designs for the examination of working models could provide a basis for understanding health promotion behavior more comprehensively, coherently, and faithfully than is currently available. Examination of personal or family expectations and intentions concerning self and others in relation to central functions of daily living (e.g., help seeking and caregiving) and criteria used for evaluating goal achievement as well as situational constraints and facilitators of behavior could put nurses in a better position to explain and predict health-promoting behaviors and activities (McLaughlin, 1982; Pill, 1991).

Discourse about activities that are important in the life of a person or family is a point of entry to health-promoting practices of day-to-day life and the nature of expectations, intentions, and criteria for evaluating these practices. Methods of exploring the internal working models of young children who symbolize experience include observation of care seeking or care receiving, or play and the use of dolls, puppets, still pictures, or videos as props for the child's narrative about their experience. Analytic methods such as dimensional analysis (Schatzman, 1991) can be used to code the units of experience (i.e., working models).

Thus far, in nursing health promotion research, qualitative methods, whether in the assessment or treatment phases of study, have had limited use, and the integration of qualitative and quantitative approaches is yet to be developed. When an organization, community, or social policy is the subject of health promotion study, interpretive methods, including participant observation, ethnographic interview, case studies, and focus group discussions, are needed to provide insight into conditions that support or hinder health promotion activities.

These insights can illuminate the results of quantitative approaches that are often used to improve the generalizability and inferential strength of the research (McKinlay, 1993).

Nurses who raise questions concerning the accessibility and usefulness of professionally organized health promotion activities for a substantial number of children and their families, specifically those who are economically and socially disadvantaged, are gaining a voice and finding expression through current research designs. Bryant (1985) claimed that complex social and environmental factors work against efforts to promote the health of children. Klerman (1991) explained the impact of poverty on the health of children and the need for, access to, and utilization of health services by poor children. Ginzberg (1994) described the progressive deterioration in the structures for and delivery of health care to the poor since the beginning of the 1980s. Pollitt (1994) documented the relatively poor health and use of health services for African American children and for children whose families had annual incomes below $10,000. Kerner, Dusenbury, and Mandelblatt (1993) explored the challenges for health promotion of both poverty and cultural diversity. Best (1989) identified marked regional variations in health behavior among youths and called for an ongoing system to monitor health behaviors in need of intervention programs. This type of information compels nurses to examine the models of health promotion they use for capacity to address economic and social hardships and how they function in relation to health promotion goals (see Huston, McLoyd, & Garcia Coll, 1994, for a discussion of the effects on health of poverty). Intervention studies, specifically designed with impoverished children and their families and children of minority families in mind, are needed. Hayman (chap. 3 in this volume) supports an ecological approach to health promotion research and practice and highlights the public policy changes that could follow from intervention research cast in an ecological framework.

Nursing research that directly targets health promotion policy is needed. One question concerns whether health promotion programs addressed to families and neighborhoods are more effective than those targeted to individual children or parents. Other questions concern how children, families, and communities could best contribute to the design and implementation of health promotion programs. Focus groups may be an important avenue to learning what health issues are for people living in a variety of circumstances and about valued, credible, and reasonable means of dealing with them.

Research Programs

Development of research programs for the study of health promotion is a critical need in nursing for several reasons. Examination of the relationships in causal or explanatory models used for either assessment or intervention research requires well-thought-out and staged investigations. Much research has stopped at assessment, as noted by Grey (chap. 2 in this volume) and confirmed by Hayman (chap. 3 in this volume) and evidenced by the greater abundance of research and the greater variability of health problems addressed by assessment research compared to intervention research. The research of Jemmott and her colleagues (Jemmott & Jemmott, 1991, 1994; Jemmott, Jemmott, Spears, Hewitt, & Cruz-Collins, 1992) is an example of a program of research in which an intervention phase follows an assessment phase. Hayman's (chap. 3 in this volume) claim of the need, prior to intervention research, for tests of theoretical models to delineate relationships among variables, identification of variables that are likely foci of interventions, and determination of the most important outcomes is a call for research programs.

■ Summing Up and Looking Ahead

Nurses are making an important contribution to the development of health promotion assessment and intervention knowledge from a number of perspectives. The strengths and potentials of nursing health promotion research agendas, questions, theoretic models, designs, and programs are apparent. Research published in the period 1989-1994 shows agendas that are oriented to health problems of high social concern. The type of questions addressed stem from all levels of scientific investigation—description, explanation, and prediction. The currently available multidimensional models provide a base for specification of moderating and mediating relationships between variables that could strengthen explanation and prediction of outcomes. Although limited to date, the investigation of processes and change through time establishes a precedent for study of learning and development of health-promoting behavior and practices. Programs of nursing research in health promotion are now available to demonstrate how knowledge grows (Lakatos, 1970).

The reviews of assessment and intervention research by Grey and Hayman, respectively, in this volume indicate that much work remains to be done to strengthen the contribution of nurses to the development of health promotion knowledge. First, nursing research agendas for the promotion of children's health can be expanded and refined to better take advantage of nursing perspectives and to serve societal needs. A nursing perspective seems ideally suited to agendas concerning behavior or activities that (a) directly reduce risks to health (e.g., avoiding toxic substances, getting immunizations, and regulating sexual behavior); (b) strengthen a protective factor (e.g., eating nutritious food and exercising for cardiovascular fitness); or (c) develop or enhance competencies for accomplishing everyday and special health-related tasks. These competencies include skills in regulating feelings and behavior—for example, reducing or redirecting impulses toward aggressive behavior. Competencies are also needed for engaging in activities of daily living or giving day-to-day care (e.g., feeding a child with energy needs, growth, and satisfaction in mind). Competencies in communicating with others (e.g., informing others of the child's needs) and problem-solving competencies (e.g., reflecting on why things happen) are also needed for accomplishing health-related tasks.

Second, development of theoretic models of nursing health promotion research that encompass the needs both of children who are generally healthy and of children with special health care needs could potentially advance the study of health promotion for both groups of children. Chronic challenges to health could productively be addressed from a health promotion perspective, for they shape and even extend the day-to-day health tasks. How these tasks are undertaken determines the health-promoting qualities of a child's life.

This section of the book deliberately focused on health promotion of healthy children. However, research relevant to health promotion for children with special health care needs is reviewed in this volume in the section on chronic conditions (Grey, Cameron, Lipman, & Thurber, 1994, concerning the coping behavior of children with diabetes). Both this research literature and the research literature addressed to health promotion of children in general have been relatively isolated from each other and could productively be examined for points of intersection in purpose, theory, and methods.

Third, theoretical models framed by an ecological perspective and that engage thinking about how the family, community, institutions, and cultural milieu are joined with health promotion activities and practices are needed. An ecological perspective advances questions about the health of children at specific ages and in specific places and environments and the processes through which health is developed or promoted (Bronfenbrenner, 1993; Sallis & Owen, 1997). These processes involve personal competencies, environmental resources, and social, political, and ideological forces. Nursing research agendas conceived from an ecological perspective demand integration of knowledge from several domains (e.g., biologic, psychologic, social, cultural, political, and economic). Furthermore, ecological models require the bridging of professional disciplines, such as health, education, and social welfare (Lavin et al., 1992).

Theoretical models for assessment and intervention health promotion studies must be equipped to examine the development of competencies, trajectories of health promotion activities through time, and changes in health outcomes such as nutritional status, physical growth, and cardiovascular fitness through time. Health promotion competencies, activities, and outcomes are likely to change with the child's stage of development (Sachs, 1984, 1986), living circumstances, and culture. They also will vary with the health promotion goal. The health promotion experience and history of a child and family channels intentions and establishes a direction and patterns for subsequent health-promoting activities.

Fourth, the types of interventions that nurses use for health promotion, whether as researchers or practitioners, often are in need of clarification, development, or expansion. Hayman (chap. 3 in this volume) called for ongoing process evaluations to clarify what interventions targeted at individuals contributed relative to those targeted at the environment.

Health teaching is an area for theoretical and research expansion. Nurses have traditionally emphasized health teaching of individuals or groups of children or parents as a health promotion intervention. For this teaching, nurses have drawn widely from the currently available medical and developmental knowledge, prevailing ideas of best child-care practice, and social and governmental policy. Recent literature in such fields as cognitive, developmental, social, and cultural psychology; educational psychology and anthropology; and the sociology of education is a source for elaboration and revision of interventions that rely on forms of teaching and learning, including anticipatory guidance and guided participation (Pridham, 1993, 1997; Pridham, Limbo, Schroeder, Thoyre, & Van Riper, in press).

Anticipatory guidance is a process of forming expectations and intentions about future events or conditions with the aim of preventing difficulties and promoting accomplishment of health tasks. This process is a little-studied mainstay of the health promotion practice of nurses (Caplan, 1959; Denehy, 1990; Pridham, 1993) and could be strengthened by attention to newer ideas and research concerning how people perceive, interpret, and act on information (Bretherton, 1995; Egeland, Carlson, & Sroufe, 1993; Main, Kaplan, & Cassidy, 1985). Guided participation is an ongoing health promotion intervention for significant life transitions in which a more expert person—for example, a nurse—supports a novice in becoming a competent participant in an activity that is socially valued and central to health. Strategies for supporting children, family members, and others in the community in helping each other to engage in health-promoting activities are needed.

Interventions designed for family, school, and community groups and are suited for use with people who have limited economic and social resources are needed. These interventions include dialogic educational strategies of the sort proposed by Freire (1973). Strategies of this type promise to support increased participation of patients or clients in health promotion services (Schubiner & Eggly, 1995).

Last, a high-priority task, made compellingly by Hayman throughout her chapter in this volume, is the mounting of programs of research with linked assessment and intervention phases and staged testing of complex, multidimensional explanatory models. The aim of this research is the development of models with high heuristic power (Lakatos, 1970).

Nursing Education for Health Promotion Research and Practice

The education of nursing students at every level and continuing education of graduate nurses must include health promotion as a central component of the curriculum (Pridham, Broome, Woodring, & Baroni, 1996). Directions for nursing education follow from attention to what health promotion for children and their families is and could be like. Health promotion concerns the day-to-day activities of children and the participation in these activities of children and their families in growth-promoting and adaptive ways. Given this perspective of health promotion, fundamental and curriculumwide changes in nursing education are needed for nurses to take the primary health promotion role they are expected to take (Gott & O'Brien, 1990; Hills & Lindsey, 1994; Maglacas, 1988; Pender et al., 1992). Pender and her colleagues (1992) outlined areas of emphasis for health promotion and disease prevention in undergraduate and graduate nursing curricula. Critical features of nursing curricula to prepare nurses for health promotion include egalitarian relationships, development of competencies for full participation in health promotion practice and for engagement in research, and collaborative and interdisciplinary practice (Hills & Lindsey, 1994). Ethical issues involved in health promotion practice (e.g., blaming the victim, marketing health promotion, and bias in selection of reduction of risks;

McLeroy, Gottlieb, & Burdine, 1987) are also important to address.

Health promotion is a multivariate phenomenon and a multidimensional activity. At all levels of education and for both assessment and intervention phases of practice, keeping several factors in mind while holding others constant could help develop a skill basic to health promotion thinking. For example, nurses who are designing a health promotion program, whether for an individual child or a population of children, need to keep in mind the health risks to which young children are vulnerable, given the child's environment and developmental accomplishments, while at the same time focusing on what family members expect and intend concerning the child's health and its support.

The multiple dimensions of health promotion refer to biological, psychological, interpersonal, social, cultural, and historical domains of living, among others. In their general education, nurses, on the whole, are oriented to all of these domains, and as a consequence are prepared to integrate information from a variety of domains. However, nurses are not likely to become and remain expert in the theory and research in all domains. At both upper-division baccalaureate and graduate levels, exercises in posing and solving health promotion problems are one approach to developing skill in obtaining and integrating information from multiple domains. Students at all levels can develop skills in seeking scholars in nursing and in other disciplines who have expertise that can be used to address health promotion issues. Interaction with peers and faculty members within and outside nursing can be structured to provide practice in collaborative problem solving.

Nursing actions to support clients in developing health-promoting behaviors and practices require a continuing relationship that permits disclosure of very personal and not easily shared expectations and intentions (i.e., the substance of a working model of an activity).

Nurses at all levels of education need opportunities to develop, reflect on, and study long-term relationships in the context of health promotion with one or more children and their families.

Because the health-relevant tasks and life functions in which children and their caregivers are engaged are variable and the working models are idiosyncratic, nurses must learn ways of constructing sensitive and responsive health promotion practice. This type of practice requires skills for efficiently learning the tasks, working models, and life circumstances of children and their caregivers and for labeling or classifying the observed or reported material. Collaboration between nurse educators, practitioners, and researchers is needed to develop theory for classification of tasks, aspects of working models, and life circumstances.

Sensitive and responsive health promotion practice requires skill in the use of media messages pertinent to health promotion. This skill includes the critique of media messages, knowledge of how children and their caregivers do and could use messages, and ways of reconstructing and shaping the messages to the needs of individual children and their families.

Health promotion activities are social, whether from the perspective of practice, learning, or maintenance. How the practices and rituals of a family or other social group (e.g., day care, school) and the expectations, standards, and customs of the community support, hinder, necessitate, or advance health promotion activities is a question that nurses must continually consider as they practice health promotion in relation to children (Russell & Jewell, 1992). Knowledge of aspects of the family, day care, school, and community that are relevant to health promotion activities of children and their caregivers, skills in eliciting information about these aspects, and skills in determining the health promotion needs of a specific child or population of children in light of their cultures are important aims for nursing education.

The social bases of health (Williams, 1989) and the social nature of health promotion activities require the engagement in problem solving of people who have a central role in the formation of expectations, intentions, and evaluation criteria concerning health (Russell & Jewell, 1992). These people include parents and other family members to whom they look for direction concerning health-promoting activities and practices. Skills in determining the sources of health practices and in involving family members and communities in constructing and reconstructing these practices are appropriate objectives of nursing education curricula. Skills in advancing ways of thinking about health, developing intentions for health promotion activities, and achieving consensus about practices through group discussion must also be an objective of nursing curricula.

Besides learning how to directly address health promotion problems, orientation to how political and economic structures affect health and how health promotion policy is created and influenced would support health promotion practice (Williams, 1989). This orientation includes learning about populations of children who lack, underuse, or have limited access to health promotion services, such as children of color, poor children, and those with refugee or migrant status (Braithwaite & Lythcott, 1989; Elder, Eccles, Ardelt, & Lord, 1995; Klerman, 1991; Kramer, 1992). Learning experiences for nurses could include participation in community organizing, coalition building, lobbying, and consulting activities. Nursing students could work with students in other disciplines to develop resource centers and examine and respond to legislation pertaining to health promotion.

Graduate students could learn to implement health promotion objectives across agencies through participation in the development of program standards, planning for shared resources, and monitoring progress (Chamberlin, 1994). Criteria of interagency or intersector collaboration and decision making, such as those proposed by Ziglio (1991), need to be part of this curriculum. A dialogic educational approach (Wallerstein, 1992) could be used to support nursing students in learning to help families and other community groups share concerns, identify problems relevant to health promotion, think critically, take collective action, and function as experts to others.

Looking Ahead

New challenges for the health promotion practice and research of nurses abound. Among these are large-scale problems that are rooted in or sustained by public and economic policy and community mores, such as unintentional injuries, violence, homelessness, substance abuse, adolescent pregnancies, environmental toxins and other health hazards, and communicable diseases, including HIV infection, sexually transmitted diseases, and tuberculosis (Cassetta, 1994). Mounting evidence of links between disease and health behavior (Green & Frankish, 1994, concerning asthma) and the influence of family, other social groups, and the environment on the development and maintenance of health behavior and practices (Cowen, 1991; Crooks, Lammarino, & Weinberg, 1987; Hayman & Ryan, 1994; Houtrouw & Carlson, 1993; Meininger, Hayman, Coates, & Gallagher, 1988; Stokols, 1992; Tinsley, 1992) compels nurses to take a multisystem and ecological perspective for health promotion practice and research. Nurses may have much to contribute to understanding and addressing the mechanisms and processes through which these links are created and maintained. How the organizations and communities in which nurses practice influence their health promotion activities merits study. Addressing such questions as the difference an exclusive focus on prevention and health promotion, provided through a nursing center (Riesch, 1992), or the broad-based knowledge contributed by an interdisciplinary team makes for nursing practice will help establish organizational environments that advance the role of nursing in health promotion.

What nurses need to develop knowledge for health promotion includes preparation and funding for research as well as opportunities to practice creatively, flexibly, and in connection with other disciplines and the people for whom the health promotion is intended. Since the 1950s, nursing research concerning health promotion has increased, supported by larger numbers of nurses with graduate degrees and funding for doctoral education in nursing and for health promotion research. Both the National Institute of Nursing Research and the Maternal and Child Health Bureau of the U.S. Department of Health and Human Services have supported the health promotion research of nurses.

Nurses have largely carried the health promotion movement forward at the level of families in the community. Now, nurse practitioners and nurses in hospitals have an opportunity to extend the health promotion movement. Nurses will offer leadership and vision through raising questions and defining goals about health promotion and thinking beyond maintenance of health to health promotion (Tripp & Stachowiak, 1992). Nursing leadership is needed for practice that addresses family and community health as well as individual health and that finds means of promoting the health of children who have special needs or who lack resources or access to health care (Meleis, 1990). To accomplish these leadership functions, nurses need an infrastructure of theoretical, research, and educational support for health promotion practice. The extent to which prepaid health care plans are geared to supporting health promotion activities will be a critical factor in what nurses can accomplish (Pender, 1987).

In a cost-conscious age, the issues involved in supporting health promotion activities for children and their families, although substantial, are not daunting. Brodie (chap. 1 in this volume) makes it clear that nurses throughout nursing's health promotion history have taken responsibility for improving the health of children in the face of massive need and limited resources. The examination of costs in relation to benefits of health promotion activities is a needed and challenging feature of nursing research. Pender (1987) documented economic incentives of health promotion, identified means of evaluating effectiveness, and called for improved measures of health status as a basis for determining the effectiveness of health promotion services. A risk is that health professionals may ask for too little regarding the promotion of children's health (Williams & Miller, 1992). The fact that nurses have always been responsive to critical health needs indicates how they will respond in the future.

In the larger scheme of health care and its costs, health promotion is critical. Careful study of health promotion agendas, their significance for specific populations, and the kind of commitment required to move the agendas forward is urgent. Nurses are better equipped than ever before with research tools and skills to advance this study. Furthermore, nurses are prepared and in a good position to provide bridges to the broad base of knowledge that health promotion requires. Nurses are skilled in bringing into their practice and research the vantage points and perspectives of other disciplines, many of which are needed for health promotion.

Health promotion is a complex process stemming from intimate knowledge of how people experience life tasks. To develop understanding of health promotion tasks and processes that people experience, nurse researchers must be well linked with clinicians who are in touch with these tasks and processes. Through the links with nurse researchers, clinicians can expand their awareness of types, manifestations, and implications for practice of health promotion tasks and processes experienced by their clients.

Practitioners and researchers must understand the implications of life experience for health-promoting thought and action. For this reason, health promotion is best carried out in the context of a relationship with clients in which expectations and intentions concerning health are freely shared with practitioners and researchers and in which health promotion goals and plans are jointly developed and tested. Again, nurses are optimally situated for this kind of relationship by an underlying phi-losophy of caring about and responding sensitively to the intimate, health-implicating aspects of life tasks.

The challenges confronting nurses who are committed to advancing health promotion warrant specifically designated educational and research resources. The theoretical and empirical means of advancing health promotion are growing. The importance to health of health tasks and the competencies and resources that individuals and groups have to accomplish them mandates concern with the conditions and processes that support the accomplishment of these tasks. This concern is central to nursing practice and research and a reason for nurses to take a major leadership role in the promotion of children's health.

PART II

RESPONSES OF CHILDREN AND FAMILIES TO ACUTE ILLNESS

■ *Marion E. Broome, Editor*

5

■

HISTORICAL OVERVIEW OF RESPONSES OF CHILDREN AND THEIR FAMILIES TO ACUTE ILLNESS

■ *Judith A. Vessey*

If nursing is ever to justify its name as an applied science, if it is ever to free itself from these old superficial, haphazard methods, some way must be found to submit all our practice as rapidly as possible to the most searching test which modern science can devise.

—Miss Isabel Stewart, Chairperson,
National League of Nursing Education (1929, p. 3)

Nearly 70 years ago, Isabel Stewart clearly espoused the need for a research-based nursing practice; the challenge is as great today. For pediatric nurse researchers, the efforts to identify and manage the responses of children and their families to acute illness remains a formidable task. This chapter presents a historical overview of these efforts. First, the early antecedents of related pediatric nursing research are described, followed by an examination of specific domains of study (psychosocial care, pain management, and care of critically ill children). The theoretical and empirical approaches and specific determinants that have influenced relevant nursing research are then addressed.

■ Early Antecedents

Just like children and families, pediatric nursing research has followed a distinct developmental course determined by evolving and increasingly sophisticated developmental theory, breakthroughs in medical science, issues in clinical practice, and maturing professional and role behaviors. To fully appreciate the maturation and contributions that nursing research has made and continues to make in improving the care of acutely ill children and their families, it is helpful to recognize its antecedents. Although records from early civilizations chronicled methods for caring for sick children, pediatric specialized medical and nursing care was not formalized for several millennia (Brodie, 1982) until the need for such care became evident by the mid-19th century. One legacy of the international industrial revolution and the shift from an agrarian to an urban lifestyle was skyrocketing childhood morbidity and mortality. Rates of infectious diseases and accidents far surpassed those of the preceding century. By 1840, approximately 30% of the population was under 10 years of age. Only 50% survived to adulthood, and mortality for infants in almshouses was as high as 99% (Cone, 1979a; Radbill, 1955). Yet less than 0.1% of hospitalized patients were children (Atkinson & Day, 1981a).

In response to these profound societal needs, Dr. Charles West founded London's Great Ormond Street Hospital for Sick Children in 1852. Pediatric nursing began emerging as a specialty, for an important part of the hospital's mission was the education and training of women in the duties of children's nursing. It is interesting to note that this occurred three years before Florence Nightingale ventured to the Crimea and a decade before the Nightingale School opened its door. Rapid expansion in the care of ill children followed when the first children's hospital in the United States, Children's Hospital of Philadelphia, was established in 1855. Similar institutions were rapidly established across the country.

Concomitant with the opening of children's hospitals was the founding of training schools for pediatric nurses preparing them to care for acutely ill children. The segregation of sick children in specialty hospitals, however, was not universally supported. Among its detractors was Florence Nightingale:

> Whatever you do, do not have children's wards in a general hospital, but mix them up with the adults for where adults are mixed with them, the woman in the next bed, if the patients are judiciously distributed, often becomes the child's best protector and nurse and it does her as much good as it does the child. (Nightingale, 1859, cited in Miles, 1985, p. 48)

Despite such views, children's hospitals and nurses' training schools, which taught them how to care for sick children, continued to flourish in response to public demands.

Early emphasis was on meeting the physical needs of sick children, although little reliable information existed. In the manner of Nightingale, nurses began recording their interventions and effectiveness. As early as 1900, nurses at Boston's Floating Hospital[1] actively engaged in feeding research. Their work, of sufficient merit to attract the attention of Dr. Simon Flexner, an architect of modern medicine, laid important groundwork for future research endeavors. Practice-related research in the 1920s and 1930s was tied to the need for systematic evaluations of nursing practice (Clayton, 1927; Gortner & Nahm, 1977). Case reports on the care management strategies for sick children began to appear in the *American Journal of Nursing*. Topics covered were Pott's disease, pyloric stenosis, and caring for the premature infant without an incubator, to name a few. Despite these early attempts, nurses' research on phenomena affecting ill children and their families was limited and sporadic.

Nursing research did not begin to come into its own until the 1940s when its development closely paralleled that of graduate nursing education. The need to connect research activity to a nursing problem was promulgated by nursing leaders (Bixler, 1942). Investigations by nurses

TABLE 5.1 Chronological Listing of Research Published in *Nursing Research,* 1952-1970

Year	Author(s) and Publication
1952	Wilkins, G. N. The role of the nurse in preparing preschool children. *Nursing Research, 1,* 36.
1953	Jacobs, C. G. A study of the young child's contacts with staff members in a selected pediatric hospital. *Nursing Research, 2,* 39.
1956	Iffrig, M. C. Nursing observations of one hundred premature infants and their feeding programs. *Nursing Research, 5,* 71-81.
1965	Mahaffy, P. R. The effects of hospitalization on children admitted for tonsillectomy and adenoidectomy. *Nursing Research, 14*(1), 12-19.
1967	Roy, M. C. Role cues and mothers of hospitalized children. *Nursing Research, 16*(2), 178-182.
	McCaffery, M., & Johnson, D. E. Effect of parent group discussion upon epistemic responses. *Nursing Research, 16*(4), 352-358.
1968	Garlinghouse, J., & Sharp, L. J. The hemophilic child's self-concept and family stress in relation to bleeding episodes. *Nursing Research, 17*(1), 32-36.
	Marrow, D. L., & Johnson, B. S. Perceptions of the mother's role with her hospitalized child. *Nursing Research, 17*(2), 155-156.
	Torrance, J. T. Temperature readings in premature infants. *Nursing Research, 17*(4), 312-320.
	Neal, M. V., & Naven, C. M. Ability of premature infant to monitor his own body temperature. *Nursing Research, 17*(5), 396-402.
1969	Seidl, F. W. Pediatric nursing personnel and parent participation: A study in attitudes. *Nursing Research, 18*(1), 40-44.
	Fuszard, M. B. Acceptance of authoritarianism in the nurse by the hospitalized teenager. *Nursing Research, 18*(5), 426-432.

in various specialties such as pediatrics ensued. For example, in the immediate postwar period, pediatric nurses were concerned with controlling communicable diseases and improving child welfare. By the early 1950s, they were questioning practices common to most hospitals, such as limited visiting hours, restricted parental roles, and open ward design and management (Fitzgerald, 1982). The need to systematically investigate these and other issues was promulgated in 1953 by the then neophyte journal, *Nursing Research,* in its column titled "Research Needed." Requests for research on caring for children with tuberculosis and on parental visitation were noted (Research Reporter, 1953). Despite this call for clinical research, studies of nurses by nurses still outnumbered clinical topics 10 to 1 (Gortner, 1983).

During the 1960s and early 1970s, the first clinical studies to investigate psychosocial care, pain management, care of high-risk groups (e.g., premature infants), and nursing strategies to reduce health risks were reported (Gortner & Nahm, 1977; see Table 5.1). Since then, nursing research directed toward improving outcomes of acutely ill children and their families has increased exponentially (Barnard & Neal, 1977). Unfortunately, changes in clinical practice have been slow and sporadic. To correct this, research utilization strategies now are being actively developed and implemented.

In summary, a growing body of nursing research that has investigated the responses of children and their families to acute illness now exists. Many of these studies validate nurses' clinical hunches, some of which have been held for centuries. However, pediatric nursing research accounts for a small percentage of all of nursing research (see Table 5.2). Moreover, expanded research activity on a particular topic has been sporadic; often several decades elapsed before findings made their way into practice. Interdisciplinary influences (e.g., medicine and psychology) and social pressures

TABLE 5.2 Percentage Published Pediatric Nursing Research Articles of Total Published Nursing Research Articles

Year	Percentage
1952-1959	1
1960	0
1970	2
1980	6

SOURCE: Brown, Tanner, and Padrick (1984).

(e.g., consumer advocacy groups), such as those fostering psychosocial care of children, appeared to be the catalysts for many of these transitions.

■ *Domains of Research Activity*

The majority of nursing research conducted over the past 40 years can be classified into three domains: (a) psychosocial care, including parental visitation, coping, play therapy, preparation, and education; (b) pain management; and (c) interventions in critical care arenas.

Psychosocial Care of Acutely Ill Children

Coping

> To keep the sick child happy; to remove from it all avoidable causes of alarm, of suffering of discomfort; . . . are duties of the gravest kind which weigh on the parent and the nurse.
>
> —Dr. Charles West, Founder,
> Great Ormond Street Hospital
> for Sick Children (1885, p. 214)

The pediatric nursing literature is replete with articles on the stresses that children en-

counter during hospitalization and the ways in which they adapt to them. Early anecdotal discussions of children's responses to hospitalization began to be replaced in the late 1960s and early 1970s by reports of systematic investigations. The deleterious effects of hospitalization on children's emotional health and the effects on their parents were clearly documented (Mahaffy, 1965; Roy, 1967; Wolfer & Visintainer, 1975). However, specific determinants of children's upset were less certain. To identify the children at greatest risk, additional studies explored pain, immobility, mutilation, and loss of control as significant concerns of acutely ill children (Lambert, 1984; Ritchie, 1977; Stevens, 1986).

Simultaneously, organized approaches to studying children's coping abilities and coping styles emerged. Children's age and developmental level, length of stay, disease severity, and predisposing family orientation were correlated with children's potential to effectively cope with hospitalization and its attendant stressors (McClowry, 1988). Other studies examined specific coping behaviors. Rose (1972) was the first to view transient changes in children's behavior as a means of coping and to propose a method for categorizing their responses. These notions were expanded by labeling behavioral changes as either self-sustaining or indicative of loss of control; the situations in which these behaviors were likely to be exhibited also was noted (Cormier, 1979; Savedra & Tesler, 1981; Youssef, 1981).

Three specific coping styles—inactive, orienting, and active—were identified (Rose, 1972), promulgated (Tesler & Savedra, 1981), and later refined by LaMontagne (1984), who integrated locus of control theory with coping styles. The relationships between these coping styles and selected child and environmental characteristics also have been studied. Parental visitation (Savedra & Tesler, 1981) and the number of stressful events encountered (Rose, 1972) did not affect children's coping behav-

Psychological Preparation

Psychological preparation for hospitalization, procedures, and surgery refers to those interventions specifically designed to help children anticipate, deal with, and gain mastery over the events they will experience. Psychological preparation is a multifaceted concept, and numerous studies have been conducted by individuals from a variety of disciplines. In general, the foci of these studies were methods of preparation, appropriate timing and settings for preparation, and parental preparation. Relevant nursing research was directed at determining the best methods for preparing children for hospitalization and procedures.

Techniques for child-specific psychological preparation have included tours (Stainton, 1974), puppetry (Bailey, 1967), play experiences (Ellerton, Caty, & Ritchie, 1985), simulations (Abbott, Hansen, & Lewis, 1970), audiovisuals (Johnson, Kirchhoff, & Endress, 1975), and a variety of other approaches. These diverse treatment strategies can be better examined by classifying them by the major behavioral approaches they have incorporated: selected procedural information, sensory preparation, modeling, and behavioral rehearsal.

Procedural information was the first preparation approach to be adopted by nurses. Specific content about hospitalization is provided for children to familiarize them with the new experiences they will encounter (Stainton, 1974; Wilson, 1987). Its primary focus is to transmit factual information; any contributions to the child's emotional state is secondary. The implicit rationale for this approach is that when children know what to expect from a situation they will initiate the appropriate coping mechanisms.

Sensory preparation expanded on procedural approaches by adding descriptions of the sensations that children were likely to experience. Johnson and colleagues (1975) compared the effectiveness of sensory preparation to procedural information in school-age children who were having orthopedic casts removed. Those that received sensory information, regardless of their fear, had significantly lower distress scores than those in the procedural information and control groups. Later studies could not replicate these findings exactly and found both procedural and sensory preparation effective (Abrams, 1982; Eland, 1981).

Modeling approaches developed in tandem with sensory preparation. These techniques are based on the premise that children can be taught appropriate behavior and coping abilities by watching vignettes of peers reacting to similar events to those that they will experience. Modeling is frequently taught by film or video, but also may occur through puppetry or direct peer interaction. The majority of the modeling research has been conducted by colleagues in other disciplines (Ferguson, 1979; Melamed & Siegel, 1975; Vernon, 1975).

Behavioral rehearsal built on modeling techniques. There are numerous similarities, but in behavioral rehearsal, children are encouraged to actually act out potential situations they will encounter. Work by Visintainer and Wolfer (1975; Wolfer & Visintainer, 1975) demonstrated that this approach was highly effective, allowing children to control the amount of input they received.

The effectiveness of any preparation approach is often modulated by parental stress levels. Parents find their child's hospitalization anxiety producing (Lynn, 1986; Schmeltz & White, 1982; Skipper, Leonard, & Rhymes, 1968); significant correlations between maternal and child anxiety have been documented (Meng & Zastowny, 1982; Vardaro, 1978). The relationship is most evident with younger children and the very sick. Methods to reduce parental stress have been explored with some success (Meng & Zastowny, 1982; Miles & Carter, 1982; Schmeltz & White, 1982).

The relationships between the type of preparation, the child's developmental level and coping style, and short- and long-term behavioral outcomes have not been reported. Further exploration of the relationships between these constructs is clearly needed. Yet nurse researchers are not actively studying psychosocial preparation for hospitalization and illness. This is unfortunate because earlier studies were conducted in care arenas and situations that in no way resemble today's hospitalization experiences and may not be generalizable to the current context.

Summary and Critique

Psychosocial care is perhaps the richest compendium of the pediatric nursing research domains for acutely ill children. Despite the fact that this topic has been widely investigated over the past three decades, there are numerous problems with the research base. Thompson (1985), in his text *Psychosocial Research on Pediatric Hospitalization and Health Care,* clearly identified several problem areas. A similar list of concerns emerged from Vessey and Carlson's (1996) research synthesis and meta-analysis. First, the majority of studies fail to give complete or even adequate descriptions of the study design, instrumentation, or analytic techniques, regardless of when they were conducted. Because of these limitations, planned replications of the earliest studies were difficult if not impossible. What ensued were a number of studies conducted in the 1970s and 1980s that did not significantly build on earlier work but, rather, examined similar constructs without correcting earlier flaws. For example, at no point during the past 40 years did studies routinely control for bias by blinding observers.

Second, in some studies it was difficult to identify the theoretical underpinnings, as these were rarely made explicit. Other studies completely disregarded key theoretical issues, such as the interaction between development and preparation strategies. For example, in the interest of obtaining adequate samples, many studies enrolled children whose age ranges spanned several developmental levels. Other studies depended on secondary measures rather than the primary measure of a construct. For example, most preparation studies only measured behavioral upset, neglecting to assess whether the child had learned anything about the experiences for which he or she was being prepared.

A third concern is methodological confusion. For example, if control groups were used, the participants often received no treatments whatsoever rather than providing the contact that would be experienced by an attentional control group. As any contact has been known to decrease anxiety, failure to address this issue in the study's design is problematic. Documentation of instruments' reliability, validity, or appropriateness were rarely addressed. Selected samples were frequently accessed, with differing age groups (infants, toddlers, and older adolescents), ethnic backgrounds (anyone but Caucasians), and range of diagnoses being severely underrepresented. Moreover, the analytic techniques employed were not always appropriate for the design.

Despite some significant limitations, this body of research has been pivotal in improving the psychosocial care of acutely ill children and their families. These findings have been used by hospitals to humanize care and by accrediting bodies such as the Joint Commission on Accreditation of Healthcare Organizations to set standards of care.

Pain Management

An hour of pain is as long as a day of pleasure.

—*Proverb*

Nurse researchers have contributed a great deal to reliably describing children's pain experiences and how they differ from adults (Beyer & Byers, 1985; Jerrett, 1985; Jerrett & Evans, 1986). Specific factors shown to affect children's pain experiences are children's cognitive level and other developmental indicators, understanding of illness (Perrin & Gerrity, 1981), and prior pain experiences (Torrance, 1986b; Savedra, Gibbons, Tesler, Ward, & Wegner, 1982). These studies provided valuable insights for research designed to objectively and accurately assess children's pain.

An extensive body of pain assessment research has been conducted by individuals from numerous disciplines. These studies have resulted in a variety of behavioral, physiological, and psychological assessment measures (McGrath, 1990), with nurse researchers primarily involved with developing the latter type of measures. Early attempts were dependent on self-report either through direct response, interview, questionnaire, or rating scale and used a variety of prompts including colors, faces, or word lists. These provided the foundation for designing and validating more sophisticated rating scales. For example, Schultz (1971) initially identified that children would describe pain by color; Stewart (1977) later developed a pain scale based on the color spectrum. This scale was tested by Eland (1981), who adapted the idea by having children color in a body outline with colored crayons, each of which represented a different level of pain intensity (Eland, 1981; McGrath, 1990). Tesler, Ward, Savedra, Wegner, and Gibbons (1983) expanded this notion in a questionnaire they developed that used both colors and words to evaluate not only children's pain responses but also their coping abilities.

Most of the rating scales that have been developed vary in design and are based on the numeric scores that correlate to various pain levels. Several direct scaling techniques use poker chips (Hester, 1979), faces (Beyer & Aradine, 1986, 1988), numbers (Beyer & Aradine, 1986, 1988), and thermometers. Unfortunately, each design type has inherent methodologic difficulties in that children must demonstrate sequencing skills. Scales using poker chips and numbers require that children relate their pain to an abstract concept. Scales based on faces overcome the abstraction issue but are confounded in that the faces may elicit an affective response rather than targeting children's responses to pain severity alone. Moreover, most scales treat their various intervals as ratio rather than ordinal data, with little supporting evidence that the indicated intervals directly correlate with pain intensity. This is not only a potential problem for clinical use but complicates using pain scale scores in statistical analyses of intervention studies (McGrath, 1990).

Only a few nursing researchers have investigated pain management strategies, despite the fact that it has long been identified that acutely ill children receive less treatment for their pain than adults do (Beyer, DeGood, Ashley, & Russell, 1983). Of those studies that have been conducted, most focus on using preparation strategies similar to those used in reducing psychological distress (Broome & Endsley, 1987; Eland, 1981; Gedaly-Duff, 1984). It is only recently that nurse researchers have begun investigating a variety of pharmacological and nonpharmacological approaches (Vessey & Carlson, 1996).

Summary and Critique

Nursing research on pain has advanced nursing science and raised health care professionals' sensitivity to children's pain, thus positively influencing pain management in acutely ill children. Despite these laudable achievements, pain research has been inconsistent, and some areas of interest remain underinvestigated.

Pain assessment has received the most attention. Most pain assessment studies, however, have focused on a limited range of assessment techniques, with little emphasis placed on physiologic indicators, behavioral observation, or multidimensional approaches. Like the research on psychological preparation, the majority of studies focus on school-age children. Although pain assessment in infants has been studied by other disciplines since the mid-1960s (McGrath, 1990), nurse researchers have only recently begun to investigate this area.

Other than studies on pain assessment, little pediatric research on the physiology of pain or on management techniques have been conducted by nurse researchers. In part, the lack of physiologically based research is likely due to having few appropriately schooled individuals able to conduct such studies. The reasons for the paucity of studies on pharmacologic or nonpharmacologic pain management and their relationships is more difficult to explain, although the cost of such studies and challenges encountered in negotiating access may be partial explanations.

It is interesting to note that research on pediatric pain is highly developed compared to the studies of other symptoms, such as fatigue or nausea and vomiting. For these symptoms, clinical practice still relies on extrapolating information from studies of adults.

Interventions for Critically Ill Children

Intensive Care Units

> I slept sounder than ever I remember to
> have done in my life . . . ; for when I
> awaked it was day light, I attempted to
> rise, but was not able to stir; for as I
> happened to lie on my back, I found my
> arms and legs were strongly fastened on
> each side to the ground. . . . I likewise felt
> several slender ligatures across my body,
> from my armpits and my thighs. I could
> only look upwards—and the light offended

> my eyes. I heard a confused noise about
> me; but in the posture I lay could see
> nothing.
>
> —*Jonathan Swift,* Gulliver's Travels
> *(1726/1983, p. 27)*

Pediatric intensive care units (PICUs) began to flourish in the 1960s and adopted many of the same restrictive visitation policies in place on general units. Conventional wisdom held that parental visitation was too stressful for children and the environment too stressful for their parents. Nurses then assumed that parental presence interfered with care and that children were not at high risk for psychological upset due to their illness acuity and altered consciousness. These assumptions were challenged by Barnes (1975a, 1975b) in her descriptive work of children's recollections of the PICU and behavioral regression on discharge. She demonstrated that children found many aspects of their PICU stay stressful, that their recollections were often distorted, and that behavioral regression was common. Carty (1977) validated many of these findings, further illuminating the stresses associated with a PICU stay. Attention was later focused on the parents when researchers assessed those situations that parents found stressful and the means by which they coped (Lewandowski, 1980; Miles & Carter, 1982; Proctor, 1987). To better capture stresses experienced by parents, instrument development was undertaken (Miles & Carter, 1982). Additional research on play behaviors and visitation by a variety of interdisciplinary colleagues clearly indicated the need for changes in PICU practices. However, liberalization of psychosocial policies involving parents has been arduous, even in the face of research findings. Why this is so is not known, although it can be speculated that PICU personnel may not place the same priority on psychosocial care as other hospital personnel do. The traffic flow, work intensity, and physical layouts of PICUs also may make it more difficult to operationalize psychosocial policies.

Neonatal Care

> Premature infants should be cared for in hospital where they could be scientifically studied, and in this way our knowledge advances and our methods of rearing them are improved.
>
> —*Mary Dabney Smith*
> *(1907/1911, p. 792)*

Despite early recognition that there was much to be studied about premature infants, early studies primarily focused on morbidity and mortality (Peebles, 1933), underscoring the need for specialized care (Lundeen, 1937; Napier, 1927). By the 1950s and early 1960s, researchers were investigating nutrition and growth (Hasselmeyer, de LaPuente, Lundeen, & Morrison, 1963; Iffrig, 1956; Kagan et al., 1955), temperature taking and thermoregulation (Neal & Nauen, 1968; Torrance, 1968a), transport (Losty, Orlofsky, & Wallace, 1950), and behavioral patterns (Hasselmeyer, 1961). Concomitant with the advent of neonatal intensive care units in the mid-1960s, neonatal nursing research began to flourish. In the 1970s and 1980s, the quality and quantity of neonatal nursing research grew exponentially. Major programs of research were developed that focused on such topics as infant stimulation (Barnard, 1972; Barnard & Bee, 1983; Katz, 1971; Kramer, Chamorro, Green, & Knudtson, 1975; Neal, 1968; Porter, 1972; Rausch, 1981; Rice, 1977; Segall, 1972), temperament (Medoff-Cooper, 1986), thermoregulation, nonnutritive sucking (Anderson, 1975; Anderson, McBride, Dahm, Ellis & Vidyasagar, 1982; Measel & Anderson, 1979), suctioning, and other measures of physiologic stability (Blackburn & Patteson, 1991; Fuller, Wenner & Blackburn, 1978;

Taquino & Blackburn, 1994), breastfeeding (Meier, 1988; Meier & Pugh, 1985), and maternal stress (Gennaro, 1988; Mercer, 1981; Mercer & Ferketich, 1988).

The landmark study by Brooten and colleagues (1988) of a clinical trial of early discharge and home follow-up of very-low-birth-weight infants significantly influenced the care of premature neonates, the role of advanced practice nurses, and the larger sphere of health services research. Many of these studies went far beyond simple description by using sophisticated designs and analytic techniques.

Neonatal nursing research has significantly improved the outcomes of infants through two mechanisms: (a) reducing the amount of complications associated with high-risk pregnancies and subsequent preterm deliveries and (b) successfully managing the care of low-birth-weight infants. Programs of research have addressed questions in a variety of biopsychosocial areas. Challenges still remain with study design, obtaining adequate samples, and having access to appropriate instrumentation. Moreover, investigators are challenged by the rapidity in which technology changes and new questions arise; findings may be virtually obsolete before a study is complete. Despite these concerns, numerous programs of research directed by seasoned researchers have produced findings that continue to shape policy, advance nursing care, and improve infants' outcomes.

Summary and Critique

Of particular interest is how differently the patterns and amounts of research activity have differed between neonatal and pediatric ICUs. Although reasons for this difference have not been clearly explicated, it may be conjectured that because the first specialized care of critically ill children was delivered in adult intensive care units it seemed only reasonable to apply the findings from adult studies to sick children. For neonatal nurses, however, extrapolating knowledge from studies of critically ill adults was not only difficult but dangerous. The lack of relevant research findings required neonatal nurses to rapidly establish a knowledge base appropriate for guiding the care they delivered to premature, acutely ill infants.

This need was clearly recognized and promoted by other groups. In 1976, the American Nurses' Association Commission on Nursing Research listed as a priority studies to improve the outlook for high-risk parents and high-risk infants. The National Center for Nursing Research's first conference on research priorities (CORP) also identified research on low-birth-weight infants as a priority area. Support and prioritization by such organizations clearly had a positive effect on related research endeavors influencing the study of acutely ill children.

■ Theoretical and Empirical Approaches Influencing the Study of Acutely Ill Children

The earliest nursing research examining phenomena of interest in the care of acutely ill children relied on case study designs or simple epidemiologic records. Over time, these expanded to include questionnaires, surveys, and interview schedules. Measures were investigator derived and not subjected to the rigors of psychometric testing. Another limitation of these techniques was that the data were virtually always collected from a secondary source other than the child, usually a parent or nurse. By the 1970s, observational techniques were used, with some of the earliest approaches employed in studies of play therapy. However, these methods were often suspect because of problems in establishing reliability and validity. The evolution of video technology in the 1980s and 1990s legitimized many observational methods by providing a mechanism for reducing observer bias and subject reactivity as well as providing direct information from the child; thus strengthening research designs.

Physiological measures have been underutilized. The most common measures, heart rate and blood pressure, have been used with limited success because of their high reactivity and difficulties in achieving measurement sensitivity. The problems encountered with these measures have lessened with the advent of the Dinamap, pulse oximetry, and other electronic devices. Other techniques for assessing stress, such as the palmar sweat test (Dabbs, Johnson, & Leventhal, 1968; Johnson & Dabbs, 1967) and urinary cortisol levels (Barnes, Kenney, Call, & Reinhart, 1972), have been used infrequently but have far superior psychometric properties.

Despite this increasing sophistication, the majority of study designs are still descriptive, many relying on interviews or surveys. Although these descriptive studies are the first step in investigating areas not previously studied, their data do little to help explain phenomena, prescribe appropriate interventions, or predict clinical outcomes. In summary, many research findings, although suggesting direction(s) for further study, have provided limited direction for clinical practice or even future research.

Another area of concern is methodologic appropriateness and congruence, as has been previously noted. It is unfortunate that the theoretical and methodological aspects (e.g., sample size, choice of statistics, and valid instrumentation) of some studies do not stand up to close scientific scrutiny. Greater advantage of the methodological or analytic techniques being used in other disciplines such as biological assays, time series analyses, and meta-analytic techniques could be taken.

Stronger theoretical support for studies is needed. For example, there has been heavy reliance on theorists such as Piaget (cited in Ginzburg & Opper, 1979) and Erikson (cited in Crain, 1980), but the works of other developmental theorists such as Vygotsky (cited in Cole, John-Steiner, Scribner, & Souberman, 1978) or the neo-Piagetians have gone relatively unexplored. Theories from other domains, such as symbolic interactionism theories or system theories, also have been underutilized. To date, various nursing theories have been used in studying the responses of acutely ill children and their families. However, these have not demonstrated much utility in describing, explaining, and predicting phenomena manifested by sick children and their families. The one possible exception is Orem's (1992) theory of self-care, likely due to its developmental focus and clinical utility.

■ Determinants of Research Activity: A Historical Perspective

Pediatric nursing has lagged somewhat behind other nursing specialties in developing a research knowledge base. There are numerous explanations for this, including the preparation of pediatric nurse researchers, the support of organized nursing associations, and the difficulty in conducting clinical studies in the acute care arena.

Preparation of Pediatric Nurse Researchers

The instruction of young women in the care and management of sick children set the pattern of development in sick children's nursing for the next 100 years.

Charles West (1854/1954, cited in Miles, 1985, p. 49)

Despite the determinants listed above, the underlying problem is rooted in the philosophy that children were considered to be "little adults." Recognizing that children have differing needs depending on their level of development has been an evolving process. It is not surprising that the developmental trajectory of pediatric nursing research has been similar. Studies related to acutely ill children and their families were not solely the purview of pediatric nurses. In many respects, this research developed on the coattails of medical specialization and medical surgical nursing (Miles, 1985). Because children were viewed as little adults, knowledge from adult studies, such as wound care and suctioning, initially was generalized to pediatric practice without further validation. Later, areas of inquiry such as saline versus heparin flushes were derived from studies of adult populations and are still being evaluated. Psychiatric nurse researchers played a major role in shaping the psychosocial care of hospitalized children while maternity nurse researchers laid the groundwork for research with premature infants until neonatal nursing became its own specialty in the 1970s (Campbell, 1990).

Advanced Education

Doctoral education in nursing and concomitant research activity has only just matured in the past two decades; a cadre of experienced researchers is now emerging (Brodie, 1986). The number of nursing doctoral programs expanded from 12 in 1974 to 62 as of 1995 (Sigma Theta Tau, 1995). Despite this rapid growth in doctoral programs, fewer pediatric nurses than those in other specialties have sought doctoral study. Although the reasons are unclear, the lack of role models, fewer master's programs, and the idea that the collective personality of pediatric nurses did not augur well with doctoral study have all been suggested as possible explanations.

For pediatric nurses who did seek doctoral study, many acquired their degrees in the related fields of psychology, early childhood education, and anthropology. Such preparation has significantly contributed to the theoretical underpinnings of pediatric practice but done little to advance clinical knowledge. Applying nonnursing models and methodology to clinical questions and working with professors and peers that did not understand nor, in some cases, appreciate problems encountered in the clinical arena was a daunting proposition for neophyte researchers. Moreover, when these nurses returned to clinical practice, they were faced with the difficult task of adapting these approaches to the clinical arena (Brodie, 1988).

The Role of Professional Nursing Organizations

Professional organizations had an early and major involvement in shaping early nursing research agendas. The American Nurses' Association (ANA) has sponsored nursing research through publication of *The American Journal of Nursing* (1900–present), *Nursing Research* (1952–present), and other specialty journals; establishing the *American Nurses' Foundation* (1955–present); sponsoring nursing research conferences (1965-1974); and last, establishing the *Committee on Research and Studies* (1956-1970), which paved the way for the *Commission on Nursing Research* (1970) and the *Council of Nurse Researchers* (1971; Brimmer, 1978; See, 1977). Although many of these activities tangentially supported pediatric nursing research, one specific initiative was a project investigating the impact of pediatric nurse practitioners (Brimmer, 1978). The National League for Nursing also was active in promoting nursing research, but most of their efforts were directed toward educational and professional issues rather than clinical topics (Johnson, 1977).

The role of specialty professional organizations in facilitating programs of clinical research has gone relatively unrecognized. However, when one examines long-standing professional organizations, such as the Oncology Nurses' Society (ONS) or the American Association for Critical Care Nurses (AACN), it is clear that they have significantly helped advance their specialized knowledge bases by developing research agendas, awarding grant monies for preliminary studies, providing outlets for dissemination of new knowledge (e.g., journals and conferences), and establishing specific research priorities. Many of nursing's noted researchers began their careers with seed monies from professional organizations, some of which, for example, the Association of Women's Health, Obstetrical, and Neonatal Nursing (AWHONN) and the American Association of Critical Care Nurses (AACN), have initiated nationwide research utilization demonstration projects that rapidly test and integrate results from collective research studies into clinical practice.

When examining the history of clinical research in acute care pediatrics, one must consider the role played by professional organizations. It is important to note that pediatric nursing did not have a comprehensive professional organization until recently. The Maternal-Child Council of the American Nurses' Association represented both maternity and pediatric interests. It can be argued that by necessity the Council adopted a compromise position between the two specialties that resulted in focusing much of its activity on the neonatal period. Moreover, promoting research activity was not one of its central purposes. The Council was dissolved during the ANA's reorganization in 1993–1994. Other pediatric nursing organizations, such as the Association of Pediatric Oncology Nurses (APON) and the National Association of Pediatric Nurse Associates and Practitioners (NAPNAP) were founded to represent the special interests of a select group of pediatric nurses; however, little research activity has been generated by these groups. The Society of Pediatric Nurses (SPN), founded in 1990, is the first comprehensive pediatric nursing organization, but it is still too new to as yet significantly influence pediatric clinical nursing research.

Over the years, pediatric nurse researchers have become actively involved in a variety of other professional organizations that helped meet their professional needs. Some of these are subgroups within nursing organizations (e.g., the Association of Operating Room Nurses [AORN]), some are subgroups of medical organizations (the Pediatric Nursing Endocrinology Society), and some are interdisciplinary organizations (e.g., the Association for the Care of Children's Health [ACCH] and the Society of Research in Child Development [SRCD]). Although these organizations provide opportunities for funding research and disseminating research results, there is no single forum for pediatric nurse researchers to discuss clinical problems or the ways in which research could address these problems.

Federal Support for Research Activity

The [NCNR] priorities will provide a systematic plan for knowledge development and a blueprint for the federal government.

—*Ada Sue Hinshaw*
(cited in Carnegie, 1991, p. 6)

The National Center for Nursing Research (NCNR), established in 1986 by congressional mandate, was elevated to full National Institutes of Health (NIH) status in 1993 when it became the National Institute of Nursing Research (NINR). The creation of the NCNR/NINR has significantly advanced and legitimized nursing research. Perhaps

those areas that have benefited the most, however, are those that have been designated as research priority areas.

The two conferences on research priorities have determined NINR priorities for the 1990s. Unfortunately, no specific priority has been set by the NCNR/NINR to address acute illness or pediatrics, unlike other areas of interest such as HIV, health promotion, or nursing informatics. Some research topics related to the responses of acutely ill children, such as pain, do fit nicely into specific priority areas, such as the one on symptom management. However, these conferences have done little to promote research related specifically to acutely ill children and their families.

Conduct of Studies in Clinical Areas

No devotion to science, no thought of the greater good to the greater number, can for an instant justify the experimenting on helpless infants, children pathetically abandoned by fate and entrusted to the community for their safeguarding.

—*Konrad Bercovici*
(1921, cited in Lederer & Grodin, 1994, p. 13)

A major barrier in clinical research encountered by virtually all pediatric nursing researchers is the difficulty in accessing adequate numbers of patients (Brodie, 1988). Along with the problems they face seeking access to acutely ill populations in academic medical centers, pediatric nurse researchers have had to deal with differing types of institutions, multiple institutional reviews, and stricter review standards than those studying adults. Unlike academic medical centers, most pediatric hospitals are free-standing institutions; their linkages with academic institutions and support for research vary widely.

At best, time delays are encountered, for researchers must obtain approval from two institutional review committees—the university's and the hospital's. At worst, researchers have abandoned their projects because the hospital's philosophy did not support nursing research, viewing research as the purview of the physician. Moreover, all institutional review boards have more rigorous standards for conducting research on dependent populations. For university-based nurse researchers, who have a limited time in which to achieve progress, these innumerable delays often force them to abandon clinical research of acutely ill children and adopt research agendas that are more expedient.

Over time, problems with access have lessened, with the value of nursing research being increasingly recognized and linkages created between pediatric hospitals and academic institutions through instituting joint appointments and establishing nursing research facilitation positions. It must be noted, however, that these recent and neophyte associations are threatened in today's climate of cost containment.

ill children and their families. Although no one determinant predominates, it is likely that a combination of them has had a synergistically negative effect on research activity. Moreover, not until pediatric nurses are socialized to the view that nursing research is the foundation of their clinical practice will the research agenda for ill children and their families be advanced.

The amount of published research directed toward children's and families' responses to acute illness has increased gradually since the turn of century, with a significant upturn during the past two decades. Despite these strides, the state of this body of research remains underdeveloped. Vision and tenacity are the critical characteristics of pediatric nurse researchers. For nurses to continually advance the care of sick children and their families, they must continue to develop programs of research that (a) are theoretically sound, (b) are methodologically rigorous, and (c) have clinical relevance.

■ *Summary and Conclusions*

Numerous determinants have limited nursing research on the responses of acutely

■ *Note*

1. Boston Floating Hospital had its origin as a barge hired to take sick infants and their mothers on a day cruise of Boston's harbor. It was believed they would benefit from the fresh salty air (Beaven, 1957).

6

■

INTEGRATIVE REVIEW OF ASSESSMENT MODELS FOR EXAMINING CHILDREN'S AND FAMILIES' RESPONSES TO ACUTE ILLNESS

■ *JoAnne M. Youngblut*

Acutely ill children have been the focus of a considerable amount of nursing research since the 1950s. Those earlier studies were generally designed to assess parents' and children's psychologic responses to the stress of acute illness and hospitalization. An increase in the number of pediatric nurses equipped with research skills and an interest in developing knowledge that could guide and inform nursing practice resulted in a broadening of the scope of the research to include assessment of children's physiologic responses to a stressor, acute illness and hospitalization. This chapter examines the research methods used to assess children's and families' responses to a child's acute illness and the findings obtained using these methods in studies published between 1989 and 1994. The chapter is organized into two major sections, parent/family responses and child responses, with child responses further divided into behavioral and physiologic responses.

A review of the nursing research literature over the past 5 years was conducted. Articles were identified through a manual search of five nursing research journals, four pediatric nursing journals, and five critical care nursing journals. Articles selected met the following criteria:

- They were studies published in an identified journal between 1989 and 1994.
- A nurse was the first author.
- Those studied were children between 1 month and 18 years of age or families with a child in this age range.
- The index child experienced an acute illness.

Acute illness was defined as a short-term health condition treated at home or in the hospital, the initial phase of a chronic illness, the exacerbation of a chronic illness that required hospitalization, or illness or injury resulting in hospitalization in an intensive care unit. Studies of children's and their families' responses that occurred within 6 weeks following hospital discharge were included. Studies were excluded if the stage of the chronic illness was not clearly described, a nursing intervention was tested, or data were collected on the target child and family past the 6-week period following hospital discharge.

Of the 65 articles selected, 25 (38.5%) focused on parents, and 40 (61.5%) focused on acutely ill children. Most of the studies were quantitative (84.6%), including 8 descriptive, 18 comparative, 25 correlational, and 4 psychometric studies. The greatest number of articles were published in the *Journal of Pediatric Nursing* ($n = 19$), followed by *Pediatric Nursing* ($n = 13$), and *Maternal-Child Nursing Journal* ($n = 12$). Few were published in the critical care journals ($n = 10$) or in the discipline's primary research journals ($n = 7$).

■ *Responses of Parents and Families*

Most studies of the responses of parents or families focused on the family's experience during a child's hospitalization in an intensive care unit rather than on their experience during a child's acute illness. Seven studies (28%) examined parents' experiences with an acutely ill child; 18 (72%) focused on parents or families with a critically ill child. This is most likely a reflection of the evolution of pediatric critical care over the past decade and the increasing acuity of children hospitalized for any length of time. Research designs included descriptive ($n = 7$), comparative ($n = 5$), correlational ($n = 9$), and qualitative ($n = 4$). Studies on both acute and critical illness focused on needs, concerns, or feelings ($n = 7$),

factors related to stress and coping ($n = 11$), parental role ($n = 5$), and family system responses ($n = 2$). The measurement tools used most often in the quantitative studies are noted in Table 6.1. All were designed to collect self-reports of parents.

Needs, Concerns, or Feelings

Kristjansdottir (1991) investigated the needs of 5 parents with hospitalized, acutely ill preschool children, and Fisher (1994) identified the needs of 15 mothers and 15 fathers of 30 critically ill children, ages under 1–17 years. Weichler (1990) described mothers' information needs in the first month after their children, ages 5–16 years, received liver transplants. Concerns about the child's experience and need for information, support or comfort, and trust were identified most frequently by parents (Fisher, 1994; Kristjansdottir, 1991). Indeed, in Fisher's study, 7 of the top 15 needs were related to information. Mothers in Weichler's (1990) study identified specific information needs related to the child's transplant, such as lab values and signs and symptoms of rejection and infection. These needs changed, however, over the posttransplant period, with information needs at discharge reflecting the parent's responsibilities in both medical and nonmedical aspects of the child's life. Mothers also expressed a need to learn ways to support their children emotionally during the posttransplant period.

Parents of acutely ill children reported needs for financial support, feelings of helplessness and guilt, vigilance and protection of the ill child, and concerns about the child's siblings (Kristjansdottir, 1991). Parents of critically ill children felt that knowing the child's prognosis, knowing that the child might be able to hear the parent even if the child was not alert, seeing the child frequently, and feeling that there was hope were important needs. Younger parents, ages 15–30 years, rated several needs higher than older parents did, and mothers rated some needs higher than fathers did (Fisher, 1994).

In a qualitative study of 13 parents of 8 critically ill children using grounded theory methodology, Turner, Tomlinson, and Harbaugh (1990) found that parents described many things about which they were uncertain. "Illness uncertainty" encompassed the etiology of the child's condition, treatment, illness severity, prognosis, and the quality of the child's future. "Caregiver uncertainty" centered on the quality of care and competence of health care workers. "Family system uncertainty" involved performing the parental role with both the ill child and children at home; juggling demands from a job, other children, and personal care with the critically ill child's needs; and thinking about the effects of the illness on themselves and other family members. Some of these uncertainties led to misconceptions that increased parents' stress or anxiety.

Parents' concerns at 24 to 36 hours after a child's pediatric intensive care unit (PICU) admission were investigated by Youngblut and Jay (1991), who interviewed 17 parents of 10 critically ill children, ages 15 months–14 years, and by Youngblut and Shiao (1992), who studied 16 mothers and 13 fathers of 16 children, ages 1 month–5 years. In both studies, parents rated concern about the child's future (survival; physical or mental impairment) highest. In the first study, diagnosis category (infection or accidental injury) was not related to parental concerns but to the admitting physician's prognosis. Fathers of children with a good prognosis had fewer concerns about the child's experience than fathers of children with an uncertain prognosis, and parents of children with a good prognosis had fewer parenting concerns at 24 hours after admission than parents of children with an uncertain prognosis (Youngblut & Jay, 1991). In the second study, higher illness severity scores (Pediatric Risk of Mortality [PRISM] scores; Pollack, Ruttimann, & Getson, 1988) were related to greater concerns about parenting and about the child's experience for fathers, but not mothers (Youngblut & Shiao, 1992).

Ferrell, Rhiner, Shapiro, and Dierkes (1994) described the effects on parents and family of a hospitalized child's pain related to cancer or its treatment. Children in this qualitative study ($N = 21$) were ages 5–22 years. Parents described frustration, helplessness, and despair with the diagnosis and their child's experience of pain. Parents' descriptions of the experience of having a child with cancer focused on wishing to trade places, trying to hide emotions, dealing with physical losses, searching for meaning, unfairness, hope versus despair, uncertainty, horror, losing control, and the community of suffering. Many parents felt the child's pain was not taken seriously by health care providers. Parents felt unprepared to deal with the child's pain at home, and some physically felt their child's pain themselves. Some parents wished for the child's death in order to relieve the child's suffering.

These studies suggest that parents continued their roles as nurturer, protector, and caregiver of their children in the hospital as in the home, regardless of the child's health status. The need for information about the child's condition, concerns about their child's experience, and the quality of care provided by health care providers during the acute phase of the illness, reflect the nurturer and protector roles. The need for information about emotional support strategies and the child's medication and treatment regimen phase reflects the caregiver role. A parent's concerns about the child's siblings and the other parent indicate that the child's illness and hospitalization occur in a family context. Thus, parents' responsibilities continue despite their child's immediate illness. Mothers, younger parents, and parents of children with an uncertain future may have greater concerns and may require more assessment and information to meet their responsibilities. These studies suggest that assessing parents'

TABLE 6.1 Instruments Used in Parent/Family Studies

Instrument	Description	Studies	Study Evidence That Supports Validity	Reliability
Critical Care Family Needs Inventory–Modified (CCFNI)	59 items; 4-point response format: "not important" to "very important"	Fisher (1994)	Mothers had higher scores than fathers on 9 of 59 needs	Alpha = .89
FACES III	10 items for Cohesion scale and 10 items for Adaptability scale; 5-point response format: "almost never" to "almost always"	Philichi (1989)	Higher Cohesion for PICU parents than published norms	No evidence
Feetham Family Functioning Survey (FFFS)	25 Porter-format items; 7-point response format: "little" to "much"	Youngblut and Shiao (1993)	Fathers: Longer length of stay related to more satisfaction with family Mothers: Longer intubation related to lower satisfaction with family	Alpha = .76 and .80
Maternal Vigilance	Single item; parent estimate of time spent with child on each of 4 previous days	Tomlinson, Kirschbaum, Tomcyck, and Peterson (1993)	Vigilance inversely related to experience of the primary nurse	No evidence.
Parental Concerns Scale	26 items, 4 subscales; 5-point response format: "not a concern" to "greatest concern"	Youngblut and Shiao (1992, 1993)	Fathers: greater concerns about parenting and child experience related to greater illness severity	Alpha = .63 to .87 for mothers, .67 to .91 for fathers
Parental Control Preference	24 items; 4-point response format: "none of the time" to "all of the time"	Schepp (1992)	Higher control preference related to younger child age, increased amount of time spent in hospital with child, fewer children in family	Alpha = .85 and .87

Instrument	Description	Source	Findings	Reliability
Parental Satisfaction Scale	7 items "Likert-type"	Tomlinson, Kirschbaum, Tomcyck, and Peterson (1993)	Greater maternal satisfaction related to greater child acuity	No evidence
Parental Stressor Scale: PICU	39 items, 7 subscales; 5-point response format: "not stressful" to "extremely stressful"	Youngblut and Shiao (1992, 1993)	No new evidence	*Alpha* = .70 to .92 for mothers, .51 to .95 for fathers
Ways of Coping	8 subscales; number of items, response format not given	LaMontagne, Hepworth, Pawlak, and Chiafery (1992)	Greater parental age related to greater use of problem-focused coping	No evidence
State-Trait Anxiety Inventory	2 scales; response format, number of items not given	LaMontagne, Hepworth, Pawlak, and Chiafery (1992)	State anxiety higher at 24-48 hours than at 72 hours	No evidence
Parent Activities Questionnaire	35 items, 3 subscales; response format not given	LaMontagne, Hepworth, Pawlak, and Chiafery (1992)	Higher parent activity score related to greater problem-focused coping, less distancing and escape avoidance	*Alpha* = .93 for total scale, .15 to .89 for subscales

expectations and performance of their parental and family roles and providing information relevant to performing these roles would address many of the parents' often unspoken concerns.

Stress and Coping

Schepp's (1991, 1992) correlational studies focused on mothers' coping efforts during their child's acute illness. In the first study, mothers of 45 hospitalized infants and toddlers provided relative ratings of 16 stressful events. The most anxiety-producing events requiring the greatest coping effort were separation from the child, uncertainty about the child's condition, and aspects of the child's experience. Greater predictability of events was strongly related to less anxiety, and lower anxiety was strongly related to fewer coping efforts (Schepp, 1991). In Schepp's (1992) subsequent study, 384 mothers of hospitalized children, ages 1–18 years, rated the degree of control wanted over their child's care. Preference for control was higher among younger and minority (primarily Hispanic) mothers, mothers of younger children, mothers who had no previous experience with a child's hospitalization, mothers with fewer other children, and mothers who spent more time with their child in the hospital.

Studies of parents with critically ill children have identified and described specific stressors and coping efforts. In a study of 24 mothers and 6 fathers of 30 critically ill children, LaMontagne and Pawlak (1990) found three main stress themes: loss of the parenting role, uncertainty over outcome, and information needs. The most frequently used coping strategies were seeking social support (problem-focused) and positive reappraisal (emotion-focused). Although parents used problem- and emotion-focused coping strategies about equally for role loss stressors, they used emotion-focused

strategies more often than problem-focused strategies to cope with uncertainty.

In a subsequent study, 47 parents of 47 children, ages 1 month–17 years (LaMontagne, Hepworth, Pawlak, & Chiafery, 1992) reported using problem- and emotion-focused coping strategies equally. However, older parents used more problem-focused and "seeking social support" strategies, and less "accepting responsibility" strategies. Parental anxiety was greater at 24 to 48 hours after admission than at 72 hours. Parents who had higher anxiety both at 24 to 48 hours and at 72 hours used fewer problem-solving and more escape-avoidance strategies. Lower anxiety scores were related to greater use of social support at 24 to 48 hours and greater use of distancing at 72 hours. The child's age was not related to parental coping, activities, or anxiety.

Several researchers investigated environmental stressors for parents during a child's PICU stay. Miles, Carter, and colleagues conducted a series of studies related to parental stress in the PICU. In one study, 324 mothers and 186 fathers of 350 children hospitalized in a PICU, timing of data collection varied from 24 to 99 hours after admission to the PICU (Miles, Carter, Riddle, Hennessey, & Eberly, 1989c). The two greatest stressors for parents were the child's behavior and emotions and alterations in the parental role (Miles et al., 1989c). However, when analyses were done separately for mothers and fathers, a different picture emerged. Mothers' top stressors were child's behavior and emotions and alterations in parental role; fathers' top stressors were staff communication and child's behavior and emotions. Mothers' stress ratings were higher than fathers' ratings for 5 of the 7 stressor dimensions measured (Riddle, Hennessey, Eberly, Carter, & Miles, 1989). Heuer (1993) studied 32 parents of 22 critically ill children, ages 6 weeks–15 years, conducting interviews after 48 hours postadmission. In this study, parental role and procedures were the two top stressors for mothers, whereas fathers' scores were highest for procedures and sights and sounds of the PICU. No statistical analyses were reported, and the dimension means in Heuer's study were considerably lower than those reported by Miles, Carter and colleagues. It appears that items rated as "not experienced" by the parent (and receiving a score of "0") were not omitted from the mean scores as suggested by Carter and Miles (1983). Thus, Heuer's results cannot be compared with those of Miles and colleagues (1989c) or Riddle and colleagues (1989).

Factors affecting parents' responses to environmental stressors include diagnosis, trait anxiety, parental and child age, illness severity, and pre-ICU preparation. Despite the greater likelihood of pre-ICU preparation, parents of children with cardiac conditions rated parental role and child appearance stressors higher than did parents of children with other illnesses (Miles, Carter, Hennessey, Riddle, & Eberly, 1989b). Higher total stressor scores were related to higher trait anxiety, lower parental age, greater perceived severity of illness, younger child age, more ICU visitation, and perception of inadequate pre-PICU preparation (Miles, Carter, Hennessey, Eberly, & Riddle, 1989a). Greater anxiety was associated with an unexpected admission, greater perceived illness severity, and greater stress about role alterations, child behavior, and child appearance (Miles et al., 1989a).

Family members of pediatric patients from a neonatal ICU and a PICU and adult patients from three adult ICUs reported that they were fearful throughout the ICU stay (Kleiber et al., 1994). They also worried or were concerned, but it was less intense than the fear. Improvements in patient condition provided temporary relief from fear and worry. PICU parents experienced exhaustion and fatigue on the first and second days after the child's admission. Family members were angry about a variety of factors, including their feelings of helplessness and the unknown etiology of the patient's condition.

Parents identified friends as most supportive, followed by nurses, then physicians. A caring attitude and providing information were viewed as supportive behaviors.

Tomlinson and Mitchell (1992) used a phenomenologic approach to study dimensions of social support for parents of critically ill children. Some attempts at support by others were negatively received by parents, particularly unwanted actions and inappropriate comments, assistance offered with an implied need for reciprocation, and a felt need to care for some visitors. Because of the way that information about the child's condition was communicated to others, a large support network was burdensome for less connected families but not for more tightly connected families. Fathers reported smaller support networks than mothers and had more difficulty expressing their feelings, which limited their ability to obtain support.

Stress brought parental dyads together emotionally; however, physical separation was associated with "a sense of isolation and lack of spousal support" (Tomlinson & Mitchell, 1992, p. 392). When a parent had to balance work and visitation demands, his or her ability to provide support for the other parent was diminished. Finally, parents felt guilt and responsibility for the chain of events that led to the child's PICU admission.

In most of these studies, parent role issues, uncertainty about the child's future, and aspects of the child's experience (e.g., pain, appearance) were consistently identified as stressors. Strategies that helped parents deal with these stressors varied across time and stressors. Social support was frequently mentioned as important to coping efforts. However, support attempts that were not consistent with the family's needs and wants or that came with obligations were negatively received. Also, the effectiveness of the social network was based on the quality of the interactions among its members rather than its size. Having information about the child's condition and upcoming events resulted in less parental anxiety and perhaps less uncertainty. This finding is not surprising given that, as noted earlier, parents frequently reported a need for information (Fisher, 1994; Kristjansdottir, 1991; Weichler, 1990).

Parental Role

Two of the 5 studies on parental role used grounded theory methodology to examine the evolution of mothers' involvement in their disabled child's care during hospitalization. Perkins (1993) described a process by which the parent, usually the mother, moved from being the child's protector to being the child's survival agent to being the central person in the child's care. In each phase, there was an increase in parents' commitment to provide for the child, in their knowledge of the child, the disability, and its treatment, and in their involvement in providing independent care.

Burke, Kauffmann, Costello, and Dillon (1991) reported the results of a series of studies designed to elucidate the experience of parenting a child with repeated hospitalizations. Parents identified the problem of "hazardous secrets," referring to negative information about the child's condition or treatment, variability in care by health care workers, and the impact of inexperienced, unsupervised health care workers performing invasive procedures. Parents dealt with problems by "reluctantly taking charge" of tasks that the health care providers could not or would not perform and by increasing their vigilance. In "tenaciously seeking information," parents believed they were perceived as collaborative when seeking information from those caring for their child but as unacceptable or too assertive when seeking information from providers at a competing or referring facility. Burke and colleagues (1991) viewed this gradual change in parental

role as allowing parents to regain control of the situation.

The third study, conducted by Rhiner, Ferrell, Shapiro, and Dierkes (1994), described the parents' role in pain management for their hospitalized children with cancer. Parents described both restricting and encouraging medication use while allowing the child as much control as possible. Parents obtained or used nonpharmacologic pain relief measures, advocated for the child regarding pain relief, and assessed the quality and intensity of their child's pain. Their involvement in pain management progressed from learning about the medication to advocating for pain relief to anticipating and trying to prevent the recurrence of pain. Parents reported that health care providers could help by listening to the parents, using a specialized pain team, and providing continuity of care together with education for the family. Parents also recommended using specific dosing regimens, such as patient-controlled analgesia, routine rather than "as needed" administration of pain medication, and larger doses or stronger medications to relieve the child's pain. These parents advised other parents to find a physician they trust, know that the pain can be relieved, maintain self-control, give control to the child, be honest with and listen to the child, and have faith.

In the fourth study, Snowden and Gottlieb (1989) observed 12 mothers in the presence of their child during the child's PICU and subsequent general care unit stay. They identified six roles that mothers demonstrated: vigilant parent, nurturer/comforter, medical parent, caregiver, entertainer, and protector. The most common role during both the PICU and general care unit stay was that of the vigilant parent (watchful observation, talking to the child); the next most common was the nurturer/comforter role (touch, verbal soothing or nurturing, relief of discomfort). Nurturer/comforter and caregiver roles were observed less often during a

nursing or medical procedure. Vigilance was more common if the child was unresponsive or if the mother was accompanied by others when visiting the child.

The fifth study examined factors related to satisfaction and vigilance of mothers with a critically ill child. Tomlinson, Kirschbaum, Tomczyk, and Peterson (1993) found that maternal satisfaction with care after a child's bone marrow transplant increased as the child's acuity increased and that mothers ($N = 20$) were more vigilant (spent more time at the bedside) with less experienced nurses. This could mean that mothers were more concerned about their child when in the care of less experienced nurses, or it might indicate that less experienced nurses were more receptive to having parents stay at the bedside. Indeed, experience of the nurse was inversely related to both mothers' time at the bedside and nurses' attitudes toward parental participation, although time at bedside and attitudes were not related.

Family System Responses

Two studies examined the effect of PICU admission on the family system; a third study described the effect of a child's pain on the family. Philichi (1989) studied family cohesion and adaptability in a sample of 50 parents of 30 children, ages 4 months–15 years, in the PICU after each child's third PICU day. Comparison of parents' cohesion and adaptability scores with published norms revealed significantly higher cohesion scores for the PICU parents but similar adaptability scores. Mothers' adaptability scores were significantly higher than fathers', although their cohesion scores were similar. However, it appears that the paired mother-father data were compared with the independent samples' t test, violating an underlying assumption of the test, which weakens the findings.

Youngblut and Shiao (1993) measured family functioning at 24 to 48 hours after PICU admission and again at 2 to 4 weeks after hospital discharge with a sample of 9 two-parent families with an ill child under age 6 years. Mothers' cohesion scores decreased significantly from Time 1 to Time 2. Both mothers and fathers rated their families as significantly more adaptable than published norms, although cohesion scores did not differ significantly. Greater length of hospital stay was related to greater satisfaction with family for fathers. The longer the child was intubated, the lower the mother's perception of family cohesion and the greater her dissatisfaction with family. The small sample size, however, means that these results may not be stable across samples, and further study with larger samples is necessary before applying these results to practice.

Parents of 21 hospitalized children, ages 5–22 years, with cancer described both positive and negative effects of their child's pain on family members and family relationships (Ferrell et al., 1994). In some families, spousal relationships were strained and distant, even if they had been strong and close prior to the diagnosis, and siblings were jealous of the increased attention the ill child received and upset by separation and the possibility of the ill child's death. However, in other families, the illness and its stressors brought the family closer together, helping them redefine priorities, and increased the maturity and responsibility of siblings. Fathers experienced role changes that were frustrating and difficult, including a lack of control over the situation and increased responsibility (perhaps total responsibility) for care of the siblings and the household.

In these studies, parental roles varied with time, the child's state, and aspects of the situation. Parents became more comfortable and expert at caregiving as time with the ill child increased. They played more active roles when the child was alert. Mothers were more vigilant during procedures, in the presence of other visitors, and with less experienced nurses. Evidence for the effect of the child's illness on the family is mixed. Compared to published norms, Philichi (1989) reported greater cohesion but similar adaptability, and Youngblut and Shiao (1993) reported greater adaptability but similar cohesion for parents with a child in the PICU. Some families in Ferrell and colleagues' (1994) study reported greater cohesion among family members; others reported less. These differences may be related to the differences in the ill child's age range and, thus, family life-cycle stage.

In summary, research on parent and family responses to the child's acute illness has focused primarily on the response of an individual parent, usually the mother. The most common response to a child's illness is change in the parental role from more active to more watchful roles. Responsibilities of parents for siblings and other family members continue, despite the child's illness and hospitalization. Uncertainty is a stressful aspect of the child's illness, and parents respond by gathering information about the child's condition and upcoming events and by seeking support from others. Few studies have assessed the response of the family unit, and those that have report inconsistent findings.

Critique of Research

The most common methodologic limitation of this set of studies is the frequent use of small samples. The designs of the studies are generally appropriate for the research questions asked. Appropriate instruments are used to measure the concepts of interest. Most of the studies included estimates of reliability for the measurement instruments (shown in Table 6.1)

calculated with the sample data rather than reporting only the original developer's reliabilities. This is a strength, for reliability is not a property of the instrument but is significantly influenced by characteristics of the sample and the testing situation (Nunnally, 1978). Statistical analyses were generally conducted with statistical procedures consistent with the research questions and the level of measurement. Exceptions to these generalizations were identified in the discussion of the specific study.

Stress theory was the predominant theoretical perspective underlying the research on parent and family responses. However, researchers who assume that the child's illness is stressful to the parent and the family generally assess for only negative effects, ignoring the possibility of positive or growth-producing effects. One gap in the research is the identification of positive responses by the parent and the family as well as the conditions under which these positive responses occur.

Previous research has focused primarily on mothers' responses, ignoring fathers' responses; this was probably due to reliance on the attachment paradigm. In contrast, most of the studies reviewed here included both mothers and fathers as respondents, reflecting a family perspective. However, many lumped mothers and fathers together into one group called "parents" rather than conducting separate analyses for mothers and for fathers. This practice ignores the differences in roles and perspectives frequently found between men and women. Given the importance of changes in role function and performance noted in these studies, this is a major limitation. Also limited is research assessing the responses of other family members, such as siblings and grandparents, or of the family unit.

The influence of family developmental theory on the research has been limited. According to this paradigm, family tasks change based on the age of the children in the family (Duvall,

1977), suggesting that family and parent responses might differ based on the age of the ill child. However, most of the studies reviewed here did not restrict the age range of the ill child, resulting in samples with families representing many or all family life-cycle stages and a wide variety of family tasks. This practice of sampling families with ill children over a wide age range inhibits researchers' ability to find parent or family issues that are germane to a specific life-cycle stage or age of the child. Thus, despite interest in family-centered care, family theories have had limited impact on research questions, study design, and data analysis strategies.

■ Children's Responses to Acute Illness

Between 1989 and 1994, 14 studies of children's behavioral responses and 26 studies of children's physiologic responses to acute and critical illness were published. Three of the behavioral studies were qualitative. The 37 quantitative studies used 6 descriptive, 4 psychometric, 12 comparative, and 15 correlational designs. In contrast to the research on parent and family reactions, 87.5% of the studies concentrated on acutely ill children, and only 5 studies focused on critically ill children. Major concepts examined in the behavioral studies were stress and coping ($n = 7$), behavior and emotions ($n = 5$), and concerns and fears ($n = 2$); the physiologic studies focused on pain ($n = 12$), temperature measurement ($n = 5$), effects of medication ($n = 2$), tubes or lines ($n = 3$), environmental stimuli ($n = 2$), pulse oximetry ($n = 1$), and feeding ($n = 1$). Measurement tools used in the behavioral studies are listed in Table 6.2; later in the chapter, Table 6.4

lists the measures used in some of the physiologic studies.

Children's Behavioral Responses

Stress and Coping

Five of the 7 studies included preschool children. In one descriptive study (Caty, Ritchie, & Ellerton, 1989), most mothers (70%) perceived coping as an outcome, with an accompanying degree of success or failure; 10% described coping as a process; and 20% described it as both a process and an outcome. Behaviors identified by mothers as coping behaviors and as being helpful to the child were primarily positive behaviors, perhaps reflecting the mothers' view of coping as an outcome. Mothers rarely identified regressive and protest behaviors as coping behaviors. Most of the children's responses were categorized as direct action, active verbal and nonverbal behaviors used to manage self or environment (see Table 6.3).

In contrast, when preschool children's coping strategies were obtained through observation of their behavior by nurse investigators, children used a greater number and a wider variety of strategies than described by mothers. However, it is possible that the discrepancy stems from the definition of coping as outcome by mothers and as process by nurses rather than from inaccurate reporting by mothers. Barnes, Bandak, and Beardslee (1990) aggregated data from 186 case studies of infants and children (specific ages were not stated) over a 20-year time span. They found evidence of defensive, adaptive, resistive, and communicative behaviors, ego-stabilizing mechanisms, and cognitive-mastery strategies. Factors related to use of the identified mechanisms were not explored. Corbo-Richert, Caty, and Barnes (1993) aggregated data from case studies (in master's

(text continued on p. 130)

TABLE 6.2 Instruments Used in Child Behavioral Response Studies

Instrument	Description	Studies	Study Evidence That Supports Validity	Reliability
Activity Scale	Single item; 5-point response format	Jones (1994)	More child activity with greater parent participation activities ($r = .91$)	No evidence
Child and Adolescent Adjustment Profile	20 items (parent report)	Grey, Cameron, Lipman, and Thurber (1994)	Diabetic children more withdrawn than healthy children	Test-retest = .78 to .89 *Alpha* = .78 to .86
Child Drawing Hospital (measure of anxiety)	Part A: 14 items; Part B: 8 items; Part C: gestalt rating	Tiedeman and Clatworthy (1990)	Decreased from hospital admission to postdischarge; related to child age	Interrater reliability = 85% to 97% *Alpha* = .58 to .73 for Part A
Child Medical Fear Scale	17 items, 4 subscales; 3-point response format: "not at all" to "a lot"	Hart and Bossert (1994)	Higher fears related to greater trait anxiety	*Alpha* = .93
Child Rating of Anxiety	Rabbit in a hole (1-10 scale)	Tiedeman and Clatworthy (1990)	Decreased from hospital admission to postdischarge; related to child age	No evidence
Children's Coping Strategies Checklist	40 items, 6 subscales; "Is this a coping strategy?" — yes/no	Caty, Ritchie, and Ellerton (1989)	No hypothesis testing	No evidence
Children's Coping Strategies Checklist–Intrusive Procedures	15-item, yes-no, observational checklist; 3 subscales	Ellerton, Ritchie, and Caty (1994)	Greater number of coping behaviors and greater use of self-protective behaviors related to higher reported pain	Kappa = .78 to .92

Children's Coping Behaviors: A Category System	40 items, 6 subscales	Corbo-Richert (1994)	Older children and those with school experience, greater information seeking	No evidence
Children's Depression Inventory	27 items; 3-point response format	Corbo-Richert, Caty, and Barnes (1993)	No hypothesis testing	Interrater reliability = 85%
Coping Orientation for Problem Experiences	54 items, 10 categories of coping behaviors	Grey, Cameron, Lipman, and Thurber (1994)	No new evidence	Alpha = .71 to .87
		Grey, Cameron, Lipman, and Thurber (1994)	Diabetic children used 3 behaviors more than healthy children: ventilating feelings, solving family problems, and investing in close friends	Alpha = .90 for total scale, .67 to .78 for subscales
Cooperation Scale	Single item; 5-point response format	Jones (1994)	More cooperation with greater parent participation activities ($r = .71$)	No evidence
Current Health Status	5 items, "Likert-type scale"	Grey, Cameron, Lipman, and Thurber (1994)	Parent rating of child's health status higher for healthy group than for diabetic group.	Alpha = .71 to .85 Test-retest = .78 to .87
Gellert Index of Body Knowledge	Structured interview to elicit structure and function of head, heart, bones, stomach, ribs, liver, skin, nerves, and lungs	Neff and Beardslee (1990)	Higher scores (better knowledge) for older children, second time point, cancer and healthy groups (versus orthopedic group)	Interrater reliability = 88.5%
Hospital Coping Scale (coping effectiveness)	Single item; word graphic rating scale: "no help" to "best possible help"	Bossert (1994)	Lower coping effectiveness related to higher trait anxiety; chronically ill children lower than acutely ill children	No evidence

TABLE 6.2 *Continued*

Instrument	Description	Studies	Study Evidence That Supports Validity	Reliability
Human Figure Drawings (color preference)	Draw 1 picture of a person and 1 of a family doing something	Fleming, Holmes, Barton, and Osbahr (1993)	Well children: Highest number of normal drawings Children with adjustment problems: Highest number of abnormal drawings	No evidence
Luscher Color Test (color preference)	8 color squares	Fleming, Holmes, Barton, and Osbahr (1993)	Differences by age and by well vs. not well status as hypothesized	Test-retest = 64% agreement
Manifest Upset Scale	Single item; 5-point response format	Jones (1994)	Less upset with greater parent participation activities ($r = -.73$)	No evidence
Parent Rating of Own Anxiety	1 item; 1-10 response format	Tiedeman and Clatworthy (1990)	Correlated with state anxiety of State-Trait Anxiety Inventory ($r = .36$ to $.71$)	No evidence
Perceived Threats to Body Integrity	Sentence completion items: 10 innocuous, 10 related to body integrity	Neff and Beardslee (1990)	Content validity with panel of judges; older children showed greater concern about body integrity	No evidence
Picture Test (color preference)	2 sets of 6 pictures	Fleming, Holmes, Barton, and Osbahr (1993)	Physically disabled children picked blue as favorite color more than acutely ill children (as hypothesized)	Test-retest $r = .26$ to 1.00 55% agreement on favorite color

Instrument	Description	Source	Findings	Reliability
Posthospitalization Behavior Questionnaire	28 items; 5-point response format: "always" to "never"	McClowry (1990)	Mood and approach temperament dimensions related to behavior at baseline, 1 week, and 1 month postdischarge	*Alpha* = .76 to .88
Self-Perception Profile for Children	36 items; response format not given	Grey, Cameron, Lipman, and Thurber (1994)	No new evidence	*Alpha* = .71 to .85
State-Trait Anxiety Inventory	20 items; response format not given	Tiedeman and Clatworthy (1990)	Higher parent state anxiety related to higher child anxiety	*Alpha* = .90 to .93
State-Trait Anxiety Inventory for Children	20 items; response format not given	Tiedeman and Clatworthy (1990)	Higher child anxiety related to higher parent anxiety; decrease in anxiety from hospital admission to postdischarge	*Alpha* = .74 to .87 for boys, .72 to .91 for girls
Strength of Body Boundaries	Freehand drawing of house, scored on 6 characteristics	Neff and Beardslee (1990)	Greater concern in cancer group than in healthy or orthopedic groups	Interrater reliability = 78.5% to 80%

TABLE 6.3 Categories of Children's Coping Responses

| | *Mother Reports*[a] | *Child Reports*[b] | |
| | *% Preschoolers* | *% Preschoolers* | *% School-Age* |
Coping Strategy	*(N = 32)*	*(n = 9)*	*(n = 14)*
Direct action	48	100	100
Seeking comfort/help	19	89	57
Information seeking	10	89	100
Inhibition of action	8	33	79
Growth/independence	8	67	64
Intrapsychic	7	100	71

a. Caty, Ritchie, and Ellerton (1989).
b. Corbo-Richert, Caty, and Barnes (1993).

theses from the University of Pittsburgh) of 9 preschool and 14 school-age hospitalized children. Most children used coping strategies from five of the six categories on the Children's Coping Strategies Checklist (Caty et al., 1989); however, more school-age children than preschoolers used inhibition of action strategies.

Two studies described young children's coping strategies during painful procedures. Ellerton, Ritchie, and Caty (1994) observed 80 children, ages 4–7 year, before, during, and after a venipuncture; Corbo-Richert (1994) observed 24 children, ages 3–7 years, before, during, and after chest tube removal. In both studies, children's coping behaviors were predominantly self-protective, defined as crying, saying "ouch," moaning, sighing, and whining. As several of these behaviors are often used to indicate the presence of pain, it is not clear whether pain or coping was being measured. The greater number of self-protective behaviors exhibited around venipuncture was related to greater reported pain, more teaching and helping behaviors by the nurse, and a higher family socioeconomic status; age, gender, acuity, hospital experience, locus of control, and parental anxiety were not related to number of coping behaviors (Ellerton et al., 1994). In Corbo-Richert's (1994) study, children who demonstrated fewer self-protective behaviors scored higher on measures of general activity level, activity in sleep, and flexibility. Older

preschool children used more information-seeking strategies. Also, children with preschool or nursery school experience showed more information-seeking behaviors than children without this experience. The number of coping behaviors did not differ for boys and girls, with parent presence or absence, or with previous hospital experience.

Bossert (1994) studied coping behaviors of 82 hospitalized children, ages 8–11 years. Most (74%, $n = 61$) had a chronic illness and had been hospitalized at least once within the previous 3 years; 26% ($n = 21$) were admitted with acute illnesses and had not been hospitalized past 2 years of age. The children described ways they dealt with a self-identified stressful event, and their responses were classified into six categories: cognitive processing; cognitive restructuring; cooperation; countermeasures, such as removing self physically or cognitively from the situation; control; and seeking support. Strategies were similar for chronically ill and acutely ill children and for boys and girls and were not related to trait anxiety, child age, parental presence during interview, or parent rooming-in status. However, chronically ill children, and those with higher trait anxiety scores, perceived their coping efforts to be less effective. Boys and girls did not differ in their perceptions of coping effectiveness. In contrast, in a study of coping among 68 school-age children and adolescents, ages 8–16 years, with newly diagnosed diabetes and 40 healthy age-mates (Grey, Cameron, Lipman, & Thurber, 1994), those with diabetes demonstrated more trait anxiety and more use of ventilating feelings, running away from family problems, and relying on close friends to deal with stress than their healthy counterparts did.

Behavior and Emotions

In-hospital and postdischarge behaviors and emotions reported in preschool children and in school-age children included anxiety, affective responses, spiritual feelings and actions. In a study of 13 preschool children with leukemia (Jones, 1994), higher parental participation in their child's care was related to greater cooperation, less upset, and more activity by the child.

Tiedeman and Clatworthy (1990) found that older school-age children and girls experienced a decrease in anxiety from admission to discharge to 7 to 14 days posthospitalization. At each time point, boys and younger school-age children experienced more anxiety than girls and older children, respectively, but their anxiety scores remained stable over time. Other factors associated with increased anxiety were no previous experience with hospital admission, shorter lengths of hospital stay, and higher parental anxiety.

Studying affective responses to different health states, Fleming, Holmes, Barton, and Osbahr (1993) found that school-age children with physical disabilities, healthy children, and children with adjustment problems chose blue as their favorite color, indicating the need for emotional tranquility or rest, more often than acutely and chronically ill children did. Ill children most often listed red as first or second in preference, indicating they "want self-activities to bring intensity of experience and fullness of living" (Fleming et al., 1993, p. 131), and they made this choice more frequently than healthy children did. However, there were no differences in colors used in drawings across groups. Healthy children had the highest number of normal drawings; children with adjustment problems had the highest number of abnormal drawings. Health status was the only significant predictor of color preferences.

To elicit hospitalized school-age children's thoughts and feelings about God and their illness, Ebmeier, Lough, Huth, and Autio (1991) showed children a series of four pictures and asked the child's help in writing a story "about a child in the hospital and God" (p. 340). Emotions varied with the phase of hospitalization. Children reported feeling sad, scared, and worried when viewing the admission-to-the-hospital picture and the child-in-the-hospital-bed picture. For the picture implying an impending injection or venipuncture, children reported fears of dying, fear of pain from the needle, and feeling sad and lonely. However, they described the nurse in the picture as helpful and supportive and the procedure as helping the child feel better or get better. For the child-leaving-the-hospital picture, children described feelings of happiness and relief. While most described God as approving of the child in the pictures, some described the hospitalization and illness as punishment from God for wrongdoing.

McClowry (1990) found a relationship between several temperament dimensions and posthospitalization behavior among 75 school-age children. During hospitalization, more mothers rated their child's usual prehospital temperament as low on approach (indicating withdrawal) than did mothers in standardization samples; however, the difference disappeared posthospitalization. Because most of the children were admitted with medical conditions, it may be that withdrawal prior to hospitalization was related to the child's feeling sick. Higher scores on predictability, approach, mood, and threshold of responsiveness during hospitalization were related to more behavior problems after discharge. Mood, predictability and approach at 1 week postdischarge and mood, intensity, and approach at 1 month postdischarge were related to more behavior problems after hospitalization. Children with acute versus chronic illnesses displayed similar posthospitalization behaviors.

Concerns and Fears

Based on their aggregation of 186 case studies, Barnes and colleagues (1990) categorized the concerns that hospitalized children experience as body related (function, appearance, integrity), identity related, and loss (control, independence, self, significant others). Fear of death, the unknown, mutilation, intrusion, and anxiety about death and separation were also present. School-age children in other studies have expressed concerns or fears about separation (Ebmeier et al., 1991; Hart & Bossert, 1994), invasive procedures or body integrity (Ebmeier et al., 1991; Hart & Bossert, 1994; Neff & Beardslee, 1990), fears of the unknown and death (Ebmeier et al., 1991), being told that something was wrong with them (Hart & Bossert, 1994), and concerns about body boundaries (Neff & Beardslee, 1990).

For school-age children, the amount of fear or concern was related to trait anxiety, family income, child age, and medical diagnosis but not to the sex of the child or acute versus chronic illness. In Hart and Bossert's (1994) study, scores on the Child Medical Fears Scale (Broome, Hellier, Wilson, Dale, & Glenville, 1988) were similar for boys and girls and for children with acute and chronic illnesses. Children with higher trait anxiety and those from lower-income families reported more fear of the environment, intrapersonal and interpersonal events, and higher total fear scores. Children with higher trait anxiety also reported more fear of procedures. Neff and Beardslee (1990) found that school-age children with cancer who were receiving outpatient treatment expressed more concerns about bounda-

ries than healthy children and children with orthopedic problems, who were immobilized for 4 weeks following surgery. Concerns about threats to body integrity were similar across the three groups. Older children (ages 11–13 years) expressed more concerns about body integrity than did younger children (ages 8–10 years).

Anxiety due to illness or hospitalization was common for preschool and school-age children; anxiety decreased with increasing age of the child (Tiedeman & Clatworthy, 1990). Parental participation in care decreased anxiety for preschoolers (Jones, 1994). Previous experience with hospitalization decreased anxiety for school-age children (Tiedeman & Clatworthy, 1990). School-age children reported feeling scared and sad in the hospital (Ebmeier et al., 1991). Concerns about body integrity, death, and separation from parents were common for school-age children (Ebmeier et al., 1991; Hart & Bossert, 1994). Types of coping strategies used to reduce anxiety differed by age of the child. Preschool children used self-protective and direct action coping behaviors (Corbo-Richert, 1994; Ellerton et al., 1994). School-age children used cognitive coping strategies (Bossert, 1994) and adolescents coped by talking about stressors with friends (Grey et al., 1994).

Critique of Research

The two predominant theoretical perspectives which have guided research on children's behavioral responses to illness are development and stress and coping. Unlike the parent/family research, investigators of children's behavioral responses have limited the age range of children in a given study, most focusing on preschool and school-age children. None of the studies included children under 3 years old, and only a few included adolescents. To their credit, most researchers obtained data about the child directly from the child rather than from the parent. Reliability estimates based on study data were not reported for 10 of the instruments. Six of these were global single-item indicators, so omission of reliability would be expected (Youngblut & Casper, 1993). However, either internal consistency or interrater reliability should have been reported in the other 4 studies.

Children's Physiologic Responses

Pain Research

Four psychometric studies reported on measures of children's pain, 4 on pain intensity, and 4 on pharmacologic management of pain. Measurement strategies in the 4 psychometric studies included body outline ($n = 2$), visual analogue ($n = 1$), or another type of rating scale ($n = 2$).[1] Use of the body outline with 8- to 17-year-old children (Savedra, Tesler, Holzemer, Wilkie, & Ward, 1989) and with 4- to 7-year-old children (Van Cleve & Savedra, 1993) has provided strong evidence for its validity. For those ages 8–17 years, the presence of tubes, operative sites, or medical diagnosis corroborated at least one pain marking for 172 (98%) children and all of the pain markings for 140 (80%) children. The amount of agreement between the children's markings and the corroborating evidence was not related to age, gender, ethnicity, or medical/surgical condition (Savedra et al., 1989).

The rating scales evaluated included the Princess Margaret Hospital Pain Assessment Tool (PMHPAT; Robertson, 1993), the Oucher (Beyer, Villarruel, & Denyes, 1995), the Poker Chip Tool (Hester, Foster, & Kristensen, 1990), and a variety of pain intensity scales (visual analogue, color scale, graded graphic, word graphic, and magnitude estimation). The PMHPAT has five categories (facial expression, nurse's assessment, position in bed, sounds, self-assessment), each with three word descriptions

of increasing intensity (Robertson, 1993), similar to the APGAR scoring system used with newborns. In a sample of 53 perioperative children (23 pre- and postoperative, 30 postoperative only), ages 6–14 years, correlations of the PMHPAT with the nurse's visual analogue rating of the child's pain ($r = .77$) and with the child's visual analogue rating ($r = .70$) were strong, supporting the PMHPAT's construct validity.

Tesler and colleagues (1991) reported a series of studies that evaluated the psychometric performance of five intensity scales (color, visual analogue scale [VAS], graded graphic, word graphic, and magnitude estimation) with children, ages 8–17 years. In the first study, 958 healthy children used each of the five intensity scales to rate the amount of pain the child in each of five cartoon-like drawings was experiencing. The VAS provided the greatest range in means for the five drawings, but children preferred the color scale most and the VAS least. The word graphic scale was preferred by older children, Chinese children, and those with a primary language other than English; younger children preferred the color scale.

Of hospitalized children experiencing pain, 175 preferred the word graphic scale (Tesler et al., 1991). Construct validity of the word graphic scale was supported by higher pain ratings for 55 children with abdominal and thoracic surgery than for those with other surgical procedures, although this conclusion was not based on statistical analysis. Thirty-five of the hospitalized children rated their pain with the five scales. Validity and reliability of the word graphic scale were supported with moderate to high correlations (.68 to .97) among the ratings from the five scales and test-retest correlation of .91. These data suggest that the word graphic scale is reliable, valid, and easy for children ages 8 to 17 to use.

Twenty school-age children interviewed on their third postoperative day (Alex & Ritchie, 1992) associated feelings of anxiety ($n = 15$), sadness ($n = 9$), anger ($n = 6$), fatigue and exhaustion ($n = 6$) with pain. Thirteen identified fears reflecting threats to body integrity and physical well-being. Coping strategies identified by 17 children included distraction, cognitive strategies, deliberate inactivity, crying, and seeking assistance.

Savedra, Holzemer, Tesler, and Wilkie (1993) found that 98% of 65 school-age and adolescent children indicated pain on a body outline in their surgical area on the first postoperative day and that 74% marked the surgical area every time they were asked to locate their pain. Intensity of pain was significantly lower on postoperative days 3, 4, and 5. Description of pain quality did not differ by grade in school, gender, ethnicity, or type of surgical procedure.

In a study by Watt-Watson, Evernden, and Lawson (1990), 71 parents of 62 children (84% under 5 years old) hospitalized for infectious conditions rated the intensity of their children's pain on a VAS ranging from 0 to 100 mm; the mean rating was 54 mm. A few parents (9%) indicated that their child had no pain. However, pain ratings provided by others may underestimate a child's pain. Indeed, pain ratings by postoperative school-age children and adolescents were significantly higher than those of nurses and physicians, even though children's ratings were moderately correlated with both nurses' ($r = .61$) and physicians' ratings ($r = .59$; LaMontagne, Johnson, & Hepworth, 1991).

Invasive procedures, such as lumbar punctures, intravenous therapy, and venipuncture, were perceived by parents to be the most painful for their children (Watt-Watson et al., 1990). Crying was the behavior most often identified with the child's experience of pain, regardless of age. The majority of parents also cited irritability, not sleeping, and being difficult to console as pain behaviors of infants under 1 year of age, a specific facial expression as indicative of pain in children, ages 2–6 years, and irritability, facial expression, not sleeping, difficult to console, being quiet, and pale color as pain behaviors for children over 6 years of age.

Four studies found that a portion of postoperative children were undermedicated for pain, regardless of age. Alex and Ritchie (1992) reported that 24 school-age children on their first postoperative day had received medication within the previous 4 hours for 12 of 25 assessments of moderate to severe pain and for 23 of 47 assessments of none to mild pain. However, in 13 of 72 (18%) assessments, children did not receive analgesics when indicated. Elander, Hellstrom, and Qvarnstrom (1993) studied 1,152 videotaped 5-minute episodes of 12 infants recovering from major surgical procedures and found that in 36% of the taped episodes pain ratings suggested inadequate pain relief.

In Asprey's (1994) chart review study, all 25 postoperative children, ages 4–8 years, had orders for nonnarcotic analgesics and 23 (92%) had orders for narcotic analgesics, but 26% of the ordered doses were subtherapeutic. In another chart review study of 75 preverbal children under 24 months of age who experienced surgery (Altimier, Norwood, Dick, Holditch-Davis, & Lawless, 1994), 5 had no prescribed analgesics, 11 received no analgesics, and 10 received only acetaminophen postoperatively. Although adequate for other analgesics, the average prescribed and administered doses of morphine were below the minimum recommended.

In Wallace's study (1989), children, ages 3–7 years, who had elective urologic surgery received from 0 to 24 doses of analgesic during the postoperative period, with a greater number of doses related to greater intensity of temperament (responsiveness and expression of emotions). However, the number of doses of analgesia appeared to be total rather than an average per day; thus, variability in the number of days included in the postoperative period could confound the results. In another study, children received only an average of 4.4 doses per day in the first 48 hours postoperatively (Asprey, 1994).

Dosages and analgesic agents administered for infants varied during a 24-hour period in Altimier and colleagues' (1994) study, but the number of doses of analgesia and infant behavior (sleep-wake states, facial expression, and verbalization) were not correlated. On 23 occasions, analgesics were administered subcutaneously despite the presence of an intravenous line. Children with caudal analgesia during surgery were less likely to have morphine and acetaminophen ordered in combination, and they received significantly less morphine and fewer total doses of analgesics postoperatively than children who did not have caudal analgesia (Altimier et al., 1994).

Children's pain has been undermedicated for some time, and unfortunately, this problem continues. As the studies reviewed here found, undermedication occurred in infants (Altimier et al., 1994; Elander et al., 1993), toddlers (Altimier et al., 1994), preschoolers (Asprey, 1994; Wallace, 1989), and school-age children (Alex & Ritchie, 1992; Asprey, 1994). In some cases, children had no orders for analgesics; in others, the ordered analgesic was either not administered, not the appropriate drug (nonnarcotic drugs rather than narcotics), or below the therapeutic dose. Perhaps this undermedication is due to (a) underestimation of children's pain by parents (Watt-Watson et al., 1990) or health professionals (LaMontagne et al., 1991) or (b) the variety of behaviors, indicating pain, demonstrated by children of different ages (Watt-Watson et al., 1990). Instruments for measuring pain intensity that were tested from 1989 to 1994 were applicable primarily for school-age children and adolescents. The body outline tested by Van Cleve and Savedra (1993) with preschool children measured pain's location, but not its intensity. Although instruments exist to measure pain intensity for children under 6 years of age, they were not used in the identified studies.

Temperature-Measurement Research

Four of the 5 studies in this group were designed to compare tympanic membrane temperatures with a variety of other sites and modes of temperature measurement. The conclusions reached by the teams of investigators differ widely, probably due to differences in the ages of the children studied and in study methodology. Erickson and Moser Woo (1994) were the only investigators to use a true "gold standard"—bladder temperature. They found that rectal temperatures were closest to core bladder temperatures, followed by tympanic temperatures; axillary were the most discrepant, had the lowest correlations with core temperatures, and had unacceptable sensitivity and specificity. In all the other studies, a variety of peripheral sites were compared, obscuring the cause of differences in readings and lower correlations. If tympanic temperatures varied, the researchers usually concluded that the tympanic reading was faulty; however, it is just as likely that the other peripheral sites were faulty. Pontius and colleagues (1994a) concluded that paper chemical thermometers were both more accurate and more precise than electronic thermometers; however, no data were provided to substantiate their conclusion. In another study, Pontius, Kennedy, Shelley, and Mittrucker (1994b) found that electronic thermometers were more accurate; however, electronic readings were affected by the child's behavior. Nurse training improved the readings obtained. Toddlers in Rogers and colleagues' (1991) study preferred tympanic over axillary measurements. Several researchers have questioned the use of tympanic temperatures in infants (Davis, 1993) and young children (Erikson & Moser Woo, 1994) due to their smaller ear canals, suggesting that smaller probes be designed for these children (Kachoyeanos, 1995).

Effects of Medication

The 2 studies in this category were designed to capture children's reactions to a particular medication (see Table 6.4). French and Nocera (1994) investigated the reaction of 12 PICU infants, ages 1–54 weeks, to withdrawal of continuous fentanyl infusion. Half of the infants receiving fentanyl for more than 24 hours showed signs of drug withdrawal. More symptoms and more severe symptoms were associated with larger total amounts of fentanyl ($r = .76$) and longer infusion times ($r = .70$). Occurrence of symptoms was not related to concurrent use of midazolam or chloral hydrate.

Lipshitz, Marino, and Sanders (1993) studied the effect of chloral hydrate administration on length of time to fall asleep and depth of sleep as well as the occurrence of side effects in 140 children, ages birth–36 months, scheduled for echocardiography. Three children did not fall asleep, and 25 (18%) experienced paradoxical excitement. Older children and those receiving larger doses of chloral hydrate were more likely to experience excitement rather than sedation. Sedation was quicker for children who were close to their usual naptimes. Age, proximity to naptime, and dosage size were positively related to quality of sleep. Ingestion of milk and more recent ingestion of solid food interfered with deeper sleep. Although the child's bedtime and depth of sleep were not affected the night of the chloral hydrate sedation, the following day most parents reported unusual child behavior, including staggering and dizziness ($n = 25$), grogginess or deep sleep ($n = 46$), irritability or silliness ($n = 46$), and decreased appetite ($n = 11$).

Tubes

Of the 3 articles in this category, 2 reported data from the same study on feeding tube placement (Beckstrand et al., 1990; Ellett, Beckstrand, Welch, Dye, & Games, 1992). The other study investigated factors that affect peripheral intravenous line longevity in infants (Smith & Wilkinson-Faulk, 1994). Both studies were conducted using chart audits (see Table 6.4).

The study on feeding tube placement was designed to evaluate prediction equations developed by Strobel, Byrne, Ament, and Euler (1979, as cited in Beckstrand et al., 1990, and Ellett et al., 1992) relating esophageal length to child height. For children, ages 1 month—4 years, the oral-referenced equation was supported, but the nasal-referenced equation was not. The sample in the Strobel and colleagues (1979) study and in the validation study (cited in Beckstrand et al., 1990; Ellet et al., 1992) contained few children older than 4 years, and oral placement was used predominantly with younger children and nasal placement, with older children; thus the equations' predictive capabilities were not adequately tested for older children.

In their study of factors affecting the life span of peripheral intravenous lines in infants, Smith and Wilkinson-Faulk (1994) found that lines lasted longer if the infant was on a general care floor rather than the neonatal intensive care unit (NICU) and if the line had been used to infuse blood. The life span of peripheral intravenous lines was not affected by insertion site, cannula size, or brand type.

Other Studies

The focus of 4 other studies was on critically ill children's intracranial pressure (ICP) response to nursing care procedures, children's allergic response to latex exposure, use of pulse oximetry monitoring in children, and infants' feeding responses to acute respiratory illnesses (see Table 6.4).

In a sample of 13 critically ill children, ages 1.5–11 years (Hobdell et al., 1989), mean ICP increased during hyperventilation, but decreased significantly to less than baseline within 15 minutes after hyperventilation. Turning, change in head position, bedside conversation, and invasive procedures did not result in significant changes in ICP. Age (younger than 4 years vs. older than 4 years) was not related to ICP values; however, receiving pentobarbital was significantly related to higher mean ICPs after hyperventilation, bedside conversations, and invasive procedures. One methodologic limitation of this study is that the data were repeatedly tested with paired and independent sample *t* tests without the use of a repeated-measures omnibus test or statistical correction for multiple hypothesis testing. Thus, the many significance tests may have capitalized on chance, and so the results may not be replicable.

Leger and Meeropol (1992) found that incidence of latex allergy was higher in children with spina bifida than in a comparison group of children with other chronic illnesses and was also higher in children with spina bifida who had a shunt in place than it was for those without the shunt. Children with latex allergy were older, on average, than children with no allergy. Gender and family or patient history of allergic reactions to a variety of substances were not related to latex allergy.

Through a retrospective chart audit, Kozlowski, DiMarcello, Stashinko, and Phifer (1994) found that on a children's medical/surgical unit, pulse oximetry was used for all children with pulmonary, reactive airway, hematologic, and infectious diseases and for more than half of those with gastrointestinal, genitourinary, orthopedic, plastic surgery, neurologic, and trauma diagnoses. About one third of the monitored children had at least one desaturation episode (< 95%); preschool-age (3–6 years) and Black children experienced more desaturation episodes than did children of other ages and White children, respectively. Most of the desaturations occurred during the first 4 days after admission.

A study of 16 infants, ages 1–4 months, found that different oral bottle-feeding behaviors were exhibited when they had an acute respiratory infection and when they were well (Conway, 1989). Mothers described their infants as feeding more slowly, being fussy, and refusing to eat or eating less. Although Conway (1989) concluded that the infants' sucking patterns were less coordinated, the seal on the nipple was looser, and their respiratory patterns were irregular during the illness phase, these data are presented only as frequencies with no statistical comparisons. Also, fine differences in sucking, swallowing, and seal are difficult to discriminate visually and generally require equipment to measure sucking pressures. Thus, the validity of the findings are questionable.

Although generally important to practice, these last 8 studies form a disparate group. Several were undertaken to address a local practice problem; some made use of existing data. Perhaps these studies are not easily categorized because they represent initial nursing knowledge development efforts in the area. In several of the studies, responses varied with the age of the child (Beckstrand et al., 1990; Ellett et al., 1992; Kozlowski et al., 1994; Leger & Meeropol, 1992; Lipshitz et al., 1993) and timing of feeds (Kozlowski et al., 1994; Lipshitz et al., 1993). These two factors are frequently important to response; however, several studies did not consider them.

The studies of children's physiologic responses were primarily atheoretical. Only 3 of the pain studies identified a guiding framework; these included the gate theory, stress and coping, and temperament. Two of the temperature studies but none of the other physiologic studies clearly cited a theoretical framework. Both of these temperature studies were conducted by Pontius and colleagues (1994a, 1994b) and used Roy's Adaptation Theory. The age range of the children in the pain studies was generally narrow, but this was not the case in

TABLE 6.4 Instruments Used in Child Physiologic Response Studies

Instrument	Description	Studies	Study Evidence That Supports Validity	Reliability
Conway-Shannon Infant Feeding Behavior Assessment Checklist (CSIFBAC)	Subscales: type of seal around nipple, suck-pause pattern, suck-swallow pattern, respiratory pattern; scored as present or absent in each time epoch	Conway (1989)	Content validity: review by two experts in infant feeding; no hypothesis testing	Pilot study: interrater reliability = 80% Current study: average *kappa* = .49 to .94
Esophageal length	Esophageal manometry with nonperfused Konigsberg motility probe and Beckman R611 dynagraph recorder	Beckstrand, Ellett, Welch, Dye, Games, Henrie, and Barlow (1990); Ellett, Beckstrand, Welch, Dye, and Games (1992)	Pressure tracings used to indicate location of tube	1st, 2nd, and 3rd readings: r = .990 to .997 nasally, .98 to .99 orally No interrater for chart audit
Intracranial Pressure	Electronics for Medicine multisystem monitor and transducer	Hobdell, Adams, Caruso, Dihoff, Neveling, and Roncoli (1989)	"Standard calibration and balancing" every shift; decrease in ICP over time after hyperventilation with suctioning	No evidence
IV Data Collection Tool (Peripheral IV life span)	5 items on IV placement, 5 items on IV infusions, 4 items on IV discontinuance	Smith and Wilkinson-Faulk (1994)	Life span longer on general pediatric units than in the NICU, if history of blood product infusion	No evidence
Latex Allergy	History of allergic reaction to rubber gloves, balloons, or catheters	Leger and Meeropol (1992)	Distinguished between patients with spina bifida and other chronic illnesses; patients with allergy were older, more likely to have a shunt for hydrocephalus	No evidence

Neonatal Abstinence Score Tool (NAST)	32-item observational scale with item weights	French and Nocera (1994)	Higher NAST score related to higher fentanyl dose, longer infusion time	Interrater reliability = 91% to 100%
Pulse Oximeter	Nellcor N-100 monitor and OXINET system.	Kozlowski, DiMarcello, Stashinko, and Phifer (1994)	No new evidence	No evidence No interrater for chart data
Undesired Effects of Medication	2 presedation behaviors, 2 behaviors during sedation	Lipshitz, Marino, and Sanders (1993)	Presedation: Excited behavior with higher total dose; sleep onset shorter if close to usual naptime During sedation: Deeper sleep if older, close to naptime, larger dose	Interrater reliability = 95%

the other physiologic studies, which often included children of all ages.

Many different instruments were used. Investigators usually described calibration procedures for the equipment used to measure physiologic parameters; however, reliability estimates were not provided for 3 of the pain studies, all of the temperature studies, and 5 of the 9 other physiologic studies. In most of these cases, the applicable reliability was interrater reliability because the data collectors in each of these studies clearly made judgments collecting the data. Also, investigators in several studies did no statistical analyses but, instead, interpreted differences in means as true differences.

Many aspects of children's behavioral and physiologic responses to acute illness remain unexplored. With the changes in child acuity during hospitalization and in the child's hospital experience, research describing children's posthospitalization behavioral responses is needed. Research on reactions to a variety of medications and nursing interventions, such as suctioning, enteral feeding, and turning, and on problems with normal body processes, such as feeding/eating, sleeping, and elimination, both during and after hospitalization is limited. For each of these topics, factors associated with children's responses must be identified. Such factors might be the child's age, sex, and race, presence of a chronic illness prior to hospitalization, parental presence, and specific diseases or illness conditions. Responses of children during and after hospitalization in an intensive care unit have received limited attention.

■ Conclusions

When research in pediatric nursing was just beginning, nurse researchers tended to focus on parental responses and, later, on parents' (primarily mothers') reports of their children's responses. Research over the past 5 years has moved away from examining parents and now more frequently focuses on the ill child, collecting data about the child directly from the child. Consistent with the recency of this trend, studies in this review that focused on parent and family responses were more well developed than studies of children's responses. Specifically, investigators of parents' and families' responses consistently cited information about the conceptual framework that guided the study. These studies also built on one another, representing a more organized effort toward developing knowledge. They tended to use similar measurement tools and more frequently included information about reliability and validity. This area of research needs to move beyond simple description to identify factors associated with specific responses and include family members other than parents.

In the child response studies, research on pain and temperature represented the most integrated efforts at knowledge development. That is, the studies used similar methods and measures making comparisons easier and built upon and extended the work in the area. However, the strengths of the parent/family studies were not always apparent in the child response studies. Conceptual frameworks were often omitted, different instruments were used to measure the same concepts, and attention to reliability issues was frequently lacking. Some investigators also interpreted differences in means and frequencies without the aid of statistical analyses. Thus, whether the observed differences were real or reflected minor sample fluctuation remains unknown. Studies of children's responses to acute illness are at the forefront of knowledge development in nursing, but future studies in this area would benefit from improved methodology.

Another issue needing attention is the age range of children studied. Studies on children's behavioral responses consistently tested measures using children who fit within a narrow age range. This was likely related to the characteristics of the measures as well as the children themselves. By their very nature, children of different ages have different verbal and cognitive abilities. To be valid, instruments must take into account that behaviors used to indicate upset or anxiety and the items or methods used to elicit children's descriptions of these concepts vary with the child's age. The result is that instruments need to be developed and used with a specific age group. Knowledge development in other areas where instrumentation is not age specific would benefit from limiting age groups or at least analyzing the data according to age group. In this way, differences in physiologic responses and parent/family responses based on the age of the ill child will not be overlooked.

From an assessment perspective, research is needed that describes children's responses to acute illness and hospitalization. Specifically, changes in behavior, mood, mental health, personality, and physiologic functioning (e.g., eating, sleeping, and elimination) of children during hospitalization and the transition to home after an acute or critical illness need to be described and factors related to these changes identified. Because many of the reported studies used a noncategorical approach to illness, research using a categorical approach would provide insight into the effect of specific aspects of the illness on children's responses. Some of these concepts currently have reliable and valid measurement strategies, but others do not. In areas where instrumentation is available but varied, knowledge development would benefit from more consistent use of a smaller group of instruments. The effects of interruption or dysfunction in one area (e.g., pain) on other functions (e.g., play, eating, sleeping, and elimination) need to be identified.

In summary, hospitalization of a child is a stressful event for many family members. Parents experience a change in their parental role toward the ill child; however, their responsibilities for other children at home and other roles continue. Hospitalized children experience anxiety, primarily concerning body integrity, death, and separation from parents. In the reviewed studies, the level of anxiety was less for older children, those with previous hospitalizations, and preschoolers whose parents participated in their care. Children of different ages used different strategies to cope with their stress. Assisting parents to deal with their other responsibilities and roles may decrease their stress levels and allow them to participate more fully in their child's illness. In turn, their increased participation and lower stress might decrease the ill child's stress response.

As for physiologic responses, children of all ages continue to be undermedicated for their pain. Nurses' interventions to prevent omission of indicated analgesic orders, inappropriate prescription of nonnarcotics, and prescription of inappropriate dosages will ensure that necessary medications are available. However, nurses must also be willing to administer ordered analgesics to prevent children's pain as well as to treat a child's complaint of pain. Because of the diversity in topics of the other research on children's physiologic responses, integration of findings is not warranted. Focusing future research efforts on children's physiologic responses to acute illness and building on existing research in those areas are necessary before prescriptions for practice can be made.

■ *Note*

1. Number of studies adds to more than 4 because some studies used more than one measurement method.

7

■

INTEGRATIVE REVIEW OF NURSING INTERVENTION RESEARCH ON ACUTELY ILL CHILDREN AND THEIR FAMILIES

■ *Janice Denehy, Martha Craft-Rosenberg, and Mary Jo Gagan*

Research in pediatric nursing has shown phenomenal growth in the past two decades. Today, not only research journals publish studies on children and families but many pediatric and maternal-child nursing specialty journals feature research articles and summaries on a regular basis. The increase in pediatric nursing research reflects the maturing of the profession, a recognition of the need for practice based on research, and the interest of nurses in examining their contribution to the health of children and families. A more recent trend in research is testing the effects or outcomes of nursing interventions. This trend is particularly timely as changes in the health care system increasingly emphasize cost-effectiveness and outcome-based care.

Pediatric nursing needs to clearly articulate its contribution to the health of children through rigorously designed intervention studies. To accomplish this, nursing interventions must be clearly specified and tested in different settings with children representing a wide range of ages and a diversity of racial and cultural groups. Only through rigorous testing will we learn what interventions work and under what conditions. Such studies will not only contribute to nursing science but will provide empirical support for practice.

This chapter provides an integrated review of selected studies reporting the testing of nursing interventions for acutely ill children and their families, discusses methodological challenges related to these studies, and identifies emerging issues related to this body of research.

■ *Selection Process*

The selection of studies included for review in this chapter was based on a number of criteria:

- The study tested a nursing intervention.
- The population targeted was children, ages 1 month–18 years, and/or their family.
- The children involved were acutely ill or about to experience hospitalization, diagnostic tests, or procedures.
- The research design was clearly stated and appropriate for testing an intervention.
- The intervention protocol was delineated.
- The outcome measures were specified.
- The findings were analyzed and reported.

Major nursing research journals—*Nursing Research, Research in Nursing and Health,* and *Western Journal of Nursing Research*—from 1985 to 1995 were searched using manual methods. Also screened for intervention research were maternal-child and pediatric specialty journals, including *Journal of Pediatric Nursing, Pediatric Nursing,* and *Journal of Pediatric Health Care,* published in the same period. The reference lists from articles identified were useful in finding additional intervention studies, and a search of Healthnet®, a computerized database, identified articles in journals not previously screened.

For the purpose of this review, a nursing intervention was defined as "any treatment, based on clinical judgment and knowledge, that a nurse performs to enhance patient/client outcomes" (McCloskey & Bulechek, 1996, p. xvii). Identified articles that did not meet the criteria in this definition were rejected. Many of these were clinical descriptions of nursing care or presented the need for a specific nursing intervention. All of the 29 articles that met the criteria for inclusion had at least one nurse author, even though this was sometimes difficult to determine in journals where nursing credentials were not noted.

In examining the intervention research, it became evident that the studies done in the acute care setting fit into two major categories:

- *Psychosocial* interventions, including those related to parents and related to preparation

for hospitalization, surgery, or procedures (detailed in Table 7.1 later in the chapter)
- *Physiological* interventions, including those related to fluid management, pain management, and positioning (detailed in Table 7.2 later in the chapter)

■ Early Research

Before presenting the integrated review of current intervention research, it is important to have a understanding of earlier studies that provide the historical context for the empirical basis in pediatric nursing. As Vessey (chap. 5 in this volume) points out, much of the pioneering research in pediatric nursing during the 1960s examined the effects of preparation for surgery or procedures. Early intervention studies demonstrated that mothers who received preparation prior to their child's surgery experienced less upset than unprepared mothers (Mahaffy, 1965; Skipper, Leonard, & Rhymes, 1968) and that children of prepared mothers showed less anxiety than children of nonprepared parents.

Children also benefited directly from psychological preparation for painful procedures they were about to experience (Vernon, 1974). Several authors (Visintainer & Wolfer, 1975; Wolfer & Visintainer, 1979) showed that children who were prepared for elective surgeries were more cooperative and exhibited less behavioral upset than unprepared children. Johnson, Kirchoff, and Endress (1975) found that sensory preparation for stressful events reduced distress during orthopedic cast removal. And Ferguson (1979), who compared a mastery model and a coping model in preparing children for surgery, found that the coping model preparation group exhibited less behavioral upset during hospitalization. These studies showed that prepared children were more cooperative and suffered less distress as a result of preparation for the event.

Both Lockwood (1970) and Clatworthy (1981) measured the effect of play interventions on children's anxiety and other behavioral parameters. Although Lockwood did not find a significant reduction in anxiety-defense scores in the experimental group, she stated that the children's anxiety/fears were more clearly perceived and realistically focused after the preparatory doll play session. Clatworthy found that children in the control group were more anxious at the time of final evaluation than those in the experimental play group. However, the intervention did not appear to reduce the experimental group's anxiety; what in fact occurred was that the anxiety of the control group increased during hospitalization, accounting for the significant differences between groups.

Denyes (1983) reviewed the mixed findings and methodological limitations of a number of other studies testing interventions to reduce distress and anxiety in hospitalized children. Beal and Betz (1992) reviewed intervention studies done during the 1980s and reported that of 319 articles determined to be research studies only 53 (16.6%) were interventions that tested the outcomes of nursing care. The overwhelming majority of these intervention studies were conducted on the topics of prematurity, parenting, or well-child care.

■ *Psychosocial Interventions*

The 12 studies of psychosocial interventions reviewed were related to (a) parents and (b) preparation for hospitalization, surgery, or procedures (see Table 7.1).

Two studies examined the effects of interventions targeting parents. They were designed to assist parents in providing support to their children in the post anesthesia area and to assist parents in caring for their children (Bru, Carmody, Donohue-Sword, & Bookbinder, 1993; Monahan, & Schkade, 1985). The samples in these studies varied by health status and age of the children. Bru and colleagues (1993) found that parents who had a tour of the recovery area prior to surgery, sat in a chair next to their child, and provided support as indicated showed a significant decrease in postoperative anxiety, when compared to a group of parents receiving standard care. However, no differences were seen in the postoperative anxiety of the 9- to 18-year-old patients. This was the only study to include both mothers and fathers. In the second study, Monahan and Schkade (1985) illustrated that care delivered by parents in acute care settings, as opposed to traditional care by nursing staff, does not compromise the outcomes of weight maintenance and skin condition. Although parent-collected, pedi-bag urine samples were more likely to be contaminated than nurse-collected specimens, this was not true for catheterized specimens. Monahan and Schkade's study is particularly timely in this era of cost containment, when there is increasing emphasis of care by parents whether in the hospital or at home. It is important to know that prepared parents can deliver comparable care that is not only more cost-effective but also more likely to be familiar and acceptable to young children. Both of these studies with parents were done to determine the efficacy of programs designed to improve the quality of care and parental satisfaction.

The main theme of the 10 psychosocial intervention studies related to preprocedural/preoperative preparation (see Table 7.1) was to examine the effects of such preparation on children's and/or parents' anxiety and coping and children's in-hospital behavior, cooperation, and posthospital behavior. Preparation interventions varied in structure and content, ranging from the provision of information about procedures, sensory information, hospital visitations and tours, introductions to nursing and medical personnel, doll play, medical equipment manipulation or play, and videotape modeling to discussions and question-and-answer periods. These included the effect of parental presence during procedures (Bru et al., 1993), audiotaped information about child behavior and the parents' role during hospitalization (Melnyk, 1994), and the effects of distraction, or therapeutic play (Clatworthy, 1981; Vessey, Carlson, & McGill, 1994). Preparation interventions have been operationalized using such a wide range of diverse activities that little standardization exists. What is described as a preparation intervention in one study might be very different from that described in another study, making it essential that authors clearly specify their intervention protocol and the conceptual framework underlying the intervention.

In a large number of studies that focused on preparing children and/or parents for hospitalization or procedures with the goal of minimizing distress and promoting cooperation, the outcomes of these preparatory interventions were examined using a variety of measures. Only 2 studies measured physiological outcomes. Broome and Endsley (1987) found no significant differences in pulse and blood pressure measures during a fingerstick procedure following preparation between treatment and control groups. Mansson, Fredrikzon, and Rosberg (1992) also found no differences between treatment and control group on pulse, blood pressure, or blood cortisol levels in children prepared for surgery and those receiving a sedative. Of the wide variety of behavioral outcome measures used, only four were used in more than one study. The Manifest Upset Scale, the Cooperation Scale, the Global Mood Scale and the Posthospital Behavior Questionnaire were used in 2 of the 12 studies reviewed (see Table 7.1). Many researchers developed instruments or observation checklists for their studies that had not previously been tested for reliability and validity.

The number of participants in the 12 psychosocial studies reviewed ranged from 23 to 138, with a mean of about 61 persons per study. Overall, the samples in these studies were fairly evenly distributed by gender. More notable, however, was the increase in racial and ethnic diversity over time in the few studies where these data were reported. Random assignment to groups was done in only five studies (Broome & Endsley, 1987; Broome & Endsley, 1989; Fegley, 1988; Mansson et al., 1992; Melnyk, 1994). A number of authors reported that parents requested to be in study groups that included parental presence or participation, thereby making it difficult to control for the effects of self-selection. One method to assess whether threats to selection occurred would be to compare data on those parents and their children with that of others in the study to see if there are any differences on key variables (Broome & Endsley, 1989). Other authors reported reasons why some individuals were excluded or dropped from the study.

A number of studies investigated children who were at varying developmental levels. For example, Caire and Erickson's (1986) study of the effects of auditory tapes on distress during cardiac cauterization involved children who ranged in age from under 1 year to 17 years, making standardization of the intervention impossible. These authors reported the responses of different age groups to the intervention (which differed for different ages), although this was not the purpose of the study. Such a wide age range can confound the results with the effects of cognitive development, experience, and coping. Researchers should strive to have children in age ranges dictated by conventional stages of cognitive development. Specification of age range is also essential in planning preparation programs that usually have cognitive components as well as activities, such as play or videotapes, that need to be tailored to different age groups. Another consideration is the timing of the intervention. Because

(text continued on p. 153)

TABLE 7.1 Psychosocial Interventions

Author(s) and Date	Purpose of Study	Sample/Research	Intervention Protocol	Outcome Measures	Findings
Broome and Endsley (1987)	To determine if a brief sensory-procedural information preparation program would lessen behavioral and physiological manifestations of a painful experience (fingerstick)	74 children, age 5 years 40 males, 34 females Preschool screening Quasi-experimental; alternate assignment to treatment or control group	*Preparation program* (15 minutes) *Phase 1*: Child asked to describe why at clinic; misconceptions corrected *Phase 2*: Demonstration of fingerstick on doll *Phase 3*: Child feedback and manipulation of equipment *Control Group*: Colored pictures in separate room for 15 minutes	Pulse and blood pressure (1 minute before and after fingerstick) Child's Pain Response Tool (during fingerstick)	No significant differences in treatment and control group on physiological measures; all children had significant (p < .01) increases in reaction to fingerstick No correlation between physiologic and behavior measures
Broome and Endsley (1989)	To investigate the effects of maternal presence, childrearing practices and the response of young children to an interview and injection	138 children, ages 3–9 years, at health screening program Quasi-experimental; alternative assignment to treatment or control group	*Group 1*: Parent absent for interview and immunization *Group 2*: Parent absent for interview, present for immunization *Group 3*: Parent present for interview; absent for immunization *Group 4*: Parent present for interview and immunization	Childrearing Practice Questionnaire Child Behavior Observation Rating Tool	Significant (p < .05) main effect; children of authoritative parents exhibited less distress than other children during immunization whether mother present or not Children were more distressed during immunization than interview but no effect by maternal presence or absence; children whose mothers were present during interview were significantly more distressed than those whose mothers were absent

| Bru, Carmody, Donohue-Sword, and Bookbinder (1993) | To determine effect of parental visitation in postanesthesia care unit (PACU) on pre- and postoperative anxiety levels of pediatric patients and parents | 68 parent-child dyads admitted for 1st surgical (minor) procedure

52 mothers, 16 fathers

42 children, ages 5 months–9 years; 26 children, ages 9–18 years

Quasi-experimental serial (nonvisitation group studied before implementation of visitation program) | All received standard preoperative teaching

Visitation group given pamphlet describing visitation policies and what to expect when child wakes up from anesthesia, had tour of PACU, and a chair next to child's bed in PACU | Demographic data
Spielberger State-Trait Anxiety Inventory completed before and after child's surgery by all parents

Spielberger State-Trait Anxiety Inventory for Children completed by children > 9 years of age before (Trait scale only) and after surgery (both scales)

Young Child Observation Checklist filled out by nursing staff for children > 9 years old before and after surgery

PACU Parent Observation Checklist completed by nurse

PACU Parental Visitation Program Evaluation completed by parents | Groups similar
Significant ($p < .05$) decrease in state anxiety postoperatively for parents in visitation group regardless of child's age

No significant differences found in older children's anxiety pre- or postoperatively in visitation groups

Frequencies of behaviors recorded; only one child was upset before implementation of visitation program

No parents were disruptive or fainted; 75% verbally consoled; 63% asked relevant questions; 38% held child

95% of parents in visitation would recommend it to others and felt it reduced the anxiety of them and their children |

TABLE 7.1 *Continued*

Author(s) and Date	Purpose of Study	Sample/Research	Intervention Protocol	Outcome Measures	Findings
Caire and Erickson (1986)	To examine effects of auditory tapes on lowering distress for children undergoing cardiac catheterization	28 children, ages < 1 year–17 years Descriptive Convenience sample	Usual preprocedural preparation: (a) tape of relaxation suggestions and soothing music, or (b) tape of nursery rhymes or stories, or (c) tape of age-appropriate popular music	Parents and children rated precatheterization for attention span, precatheterization play, restlessness, agitation, and anxiety Child observed during procedure for signs of distress or need for medication Child interviewed after procedure (when possible)	Inverse relationship of precatheterization anxiety and response to tape Greatest effect < 1 year old; 1- to 3-year-olds had variable response; 4–6-year-old group too small to generalize; 7- to 12-year-olds benefited from music 18 of 28 children appeared to benefit (no data presented on outcome measures; no control group)
Fegley (1988)	To examine effects of choice of information in preprocedural instruction on children's responses to selected radiologic procedures	61 children, ages 4–12 years, scheduled for routine urological, radiological procedures Quasi-experimental Random assignment	*Contingent Instruction Group:* Information based on questions asked by child *Noncontingent Instruction Group:* Formal presentation	Demographic data Search for Information Protocol (measured 3 times) Manifest Upset Scale (measured 2 times) Cooperative Scale (measured 2 times) Self-Report of Distress (measured after test)	Equivalent groups Contingent group significantly ($p < .05$) less information seeking during procedure than noncontingent group Older children spent more time searching for information, were more cooperative, displayed less upset, and reported less distress

	Purpose	Sample/Design	Independent Variable/Intervention	Dependent Variable/Measures	Findings
Kennedy and Riddle (1989)	To explore influence of the time of preparation on young children's adjustment to an ambulatory surgical experience	23 children, ages 3–6 years; 17 males, 6 females; Admitted to ambulatory surgery area; no preoperative medications required; Quasi-experimental	*Group 1:* Prepared the afternoon prior to day of surgery; *Group 2:* Prepared the morning of surgery; *Preparation Program:* Storybook with 15 pictures and sensory experiences of children going through ambulatory surgery; Investigator put on surgical scrubs and mask and child given anesthesia mask to handle	Global Mood Scale (measured 6 times during surgical experience); Post Hospital Behavior Questionnaire	No significant difference between times of preparation on anxiety; Significant ($p < .05$) time effect on anxiety (between Times 1 and 3, Times 4 and 5, and Times 2 and 4) for total group; No significant differences in anxiety of children in both groups; No significant differences
Lynch (1994)	To evaluate effects of preoperative teaching program on children's distress during day surgery	30 children, ages 3–10 years; 19 males, 11 females; Quasi-experimental; Participants self-selected	*Experimental Group:* Attend group program with procedural and sensory information within 2 weeks of surgery; *Control Group:* No instruction	Demographic data; Manifest Upset Scale; Cooperation Scale; Self-Assessment Faces Scale	Equivalent groups; Children attending program were significantly ($p < .0001$) less distressed and more cooperative than control group; Children in experimental group reported less distress ($p < .05$) than control group
Monahan and Schkade (1985)	To determine if quality of nursing care is compromised by allowing parents to assume total responsibility for their child's care; also examined effects of parental involvement in gait training in first time ambulators (not reported)	44 mother-child dyads; Children, ages 14 months–4.5 years, requiring orthopedic surgery; 2×2; Nonrandom sample	*Independent Variable 1:* Care by parent unit (CBPU); Care by nurse (CBN); *Independent Variable 2:** Special therapy; Regular therapy; * Article did not address therapy findings	*Dependent Variables*; Weight; Skin integrity (5 categories with a 3-point scale); Contaminated urine specimens (quality of care measure); Parent anxiety (semantic differential item scale)	Significant weight loss in all groups; no differences between CBPU and CBN; Significant skin improvement for all groups ($p < .0015$ at Day 5; $p < .0277$ at discharge); no difference between CBPU and CBN; Fewer ($p < .029$) in CBN; CBPU parents in special therapy had more anxiety ($p < .0387$) over time

TABLE 7.1 *Continued*

Author(s) and Date	Purpose of Study	Sample/Research	Intervention Protocol	Outcome Measures	Findings
Mansson, Fredrikzon, and Rosberg (1992)	To investigate value of psychological preparation program compared to conventional premedication alone	30 children, ages 7–15 years 12 males, 18 females Admitted with acute pain and subsequently operated on for appendicitis Experimental Random assignment	*Experimental Group:* Information about procedure, equipment handling, doll play, meet medical personnel, discussed fears, reviewed information; given preoperative medication (atropine) *Control Group:* Usual instruction and preoperative medication (atropine plus narcotic)	Demographic data Visual Analog Scale (Anxiety) (child and parent) Pulse and blood pressure Pediatric unit need for analgesic Blood Cortisol Interviews 4 and 15 months postsurgery	Equivalent groups No significance between groups; significant ($p < .05$) between pre- and postoperative units No differences between groups No significance differences between groups No significant differences between groups Children in experimental group had realistic memories of symptoms and procedure, asked more questions and remembered answers Children in control group were more likely to remember fears, and parents stated more fearful

Study	Purpose	Sample	Intervention	Measures	Results
Melnyk (1994)	To evaluate the effects of child behavioral information and parental role information (separately and together) on maternal and child coping during an unplanned hospitalization (mostly nonsurgical respiratory, gastrointestinal and orthopedic problems)	108 mother-child dyads Mothers, ages 21–44 years; children, ages 3–6 years (91 medical, 17 surgical) Experimental Random assignment to 4 groups	Mothers listened to audiotapes and given some information in writing: *Group 1:* Child behavior information *Group 2:* Parental role information *Group 3:* Combined information (from Groups 2 and 3) *Group 4:* Control information	Demographic data Spielberger State-Trait Anxiety Inventory (given to mothers during and following hospitalization) Index of Parent Participation/ Hospitalized Child (48 to 72 hours) Index of Parental Support During Intrusive Procedures (8 days after discharge) Posthospital Behavior Questionnaire 2 Visual Analogue Scales measuring mother's knowledge after receiving information	Equivalent groups Significant ($p < .05$ main effect; mothers in all treatment groups reported less anxiety than control group) Mothers in treatment groups had greater participation ($p < .001$) Mothers in treatment groups supported children more ($p < .001$) during intrusive procedures Children of mothers in treatment groups exhibited less ($p < .05$) behavioral upset after discharge Mothers in treatment group had more knowledge ($p < .05$)
Spicher and Yund (1989)	To examine effects of preadmission preparation on parent and child psychological upset at time of tonsillectomy, child postsurgery behavior, and parental compliance with home care instructions	40 children, ages 3–11 years, and their mothers Outpatient tonsillectomy Quasi-experimental Convenience sample	*Experimental Group:* Preadmission program of slide-tape presentation, directed play, hospital tour, and question-and-answer period with parents *Control Group:* No preparation	Outpatient Experience Questionnaire Posthospital Behavior Questionnaire Parental Postdischarge Care Questionnaire	No significant differences in experimental or control group in parent or child behaviors No significant differences between groups No significant differences between groups; majority of parents did not follow at least half of home care instructions

151

TABLE 7.1 *Continued*

Author(s) and Date	Purpose of Study	Sample/Research	Intervention Protocol	Outcome Measures	Findings
White, Williams, Alexander, Powell-Cope, and Conlon (1990)	To evaluate strategy to promote sleep in hospitalized children	94 children, ages 3–8 years, hospitalized for 2 nights and on no medications that would affect sleep First 3 groups randomly assigned; Group 4 was convenience sample	*Group 1:* Parent-recorded story; parents absent *Group 2:* Stranger-recorded story; parents absent *Group 3:* No recorded story; parents absent *Group 4:* No recorded story; parents present	Demographic data Sleep Onset Latency Behavior Catalog Distress: Behaviors observed by researchers Self-soothing behaviors: Behaviors observed by researchers	Equivalent groups Group 1 had longer ($p < .05$) sleep onset than Group 4; Groups 1, 2 and 4 had longer ($p < .05$) sleep onset than Group 3 Group 1 had higher distress ($p < .05$) than Group 2 No significant differences among groups

hospitalization and illness in themselves are stressful to children, measuring the effects of a preparation program when the child is about to be or has been admitted to the hospital or is seriously ill may make it difficult to demonstrate treatment effects when the child is already distressed. This might explain why many of the studies in this group showed no treatment main effect.

Six of the 12 studies added control groups (Broome & Endsley, 1987, 1989; Lynch, 1994; Mansson et al., 1992; Melnyk, 1994; Spicher & Yund, 1989), 3 compared different intervention protocols (Caire & Erickson, 1986; Fegley, 1988; White, Williams, Alexander, Powell-Cope, & Conlon, 1990), and 1 examined the effect of time of intervention delivery—the day before surgery versus the day of surgery (Kennedy & Riddle, 1989). Lynch (1994) studied the effectiveness of a group preoperative teaching program for day surgery that used a videotape of a 5-year-old male going for surgery. Both procedural and sensory information were integrated in the videotape. The dependent measures included a self-reported anxiety scale and a cooperation scale. Children in the experimental group were significantly less distressed and more cooperative. Mansson and colleagues (1992) conducted a unique study that compared the effects of usual instruction and sedation to the effects of detailed explanation and use of realistic images (doll and picture book) on the outcome of postoperative analgesia use. Although no significant differences were found, this study tested an alternative to medication, which merits further exploration. Melnyk (1994) investigated the effect of different forms of information provided to parents, with the goal of reducing anxiety about the illness or hospitalization experience. She found that parents who received taped information about (a) children's behavior posthospitalization and/or (b) the parental role in caring for hospitalized children reported less anxiety and greater

participation in their child's care than parents who did not receive information. Children of mothers in the experimental groups displayed significantly less behavior change postintervention. This study is particularly timely, as the intervention consisted of two carefully prepared 7-minute audiotapes, an intervention that is cost-effective and consistent and can be used routinely by staff nurses on any shift or prior to admission.

■ *Physiological Interventions*

The 9 physiological intervention studies (see Table 7.2) cover (a) fluid management, including studies on the effect of heparin on vessel patency, (b) pain management, and (c) positioning interventions.

Three studies that compared the effects of heparin versus normal saline on maintenance of vessel patency were done because findings on adults were not viewed as applicable to children for two major reasons:

- The smaller lumen of children's vessels and lower blood pressures can influence the likelihood of clot formation around the tip of the catheter
- The standard practice of changing intravenous catheter sites every 48 to 72 hours to prevent phlebitis

Children do not have the same high rates of phlebitis as adults do when catheters are left in for long periods of time. Therefore, the standard of care is to leave the catheter in as long as it is patent and there are no signs of inflammation or induration (see Table 7.2).

The studies comparing effects of heparin and normal saline on vessel patency are unusual in the sophistication of their designs and methods. The prospective study by Kleiber, Hanrahan, Fagan, and Zittergruen (1993) used

TABLE 7.2 Physiological Interventions

Author(s) and Date	Purpose of Study	Sample/Research	Intervention Protocol	Outcome Measures	Findings
Danek and Noris (1992)	To compare effects of normal saline and heparin for maintaining patency of "heparin locks"	160 catheters: 40 #22 gauge, 120 #24 gauge Children, ages 0 to 18 years; 69% < 1 year old Double-blind using 2 groups of hospitalized children (group assignment procedure not described) Quasi-experimental	1 ml normal saline or 10 u/ml heparin flush following catheter use or every 8 hours, which was standard procedure	Length of time catheters were functional, or longevity, measured in hours	#22 gauge catheter: No significant difference in longevity (Wilcoxon: $p = .43$) #24 gauge catheter: Statistically significant longer duration for heparin (Wilcoxon: $p = .03$) than normal saline
Kleiber, Hanrahan, Fagan, and Zittergruen (1993)	To determine efficacy of saline versus heparin solution to maintain peripheral (intravenous, or IV) locks in a pediatric population	124 children for IV locks: 68 saline, 56 heparin Children, ages 28 days–22 years Prospective randomized Double-blind Nurse pretested on standardized method for locking on IV and on complications necessitating discontinuation.	Routine flushing before and after every medication or every 6 hours if no medications given	Duration of intravenous (IV) locks in hours	No significant difference between mean duration of IV locks (χ^2 value = 1.55, $p = 0.4$) No significant difference in incidence of complications ($\chi^2 = 0.76$, $p = .38$) Information on needle gauge size not available on some recipients for comparison to other studies

Author (Year)	Purpose	Sample/Design	Intervention/Instrument	Measurement	Findings
McMullen, Fioravanti, Pollack, Rideout, and Sciera (1993)	To compare efficacy of normal saline and heparin solution in pediatric population and other variables that may affect patency of IV in intermittent infusion sites	142 children, ages 0–18 years Mixed acute/chronic illnesses Double-blind experimental Random assignment to groups	Normal saline versus heparin solution flush to first line started on client Met with medical and nursing staff Trained nursing staff	Intravenous patency in hours recorded on flow sheet	No significant difference between normal saline and heparin solution Older children had longer patency ≤ 3 years: Normal saline longer than heparin solution ≤ 3 years: Type of medication did not affect patency Number of times line accessed affected patency no matter what flush was used
Carabott, Javaheri, Keilty, and Manger (1992)	To test effects of two interventions to maintain adequate hydration following tonsillectomy and adenoidectomy: (1) forcing fluids; (2) not forcing fluids	74 children, 1–18 years, admitted for same-day tonsillectomy and adenoidectomy Experimental Random assignment to experimental and control groups	Group 1: Received oral fluids, forced if necessary Group 2: Offered liquids but allowed to choose rate of consumption	Mean oral fluid intake measured in milliliters (ml) Data collection at 6 hours and at 8 hours Every hour by parent on alertness/comfort	At 6 hours, 20 in Group 1 and 7 in Group 2 had received 500 ml of fluids At 8 hours, 26 in Group 1 and 19 in Group 2 had received 500 ml of fluids No significant relationship between comfort or alertness and fluid levels
Webb, Stergios, and Rodgers (1989)	To determine if patient-controlled anesthesia (PCA) is an effective postoperative pain relief method for children, ages 11–18 years	30 children, ages 11–18 years: 15 in treatment group undergoing elective general surgery; 15 in control group Descriptive, with control group Convenience sample	Pretest of child understanding of PCA: Explain PCA to parent and child; teach child use 6 hours before surgery; and teach parents about PCA Life Care system PCA Infuser	Amount of pain measured by Verbal Self-Report of pain (0 = no pain, 10 = worst pain) and Visual Analog Scale (VAS) Amount of medication required (morphine: mg/Kg)	*Pain:* Mean pain assessment ratings by verbal report and VAS was 4.01; children were satisfied *Analgesia/Pain Medications:* PCA group tapered slightly faster than control group and remained less after Day 3 *Safety:* PCA safe for narcotic administration in this age group

TABLE 7.2 *Continued*

Author(s) and Date	Purpose of Study	Sample/Research	Intervention Protocol	Outcome Measures	Findings
Gureno and Reisinger (1991)	To describe use of patient-controlled anesthesia (PCA) for children ≥ 3 years of age	15 charts of children, ages 3–12 years, undergoing urologic surgery Retrospective chart review to determine effects of PCA for pain management as compared to current institutional practice	1. 2 RNs check and machine functioning 2. Initiate pump; stay with child for 20 minutes 3. RN stays with child for 20 minutes after loading dose or bolus 4. Naloxone drawn up and attached to pump 5. Rechecked child every 1 to 2 hours for pain control and attempts (buttons pushed) versus actual doses received 6. Parents instructed on pump function safety features 7. Monitoring by staff on medications and placebo effect	Pain control as measured by patient behaviors, self-report, and FACES rating scale Survey of parents by written questionnaire for their view of pain control	All children maintained excellent pain control Parents satisfied with patient-controlled anesthesia and would request PCA pump for their children if future surgery needed
Vessey, Carlson, and McGill (1994)	To determine the effectiveness of distraction technique (use of a kaleidoscope) in reducing a child's perceived pain and behavioral distress during acute pain experience (needle stick)	100 children, ages 3–13 years 62 males, 38 females Posttest 2 groups randomly assigned from convenience sample	*Experimental Group:* Illusion kaleidoscope to look through during blood draw; children encouraged to concentrate on what they were seeing Following blood draw, FACES and CHEOPS were completed	Pain perception as measured by FACES (Wong-Baker) pain rating scale, following needle stick Children's Hospital of Eastern Ontario Pain Scale (CHEOPS), following needle stick	Groups equivalent on demographics and prior knowledge and experience Younger children reported experiencing greater pain intensity than older children; age was a significant covariant ($p < .004$) Experimental group significantly different on FACES ($p = .004$) than control group Distraction an effective strategy in ameliorating child perception of pain during needle stick

Hader and Sorenson (1988)	To compare transcutaneous oxygen tension effects of 3 body positions: (a) supine, (b) prone, and (c) Fowler's on T_c PO_2 levels of patients in intensive care	12 children, ages 2 weeks–2 years 9 males, 3 females 1 diagnosis of infection	T_CPO_2 airshield monitoring system used	Transcutaneous oxygen tension (T_CPO_2) after stabilization and calibration of the probe	No difference in position as determined by a repeated measures ANOVA ($f = 2.98$, $p = .0883$)
		Quasi-experimental: control with 3 independent variables Convenience sample	Child positioned in one of three conditions	All T_cPO_2 monitoring performed with airshield Model AS301	Possibility of Type II error with small sample
			Values allowed to stabilize 15 to 20 minutes at reading		

random selection and was double-blind to both nurses and patients. Pilot work conducted prior to the study enabled the investigators to calculate power using a known effect to determine sample size. Nurses in this study were pretested for their use of standardized methods in care of equipment. The study design and procedure were rigorous, which makes the findings of no statistically significant difference between the treatment groups more credible. Similarly, the study conducted by McMullen, Fioravanti, Pollack, Rideout, and Sciera (1993) used random assignment and was double-blind. Danek and Noris (1992) used a two-group comparison, and the intervention was blind to the nurses participating. The investigators of these last 2 studies raised questions as to whether the extraneous variables of needle gauge and the number of times that lines were accessed need to be considered as explanatory variables in future studies.

A nonpharmacological intervention for pain experienced during venipuncture was reported by Vessey and colleagues (1994), who studied a distraction intervention that used an illusion kaleidoscope. Nonpharmacological interventions are needed to assist children during short, moderately painful procedures that do not warrant the use of analgesics. The findings of this study are encouraging (see Table 7.2), and more research is suggested on the use of distraction and other nonpharmacological pain control interventions (Vessey & Carlson, 1996). The investigators also used the method of pooling the variance estimates for extraneous variables in the two treatment groups. This method allowed them to compare groups that may have been dissimilar. The study of dissimilar groups is a reality to most clinical investigators, and this method is a possibility for many who do clinical research.

Other physiological intervention studies examined the topics of fluid management following tonsillectomy and adenoidectomy (Carabott,

Javaheri, Keilty, & Manger, 1992), and the effects of positioning (Hader & Sorensen, 1988). These studies represent interventions that promote self-care to prevent complications, promote healing, and enhance the quality of life in illness. This is an exciting direction for nursing intervention research.

Other investigators chose to study the interventions of distraction and the child's use of patient-controlled anesthesia (PCA) and examine the effects of appropriate child control over one's own health and illness. The use of pain control pumps was evaluated in studies done by Webb, Stergios, and Rodgers (1989) and Gureno and Reisinger (1991). The descriptions of the intervention protocols for these studies were abbreviated in the research reports, illustrating the need for more specificity. Both studies supported the safety and effectiveness of PCA pumps for children. However, the Gureno and Reisinger (1991) study did not use a control group. These data are significant because they provide evidence that children can provide control over their pain in a manner that is safe.

■ *Methodological Challenges in Intervention Research*

Although still limited in number and scope, studies seem to be increasing in sophistication. The appearance of experimental designs, randomized clinical trials, and the addition of double-blind procedures speaks to the continued development of researchers in nursing and their contributions to nursing knowledge. Similarly, nursing intervention studies on acutely ill children and their families more commonly use outcome measures with strong psychometric properties. These advancements are encouraging. However, there are several concerns that need to be addressed to continue refinement of intervention studies for children.

Programs of Research

Tables 7.1 and 7.2 show clearly that research topics are diffuse and scattered and that programs of research are difficult to identify. Research programs conducted by research teams are important to maximize investigator expertise and refinement of research methods that can contribute substantive work relative to nursing science and practice. Such teams should include both researchers and clinicians to facilitate identification of problems relevant to nursing practice and interventions that are appropriate for the skill level and time availability of practicing nurses who might use these interventions. Nurses also need to invite professionals from fields outside nursing to participate as members of multidisciplinary research teams, as they can provide additional perspectives on the effects of acute illness on children and their families and on the interventions to mediate these effects.

Replication Studies

The study of heparin versus saline effects is one example of a single topic being studied by more than one investigator in three settings. However, this example is unusual. There is a need for such studies conducted in both simultaneous and consecutive sequences. Simultaneous studies conducted in different settings can increase the external validity of the findings. A sequence of consecutive studies provides opportunities for investigators to raise and answer important research questions. The number and extent of replication studies needed on a given topic is a judgment made by investigators and depends on whether a pattern

of similar findings emerges over time in differing settings and with a culturally diverse range of participants.

Randomization Procedures

Randomized clinical trials are central to the study of nursing interventions, but randomization is seldom specified, and the rationale for the choice of randomization often is not given (Vessey et al., 1994). Few reports of clinical trials provide adequate descriptions of randomization procedures used (Altman & Dore, 1985; Williams & Davis, 1994). Descriptions do not need to be lengthy, but they should clearly indicate the type of randomization method and how the randomization was implemented. Both fixed and adaptive procedures can be used. Fixed allocation procedures assign the intervention to participants with a prespecified probability, and that allocation probability is not altered. In contrast, adaptive procedures change the allocation probabilities as the study progresses (Friedman, Furberg, & DeMets, 1996). The concern with adaptive randomization and simple randomization procedures is unequal treatment-group size, which reduces power and should be avoided (Brittain & Schesselman, 1982; Peto, Pike, & Armitage, 1976). For example, Carabott and colleagues (1992) used day of admission to randomize but did include a rationale or cite a reference justifying their choice (Friedman, Furberg, & DeMets, 1996). Further, the use of unequal numbers in treatment groups in some cases needs to be justified. Calculation of sample size was done through power analysis for several studies, and some authors were able to use preliminary work to determine effect sizes (Kleiber et al., 1993). However, the study by Vessey and colleagues (1994) used a medium effect size. The rationale for decisions made during the planning stage of studies needs to be described.

Size of Samples

Intervention efficacy can be determined only if the size of the sample is adequate. Often, small samples contribute to Type II errors due to the difficulties in achieving statistical significance in treatment efficacy between groups (Schmidt, 1992). Small samples usually result in unequal distribution on selected variables across and within groups. One possible solution to this problem being recommended currently is the use of several data collection sites to increase the size of a sample, but this approach is costly and fraught with quality control issues as well as issues of reliability and internal validity. A second solution is the integration and combination of findings from many studies on the same topic through the use of meta-analyses. This approach emphasizes effect size. Thus, findings from studies in which no statistical significance is found between treatment groups due to small samples are not lost but become another data point among several in the meta-analysis (Schmidt, 1995).

Even though the randomized clinical trial is still the "gold standard" for the study of some research questions, integrative reviews and meta-analyses are being used with increasing frequency for effectiveness research (Lewin, 1996). One such meta-analysis, which was conducted on 27 studies of pain management interventions with children, used two decades of research in five disciplines (Broome, Lillis, & Smith, 1989). The authors reported significance in addition to effect size but also noted limitations among studies in (a) reported estimates of reliability and validity, (b) intervention types and procedures, (c) effect size, and (d) conceptualization and assumptions in the body of pain studies used. In spite of these limitations, meta-analyses provide investigators with a mechanism to describe the field, the underlying assumptions of the research in the field, and the methods and instruments used to examine responses and to examine intervention effectiveness over many studies.

■ *Emerging Issues*

Several issues regarding nursing intervention research emerged during this integrated review. First, complete specification of the intervention studied is necessary for replication in research and for implementation of the intervention in practice. The authors of the articles reviewed here used different styles and methods of describing their intervention, ranging from a very detailed account to a simple outline.

As investigators on the Nursing Interventions Classification (McCloskey & Bulechek, 1996), we looked carefully at the language and detail provided in describing the intervention. It is essential that researchers explicate and document both the intervention protocol during the planning of their study, which includes training their research team, and the procedure for its implementation and monitoring.

A second issue is the need for and use of a standardized language to describe nursing interventions in a language with common meaning. This issue is reflective of a larger professional mandate to develop and use standardized language for nursing diagnoses, interventions, and outcomes. For example, the use of standardized language would enable investigators to use the term or intervention label *preparation,* knowing that the meaning of the label was shared by other nurses.

Another emerging and highly significant challenge is the cost-effectiveness of interventions. Cost was not discussed in the studies reviewed; however, readers can identify cost implications. Effectiveness can no longer be evaluated apart from cost considerations, and investigators are urged to discuss costs as well as risk and benefits in their research reports.

Other cost considerations are the time involved in carrying out the intervention, the time needed for training data collectors and interventionists, special equipment needed, and the development of skills needed to carry out the intervention in the practice setting. It is important to develop and test interventions that are realistic for the practicing nurse in today's cost-conscious environment.

Preparation interventions illustrate the dilemma faced by many researchers when selecting interventions: Existing data may indicate the effectiveness of preparation, but the cost as measured in terms of nursing time can be high. In this case, however, one could hypothesize that the cost invested prior to the event would prevent other costs in nurse time needed to comfort the child or to prolong or repeat the procedure. In the future, this hypothesis needs to be tested using appropriate designs and methods.

A final issue has to do with updating our current body of knowledge about children with acute illnesses and their families. Many of the studies described previously were done when children were routinely hospitalized the night before diagnostic procedures or surgery, the time when preparation was traditionally done. Children also were often hospitalized for a number of days after the procedure or surgery, which may have added to the distress or upset of the child, and provided an opportunity for nurses to study the effects of interventions prior to and during the hospitalization.

However, changes in the health care system have dictated a new focus for preparation research because many surgical and diagnostic procedures are now being done on an outpatient basis. Questions about the timing of preparation and by whom it is given are important questions for future nursing research. Another challenge is the need to prepare children who have surgery or procedures on an outpatient basis. Interventions also are needed that assist parents to care for their child at home and to understand both the psychosocial and physi-

ological changes their children may experience as a result of illness, diagnostic procedures, or surgery. Because both fathers and mothers are likely to be involved in the care and support of their children in the home, it is important to include both the mother and the father in studies focusing on parents as well as looking at the effects on the entire family unit.

■ *Conclusion*

As nurse researchers become more knowledgeable about conducting research, more carefully designed studies are being reported in the literature. Carefully constructed intervention protocols based on prior studies, child development, educational and nursing theory will be developed and tested. Use of the NIC (McCloskey & Bulechek, 1996) as an intervention model is one way to identify interventions for testing; the activities listed for each intervention in the NIC can be used to develop and test interventions. These activities form the basis for an intervention protocol to be tested on a specific population or age group. NIC interventions are designed to apply to clients of all ages and in a wide variety of settings (McCloskey & Bulechek, 1996). This application needs to be empirically tested. As nurses look to intervention models to guide their practice and research, the use of standardized language could facilitate development, communication, and dissemination of nursing knowledge not only in pediatric nursing but among other specialty areas.

Programs of research are needed to replicate and extend previous studies, utilize control and comparison groups, and apply interventions to different populations or age groups. Although many are built on similar theoretical frameworks, there is little acknowledgment of previous work in planning intervention protocols or building on past studies to advance practice models. As nursing enters a phase of development where intervention testing becomes a major research focus, teams of researchers will need to work together to form research programs that can be funded and carried on over a period of years. Such programs also invite the participation of graduate students and collaboration with other researchers on multisite studies so that samples can be increased, ethnic and regional diversity ensured, and a wide range of children studied. Such research is time consuming and costly but has the potential of generating results that will be generalizable to the practice arena. Intervention protocols need to be standardized, outcome measures need to be sensitive to the effects of the intervention, and researchers need to be trained so their instructions, interventions, and observations are reliable over time and settings.

Current research studies reflect the influence of pioneers in pediatric nursing research and show an increasing level of sophistication. However, as we move toward the next century, we as a profession have little knowledge of the outcomes or effects of nursing interventions on children and families. The increasing emphasis on outcome-based care and the need for nurses to clearly show their contribution to the health of children and families will require more intervention research. Intervention studies are the most challenging and time-consuming type of research. They require knowledge, skill, cooperative settings, adequate samples, and most important, adequate funding. It is hoped that the increasing number of investigators graduating from doctoral programs in nursing will receive the needed postdoctoral training and mentoring to prepare them to become competitive in receiving the funding needed to perform studies that determine the outcomes of nursing interventions—the essence of nursing practice.

8

■

ACUTELY ILL CHILDREN AND THEIR FAMILIES

Implications for Research, Practice, and Education

■ *Marion E. Broome*

The experience of acute or critical illness and hospitalization has long been acknowledged to be a significant event for children and their families (Thompson, 1985; Vernon, Foley, Sipowicz, & Schulman, 1965). Although institutional practices related to family-centered care have made significant progress this past decade (Johnson, Jeppson, & Redburn, 1992), children and their families are still exposed to multiple stressors during an acute/critical illness. These stressors include separation from friends and family, financial concerns, painful procedures and treatments, uncertainty about their prognosis, and interruption of daily routines that lend structure and predictability to a child's life. Hospitals and other acute care agencies vary in their commitment to supporting families and in the type and amount of resources they commit to this support. These stressors can be expected to increase in number and intensity as the acuity level of children admitted to inpatient settings

increases, the time for hospitalization compresses, and the consistent presence of a professional nurse who is immediately accessible to the family becomes less likely.

Heightened levels of fear, anxiety, pain, and the decreased ability to attend to self-care instruction all delay recovery time and increase both financial and psychological costs. Interventions that nurses have implemented in the past may or may not be effective in the new health care environment. Now more than ever, research is needed to determine how to most effectively intervene to ameliorate the stress of acute illness, mobilize strengths of children and families, and facilitate their adaptation. Nursing has a rich history of inquiry that future researchers can build upon.

In this chapter, the assumptions, theoretical and empirical models that have influenced the study of acutely ill children and their families are discussed. Both future directions for research and the methods that nurse researchers must employ to study the complex phenomenon of the acute illness experience for children and their families are presented. The implications that this research has for nurses who practice with acutely and chronically ill children are identified, followed by a discussion of changes needed in nursing education to adequately prepare nurses to care for children and their families in the 21st century.

■ *Theoretical Perspectives in the Study of the Ill Child and the Family*

Assumptions Influencing Past Inquiry

In general, studies of children experiencing acute/critical illness and hospitalization have reflected several common assumptions that researchers held about children and families. As Vessey (chap. 5 in this volume) points out, the research training of nurses influenced tremendously the questions that nurse investigators asked, the methods they used to observe phenomena of interest and their interpretation of the data. Until recently, nurses were socialized at the doctoral level in disciplines outside nursing. Therefore, many of the assumptions they held and theories they applied and tested often provided less than optimal fit with the phenomenon they were studying.

Some assumptions that have influenced the study of the acute illness experience in children include the following: (a) illness is always a negative stressor for children, (b) mothers are the primary caretaker and sole influence of how a child responds to illness, and (c) adolescents respond to illness like adults. Although all of these assumptions are intuitively appealing, they lack consistent and cohesive empirical support. Yet they often influenced the perspective and methods investigators chose to study the phenomenon of illness in children. For instance, illness has not always been found to be a negative stressor for children, especially long term. Early studies of children's responses to illness and hospitalization did not follow children posthospitalization, and later studies that did reported inconsistent results (Thompson, 1985). For selected groups of children, the very young or those hospitalized for emergent conditions, hospitalization was associated with greater upset (Thompson, 1985). Yet others, especially children experiencing elective admissions, were not necessarily distressed, and in fact, the experience of hospitalization was found to provide an opportunity for growth and challenge for the family. In Knafl, Cavillari, and Dixon's (1988) qualitative study of children and families who were hospitalized, half of the families defined their role actively and felt they were essential to successful management of their child's hospitalization. Some of the children in that study even found some aspects of their hospitalization positive, such as extra attention and gifts from adults.

The second assumption, that mothers are the primary influence over how their child responds to acute/critical illness, often artificially restricted nurses' studies of family response to only mothers. Although mothers are usually the primary caretaker for ill children and do exert significant influence, other members of the family who are involved in and affected by the illness also play major roles in how the illness affects the child/children. In a recent study, for instance, Fisher (1994) found mothers and fathers with a child in the pediatric intensive care unit (PICU) rank their needs differently and place emphasis on different aspects of care. This is similar to differences that Riddle, Hennessey, Eberly, Carter, and Miles (1989) and Heuer (1993) found in mothers' and fathers' perceptions of stressors in the PICU.

Siblings' reactions have also been documented, with some beginning attempts at supportive, educational interventions (Klieber & Montgomery, 1995).

Family- and/or father-centered interventions aimed at reducing stress through involvement in the child's illness are important areas that require continued exploration. These studies will become even more of a challenge as care and health delivery systems become more fragmented and narrow in scope. Parents do not feel prepared to care for their acutely ill child at home (Maligalig, 1994). Prior to the development of these family-centered interventions however, a mid-range theory that reflects the recent changes in care delivery as they affect the entire family's response to a child's acute illness and hospitalization is needed.

More family-oriented (and less individual-focused) models, such as the Resiliency Model of Family Adjustment and Adaptation (McCubbin, Thompson, & McCubbin, 1996) could be very useful in guiding researchers to examine multiple variables that would influence child and family response to acute/critical illness from a family perspective.

The third assumption, that adolescents who are acutely/critically ill are physiologically and psychologically similar to adults, accounts in part for the minimal number of research studies with adolescents and their responses to acute/critical illness. The dearth of research is also related to the lack of measurement tools specific for adolescents, the interest of pediatric researchers in young and school-age children, the challenge of recruiting and retaining adolescents in studies, and the small numbers of adolescents who are admitted to acute care institutions for illness care. Developmentally, adolescents are very different from adults, and their responses to illness and hospitalization, as well as to interventions, are different. It cannot be assumed that the experience of acute illness and hospitalization is any less stressful/threatening for the adolescent. In fact, theoretically it could be considered to be more so (Elkind, 1985; Warady, Mudge, Wiser, Wiser, & Rader, 1996). Therefore, more exploration of adolescents' responses to acute/critical illness is necessary before meaningful intervention research can be conducted.

Nurse researchers must examine their own assumptions and biases about children, adolescents, and families as they plan their research programs. These shape our perspectives about what is important and how we study phenomena. The critical mass of pediatric nurse researchers is relatively small and the funding resources limited, so it is even more crucial that there is continual dialogue about what knowledge is important as we strive to understand children and families experiencing illness and hospitalization.

■ Models of Child and Family Response to Illness

A significant amount of progress made in the development of the knowledge base in the nursing of acutely ill children and their families. There seems to be an adequate amount of data, both quantitative and qualitative, about the needs, coping, and stress of parents and the critically ill child that nurse investigators could use to develop a mid-range theory about the phenomenon. As Youngblut (chap. 6 in this volume) points out, parents do not leave their role of protector and nurturer at the door of the hospital. In fact, parents view their child's illness as part of "a seamless continuum." Parents have told researchers that they feel a need to be vigilant and protective when their child is ill. Yet some health professionals, despite all recent rhetoric, are still having difficulty understanding the stressful and threatening nature of a child's illness and the families right to be an integral part of decisions that are made. Entire populations of children, such as the medically fragile infant and the child/adolescent with cancer, enter and leave inpatient settings frequently over the course of their treatment. Nurse researchers have an obligation to develop theory that will assist clinicians to "see how the parent sees," using existing data from the studies reviewed by Youngblut.

Parents have made dramatic adjustments in family life so as to successfully support their child during illness. Some parents are better able than others to master the additional role of parenting a child for whom illness is a major part of their life. Nurses are in a unique position to theorize and study these parents (Miles & D'Auria, 1994). Only with adequate and explicit theories guiding our intervention research will continued progress in knowledge development that impacts practice proceed. For instance, we need to know if parents and children experience less stress and recover sooner in systems in which family-centered care is a reality. For instance, there is some very interesting research on how nurse-parent interaction influences children's and families' experience of illness (Dixon, 1995). This particular line of inquiry shows promise for assisting nurses to guide their practice and improve support for families.

In summary, the research that Youngblut reviewed (chap. 6 in this volume) provides a rich field of data to be used to develop theories of family response that could then be applied by clinicians working with families. Utilization of structured models to assess families and children's responses across institutions will facilitate the collection of data to determine patterns of response and how different nursing practices affect (support or hinder) family adaptation to the illness of a child. Health care providers can have a tremendous influence on supporting (or not supporting) children and families during

this very stressful time (Doherty & McCubbin, 1985). Areas for future research include the following:

- How families and children from different cultural backgrounds negotiate the experience of illness
- How the dynamic and compressed time environment of today's health care arena affects the ways families view their role in the child's illness
- What self-care practices children, adolescents, and families use to manage the stress of the acute illness and hospitalization

■ *Models for Intervention With Acute/Critically Ill Children and Families*

Over the past 40 years, nurse researchers have attempted to build a body of knowledge to guide nurse clinicians toward effective and efficient interventions for acutely/critically ill children and their families. Even some of the earliest research was focused on nursing interventions with parents whose child was hospitalized (Wolfer & Visintainer, 1979). Studies conducted by nurses testing interventions to ameliorate the effects of hospitalization mirrored many of those by researchers in other disciplines, particularly psychology. Even the focus of inquiry has been quite similar to that conducted in psychology, for instance, the areas of play and preparation (Peterson & Brownlee-Duffeck, 1984).

Nurse investigators have made major contributions to the pain measurement and intervention literature over the past 10 years (Hester, Foster, & Kristensen, 1990). Unfortunately, other symptoms such as nausea, fatigue, and anxiety have received far less attention. To date, the majority of interventions tested have been psychosocial, although more recent studies have examined the effectiveness of nursing interventions related to temperature taking (Kachoyeanos, 1995) and the use of noninvasive monitoring of oxygenation in infants and children (Poets & Southall, 1994). This trend is a welcome one that should become even further developed with the current emphasis on patient outcomes effectiveness initiatives (National Institute of Nursing Research, 1992; Wojner, 1996).

Over the next decade, nurses must continue to focus their interventions on both physiologic and psychologic phenomena. Cost-conscious acute care facilities demand that all care delivery be scrutinized for efficacy and efficiency. For instance, programs designed to reduce anxiety in children and families prior to hospitalization, commonly referred to as value-added programs, are often threatened with elimination in the absence of data that clearly supports that they make a difference in patient outcomes. Many aspects of physical care and treatment of the acutely ill child/adolescent have to be evaluated not only for cost-effectiveness but for the contribution that each nursing action makes to patient recovery and/or satisfaction. All nursing policies and procedures are required to be research based (Joint Commission for the Accreditation of Healthcare Organizations, 1996), but the processes used to assure this are less than clear or consistent. Important questions to answer include the following: What process of literature review is used, and who critiques the existing research? When the research is conflicting, how are nursing trials developed to ensure that the policy and procedures are valid?

As Denehy and colleagues (chap. 7 in this volume) point out, some progress has been made in identifying and describing nursing interventions, primarily through the Nursing Interventions Classification Project (NIC; McCloskey & Bulechek, 1996). Standardized language for selected nursing interventions is available, and work has begun on testing some of the interventions. Pediatric nurse researchers should make a concerted effort to examine the validity and effectiveness of interventions already identified.

Intervention research in pediatrics poses several challenges that nurse researchers will have to address as this body of research proceeds. These challenges can be characterized as issue related: (a) theoretical adequacy, (b) design and methodology, (c) adequate sampling strategies, (d) instrument development, and (e) innovative analyses.

Theoretical Adequacy

It is crucial that work continue related to the delineation and testing of interventions for children and their families. Nurse researchers in acute care settings must work closely with nurses in practice and other health care professionals to develop innovative models of intervention research. As Denehy and colleagues (chap. 7 in this volume) point out, intervention models have rarely been clearly explicated. This is not unique to nursing science. Often, nurse researchers have "borrowed" and adapted interventions from other disciplines and yet have not described the interventions in such a way as to facilitate reproducibility and close examination. Theoretical bases for interventions that are borrowed sometimes fall short. The original theory may not provide as good a fit in the new context in terms of its ability to predict the new phenomenon of interest. One example would be a child's cognitive ability to use preparation techniques when experiencing the stress of a short-stay hospitalization.

We also need to know much more about how interventions and intervention research affect acutely ill children, adolescents, and their families. Quantitative data are limited in their ability to examine the process of why families chose to be involved in research, the difference in those who do not participate, emotional and psychological effects of research participation, and how research changes how families manage the experience of illness (Committee on Bioethics, 1995). This knowledge can be gained only by talking to children and families. And "knowing children" requires investigators to use a variety of creative approaches when conducting research with children (Fine & Sandstrom, 1988).

More of our theoretical frameworks in nursing must be further developed by students and researchers in nursing to better address research concerns posed when studying children, adolescents, and families. Few pediatric nurses believe that children are only dependent-care agents (Orem, 1992) or are incapable of setting goals for themselves related to their illness (King, 1981). The focus of most nursing models on the individual (versus the family) limit, somewhat, their applicability to children within families. Until nursing models are further developed, family-centered models, such as the Family Adjustment and Adaptation Response Model (FAAR; Patterson, 1995), might provide a more useful framework for examining the complexities of child and family responses to illness and interventions (Patterson, 1995).

Designs and Methods

Intervention research with acute/critically ill children has primarily employed cross-sectional designs and pretest-posttest methods of measurement. These cross-sectional designs are limited in that they give only a snapshot of how the child and/or family is responding at one point in time. The issues of using cross-sectional designs are even more timely now that the average length of stay in inpatient settings is 3.2 days (National Association of Children's Hospitals and Related Institutions, 1996). Because discharge from the hospital does not necessarily signal the end but, rather, only one point on a continuum of illness care, testing interventions for their long-term efficacy and their feasibility across settings is an important area on which to focus inquiry. Yet crossing settings becomes a challenge for any investigator. Control over access to participants, the need for multiple Institutional Research Review Board (IRB) approvals when the research is implemented in more than one setting, and the need for closer supervision of data collectors become central issues for the research team.

Not only should interventions be standardized, but describing how research participants actually use interventions is necessary (Broome, Rehwaldt, & Foley, 1995). This is especially important when self-care activities and programs for children and families are developed and tested. Clearly outlined and articulated concepts and skills, the use of methods and materials that parents and children can use to reinforce their learning, and consistent plans for reinforcers and follow-up are all necessary components of a sound intervention model (Egan, Snyder, & Burns, 1992).

Although it is necessary to clearly describe the intervention being tested, once implemented, it may not always be possible (or even desirable) to adhere strictly to the intervention procedure, in spite of what participants in our studies tell us. Researchers must have clearly defined aims and goals for the interventions and do the necessary groundwork and exploration to find the best fit possible with the participants they will study and the goals they have for managing this investigation. Most important, investigators must then carefully listen and document what happens during implementation of the intervention. Researchers can no longer afford to ignore the process of intervention implementation while we are busy evaluating the outcomes if we are to develop meaningful, reproducible, and generalizable interventions for children and their families.

Measurement Issues

There was, until recently, few developmentally appropriate instruments designed for use with children and adolescents. It is challenging to measure variables associated with children, especially if that measurement requires a rapport and interaction with the child. Many nurse researchers were trained in fields other than nursing and brought back skills in interviewing adults along with theories that may or may not have translated well for children. Nurse researchers should consider developing networks with researchers in other fields, such as psychology, child and family development, and education. Investigators in these fields have a wealth of measurement expertise to call upon, complement nurse researchers, and strengthen research teams in health care.

Measurement burden also becomes an issue, especially when working with ill children and their families. Completing numerous questionnaires, being videotaped during invasive procedures, and submitting to multiple interviews can be very intrusive for families with an ill child. Many of the naturalistic settings in which we find ill children and families are highly charged emotionally and require a sensitive, compassionate approach to the child and family. This means that all members of the research team must be socialized and trained to be constantly aware of the burdens families carry in these settings and the tremendous debt that researchers owe to those who share their experiences with them.

Sampling Strategies

Children and families in most nursing intervention research have typically been small, primarily middle class, and Caucasian (Beal & Betz, 1992, 1993). Although a great deal of knowledge has been gained that can be used to build future research (Broome & Knafl, 1994), these findings may or may not be generalizable. Children and families seen in the health care system now are much more likely to be culturally and economically diverse. Just as nurses' training as researchers has colored their perspective about what questions, methods, and interpretations of investigations influence their work, so will their cultural and economic backgrounds influence that work. Nursing research in general is not culturally competent yet, although many investigators are struggling with some very complex and difficult questions (Villarruel, 1995).

It is not just the composition of samples that has to change, it is the approaches used to study children's and families' responses to health and illness. To expand research to other than Caucasian, middle-class samples, nurse researchers must become culturally competent. Cultural competence has been defined as "the capacity to function effectively in cross-cultural settings" (Cross, Bazron, & Dennis, 1989, as cited in Villarruel, 1995, p. 38). Villarruel (1995) developed a set of criteria for critiquing whether a research study has reflected characteristics of cultural competence and made the important point that assembling a multicultural research team is only the first step in successfully implementing an investigation with culturally diverse populations.

Another sampling issue that plagues pediatric nurse researchers is small samples (Beal & Betz, 1992), which is most likely a reflection of the small numbers of ill children seen in any one health system. Also, chronically ill children represent various ages and diagnoses and are on different treatment regimens. This presents a great deal of extraneous variability that threatens researchers' ability to generalize or even to find differences. To obtain sufficient numbers of children and families in studies, infrastructures must be built that facilitate multisite trials, a relatively new phenomenon in nursing that will require leadership from experienced researchers if it is to be successful. The

Society of Pediatric Nursing (SPN) built such a structure in 1996 and is currently testing a distraction protocol to reduce pain distress in children during moderately painful procedures (Broome, Carlson, & Vessey, 1997). The focus of this multisite trial is research utilization rather than original research; however, the infrastructures will be available in the future for clinical trials of nursing interventions. The SPN is also collaborating with other organizations, such as the American Association for Critical Care Nurses (ACCN) on the Thunder Project (AACN, 1997), an original research project designed to generate more knowledge about how children in critical care (as well as adults) respond to painful procedures. Advantages of these multisite trials are accessibility to a large pool of participants, increased ability to generalize findings based on a broad-based pool of participants, and the collective wisdom of experienced researchers working in a variety of settings. Costs in terms of money and time associated with the need to meet frequently to ensure consistency of data collection policy and procedures, the potential for team conflict and varying interpretations of data collected by the numerous teams are some of the challenges that must be addressed. However, there is great potential for progress in knowledge development.

Analysis Strategies

Nurse researchers have traditionally focused much of their attention on looking for group differences effects and not at the phenomenon of intragroup variability. Given the nature of human beings and the wide diversity and complexities that each participant brings to a study, it should not be surprising that variability within groups on variables of interest can be even greater than that between groups. One traditional approach to handling variability within and across groups is to randomly select and assign individuals to treatments. Randomization assumes that the researcher is aware of all important variables. However, even randomization does not always assure equal distribution of all variables, so examination of within-group effects is essential. In the future, one of the most important challenges will be to develop individualized interventions that can be tested with groups of children. To understand how individual differences in children influence an intervention, more descriptive and qualitative work is needed prior to testing. This kind of work will provide nurse researchers with the knowledge they need to decide, a priori, how to tailor and test their interventions.

■ *Future Directions for Inquiry*

The priorities for research in children with acute/critical illness and their families have changed markedly over the past decade. In two studies on the development of nursing research activities in children's hospitals (Frink, Feeg, & Dienneman, 1992; Feetham, Keefe, & Barnsteiner, 1987), two thirds of the respondents reported nurses were engaged in the utilization of research findings in practice, the systematic collection of data to make nursing decisions, and the design and planning of nursing studies. Hospitals who employed a doctorally prepared nurse with research in her job description and who had a research committee were more likely to have more complete research programs in place. Quality of care, patient care delivery, and fiscal issues were listed as the top three priorities.

In the clinical arena, a Delphi study by Broome, Woodring, and O'Connor-Von (1996) found that priority topics listed by pediatric nurse experts reflected a strong shift toward testing interventions, family responses, and community-based interventions for ill children. For instance, interventions designed to reduce the stress of illness and hospitalization are offered by schools and churches to well and chronically ill children. The effect of these intervention studies needs to be evaluated. Another example is the use of "just in time" interventions delivered where parents are and when they need them. Shorter stays can result in more anxiety and lower levels of pain and less information for parents, due to compressed time for preoperative and discharge planning. Researchers should also consider using technology, such as videotapes or the Internet, to provide information and reinforce concepts after discharge when parents need them.

Research models must facilitate out-of-the-box thinking that will enable researchers and clinicians to develop and test new approaches to caring for children and families. Researchers should remain skeptical about whether old data and knowledge obtained when the health care system provided services in a slower paced environment are still valid. Although it seems intuitively plausible that parents will be highly anxious about taking their child home sooner than in previous years, it is also theoretically possible that the level of anxiety is a result of the time of exposure to the stressor and that decreased exposure to hospitalization reduces anxiety. It is also possible that parents learn more about their child's illness when they realize they will be assuming much of the traditional nursing care their child would have received in the hospital.

Studies across settings are very complex and require a great deal of attention to the logistics of collecting data. Once a researcher moves out of the health care system and into a family's home, control over timing and collection of data lessens. Negotiations with families, built on relationships established between participants and the research team, are important for successful implementation of a project. Research teams are often at the mercy of very busy families' schedules. Researchers need to adopt the concept of following the families and

adapting to their schedule (Huttlinger, Wesley, & Kulwicki, 1996). In these community-based studies, funding becomes even more important, as travel time and costs are involved. Incentives for participating should be considered. Compensating the child and family for their time spent in a research study, their effort and energy, and their thoughts and experiences should be reflected in all funding proposals. Incentives send an important message to children and families about the value of their time and knowledge.

Research utilization, patient outcomes studies, and clinical practice guidelines testing will consume more and more of the acute care researcher's time and attention in the future. A number of guidelines and standards documents available to nurses in acute care settings provide direction for priority setting and care delivery (Agency for Health Care Policy and Research, 1992; National Association of Children's Hospitals and Related Institutions, 1996). These documents reflect the consensus of clinical and administrative experts about the level of care that should be available to all children and their families when being treated for an acute/critical illness. For some, the shift from generating knowledge to developing ways for nurses and other health professionals to use existing knowledge to improve practice will be a challenge. Early literature on research utilization required a great volume of research on a specific topic before a utilization study was done (Horsley, Crane, Crabtree, & Wood, 1983). Although in many areas the volume of studies has increased, the rigor has not necessarily followed. Whether the health care system, with its demanding and rapidly changing dynamics, is ready to wait to change practice until enough studies are done is questionable.

Nurse researchers will face pressures from a variety of sources to promote changes in care delivery models without sufficient data to support some of these changes. These researchers must develop mechanisms to measure the effectiveness of these changes on quality of care and cost. Because the delivery system is in a state of flux, rigorous studies will be a challenge to implement. Yet it is crucial that nurse researchers develop "think tank" networks within and outside their institution to support their own ability to implement relevant and rigorous investigations. In the past, children's hospitals that were actively involved in research had an infrastructure in place that provided support, including a chief nurse executive officer, a core group of individuals committed to research activity, and a support staff (Davies & Eng, 1993). Cost containment and budget reductions have increased demands on clinicians' time, and many of these resources have been reallocated. Yet they are critically needed if nurses are to base their practice on research.

■ Implications for Practice

The emphasis on patient outcomes effectiveness began several years ago (National Institute of Nursing Research, 1992) as costs became unrestrained and demands for measurable progress in patient status based on treatment increased. As clinical practice guidelines development proceeds, usually under strong leadership from nurses, patient outcomes research will be commonplace. The National Association of Children's Hospitals and Related Institutions (1996) focus group project provides an excellent model for bringing together expert clinicians and researchers to define practice parameters, patient outcomes, and standards of care. Now is the time to test these standards and measure their effectiveness on outcomes.

Nurses have been active and knowledgeable participants in this process. It is through concerted sharing of knowledge and experience that cumulative progress occurs. Although progress is evident, challenges to progress remain.

Research in acute care facilities requires political skills and a high level of credibility across disciplines. Priorities for care in inpatient settings focuses on physiologically and psychologically supportive care. Research and data collection is sometimes viewed by clinicians in those settings as intrusive and burdensome for children, families, and themselves. The disparate worldviews of the clinical and research world can lead to a system in which researchers enter and leave the acute care setting as a guest. Meaningful partnerships between researchers and clinicians are necessary if relevant, rigorous research is to continue. Researchers, for their part, can decrease some of the tension by viewing clinicians as expert members of the research team, whose role can inform the implementation of the design and interpretation of the data. Clinicians have the responsibility to provide input in a timely and assertive fashion, seeing themselves as important members of the team, and be willing to remain invested for often protracted periods of time as the research unfolds. In systems that are successful, there is the clear expectation that all professionals base their practice on research and be active participants in ongoing systematic research.

Another challenge will be related to how research, quality improvement, and program evaluation are defined. Outcomes research has blurred many of the traditional distinctions. Many current discussions still revolve around philosophical distinctions of the past, which often appear meaningless in today's rapidly changing environments that make changes based on no data, much less data collected in a systematic fashion. Program evaluation, or impact analysis in outcomes research, has become even more essential as institutions scrutinize all initiatives and programs within the system, especially those perceived by some to be value added and not having direct linkages to increasing quality, efficiency, or decreasing cost.

Nurse researchers can make valuable contributions, based on their knowledge of design and analyses, to the evaluation of programs. One useful model is the CIPP model, first described by Stuffelbeam (1983), that focuses on the formative evaluation of context, input, process, and product (Kennedy-Malone, 1996; Stuffelbeam, 1983).

Program evaluation used to be viewed as a less rigorous form of research in many nursing programs. Yet many advanced practice nurses and researchers in health care agencies find themselves responsible for evaluating the effectiveness of a variety of programs and projects. Ideally, the elements of program evaluation are built into the program as the project is conceptualized. Retrospectively collecting data can be cumbersome and, in many cases, results in an inadequate and incomplete database from which to draw conclusions about the cost and efficacy of the program (Fink, 1993).

Finally, another important challenge will be to assist clinicians to use the knowledge gleaned from research. There is a vast amount of research on many clinical topics and researchers can provide valuable support in assisting clinicians to synthesize and interpret existing research.

Even graduate nurses who have developed skills and competencies related to research will find it challenging to access, read, and reflect on the literature. Most professional nurses have little time for library searches or reading articles. Yet there are clear expectations set for research behaviors in most evaluations currently used in institutions. Nurses who are critical thinkers, who actively and continually evaluate the care they deliver, and who are open to new ideas are outstanding resources for any institution. Resources must be provided that enable these nurses to maintain these skills. The work of care delivery must be restructured

to free up the professional nurses' time to evaluate and plan care that is responsive to children's and families' needs and is cost-effective for the system.

The collection of data on the health status and outcomes for groups of patients has become a major responsibility for advanced practice nurses (APNs) as well as nurse managers in today's health care agencies. Analysis of these data for trends and factors that influence different outcomes requires a certain degree of skill and experience in research methods and statistical analyses. In a recent study of APNs' perceptions of their future role, many believed that more emphasis was being placed on the research component of their role in order to document outcomes (Hester & White, 1996). Examples cited were the development of critical pathways and outcomes management. Research content, over and above the required research courses, was rated very important by the APNs in that survey, suggesting they believed that competency in research was just as important as other components of their role.

■ *Educational Mandates*
   for the 21st Century

For the past two decades, the nursing literature has called for clinicians to base their practice on research. One major impediment to this has been the predominance of nurses who are prepared in preliscensure programs that do not include research courses. This lack of exposure hampers the graduate nurse who is interested in using the latest research to guide practice. Even in baccalaureate degree programs, research content is often isolated within a single research course, and few readings required for clinical courses include original research articles (Broome, 1995). Educators often rely too heavily on textbooks for reading assignments and, due to large class sizes, base their evaluation of learning on multiple-choice tests. These strategies, although useful for some type of content and for some students at selected points, do not produce critical thinkers who will later be excited about accessing current research while providing care for children. Educating young students in nursing to learn to think critically, analyze existing knowledge, and integrate that knowledge into practice requires the use of a variety of learning strategies, many of which are delineated in "Standards and Guidelines for Prelicensure and Early Professional Education" (Pridham, Broome, Woodring, & Baroni, 1996).

Graduate programs across the country have cut their requirements for research in the master's program, leaving many concerned that there will be no new generation of nurse researchers in child health/pediatrics. The transition of many graduate programs to practitioner programs and the addition of doctoral programs have crowded out much of the content and time devoted to research activities in master's programs. This is very unfortunate and must be reconsidered. Advanced practice nurses must possess adequate knowledge and skill to conceptualize and evaluate the effectiveness of clinical interventions and programs. They also will be expected to actively collaborate with other health professionals on research projects. Active collaboration requires that all members of the team bring unique skills and knowledge to a study. Successful collaboration requires a great deal of skill and experience, usually acquired after years of working with teams. Essential skills for successful collaborative research include a willingness to actively seek and use feedback from team members, strong communication and organization abilities, an awareness of group process dynamics, and the ability to clearly explicate goals and methods and a strong sense of accountability

to the research project, the participants, and the team itself. The groundwork for this knowledge and skill base in research must be built in graduate programs of nursing in pediatrics, or the already existing shortage of individuals prepared to conduct, implement, and evaluate research will shrink even further. Ultimately, the care of children and their families will suffer.

■ *Summary and Conclusions*

Research in acute care pediatric nursing will change dramatically over the next decade. Three major foci will become evident:

- Generation of basic knowledge about children's physiologic and psychologic responses to acute/critical illness and how their families manage these episodes
- Evaluation of nursing and patient care interventions on patient and family outcomes
- Study of patient care delivery models and how they influence the cost and quality of care delivered to acutely/critically ill children and their families

Methods also will change. More repeated measures, longitudinal designs that enable teams of investigators to cross settings will become the norm. Parents and children will be major players in research programs. No longer will their consent alone be sufficient. Instead, they will help researchers (a) shape the questions asked, (b) decide what strategies to use for collecting information, and (c) interpret the results.

To do meaningful research that will shape health care practices focused on children and their families, nurse researchers have some important groundwork to do. Pediatric nurses should not only test the intervention taxonomies already in place but develop clinical trials in which these interventions are then evaluated for their efficiency and effectiveness in facilitating the child's and family's return to optimal functioning. New research models should be built on what has been learned from the past (Broome & Knafl, 1994), and the research must be extended to encompass families from diverse cultures and across settings. Children and families come to the health care delivery settings at a time when they are vulnerable and seek essential services that hopefully build on their family strengths to improve their child's health and well-being. Nurse researchers have an obligation to use valid, reliable, and relevant information to guide practice. These children and their families deserve no less.

PART III

RESPONSES OF CHILDREN AND FAMILIES TO CHRONIC ILLNESS

■ *Kathleen A. Knafl, Editor*

9

■

HISTORICAL OVERVIEW OF RESPONSES OF CHILDREN AND THEIR FAMILIES TO CHRONIC ILLNESS

■ *Sandra A. Faux*

The mother, torn with anxiety, without the special knowledge which the nurse has, steps aside and into her place . . . giving that affection which the child needs but without that emotional tension which might make her unwise. . . . Possibly the methods used by his parents have hardly deserved the name of method, so inconsistent have they been. She may find that she has to deal with a child who has constantly been deceived by false statements . . . for she [the nurse] must counteract methods to which the child has been subjected, methods which according to her training are founded on reason and understanding.

—P. C. Jeans, W. Rand, and F. G. Blake (1946, p. 8)

Since the 1950s, nurses have been actively involved in examining their practice through research; for pediatric nurses, there has been a shift in the focus of their practice over the past 40 years. In 1950, acutely and chronically ill children were cared for in hospitals and other institutions with severely restricted parental visiting privileges; moreover, children with chronic illnesses rarely survived. Today, advances in health care have prolonged and improved the lives of children with chronic illness, and the majority of children are cared for by their families in their homes and communities.

This chapter provides an overview of nursing research on children with chronic illness and their families. The review encompasses studies done from 1950 to the present and is grounded in an initial discussion of the major societal and health care trends that have shaped the experiences of chronically ill children and their families over time. The discussion of research is organized around three major domains reflecting the major foci of nursing research: the individual experience, the family experience, and the family-provider interface.

■ *Societal and Health Care Trends*

Chronicity

Medical advances over the past 40 years have dramatically reduced the number of children who die from acute and chronic conditions. Consequently, there is an ever-growing population of children living with chronic conditions, some of which they are born with and some of which develop over time. A chronic health condition is one that is long term and is not curable or involves limitations in daily living requiring special assistance or adaptation in function (Perrin, 1985). These ongoing health problems also include sequelae such as limitations of functions appropriate for age and development, disfigurement, dependency on medication, special diet, or dependency on medical technology, need for medical care or related services greater than usual for the child's age, and/or special ongoing treatments at home or in school (Jessop & Stein, 1988; Stein, 1992).

It has been estimated that 31%, or approximately 20 million American children under age 18, have one or more chronic conditions. Of these, two thirds have mild conditions with minimal activity limitations, and 5% have severe conditions that constantly limit their activities (Newacheck & Taylor, 1992). Currently, an estimated 1% to 2% of the childhood population has a severe chronic illness (Perrin, 1985). Several factors have contributed to these trends: improved early diagnosis and treatment of chronic health conditions, increased empha-

sis on health promotion and maintenance, and the identification of new groups of children with chronic illnesses or disabilities.

Improved diagnosis and treatment have increased the life expectancy of children who previously died in infancy or childhood. For example, in 1966 the median survival age for a child with cystic fibrosis was 11 years; in 1993 it was 29.4 years (Cystic Fibrosis Foundation, 1992). Also, with more health promotion and maintenance measures available within the health care system, chronically ill children experience less morbidity (i.e., fewer acute illness episodes and missed school days; Turner-Henson & Holaday, 1995).

In addition, entirely new categories of chronically ill children have been created through the use of advanced technology or the appearance of new conditions. These include low- and very-low-birth-weight infants with permanent physical and neurological sequelae, children with organ transplants, cancer survivors, technology-dependent children, children who are HIV positive or have AIDS, and those with prenatal drug and alcohol exposure. Consequently, a larger proportion of families and children in the population are confronting and coping with illnesses that extend over substantial periods of their lives and may involve continuous, complex care.

Chronic childhood illness continues to be defined as an ongoing stressor for children and families, resulting in a variety of problems. For example, some researchers have found that children with chronic illness are almost three times more likely to have behavioral or emotional problems, particularly if they are from poorly functioning families (Thompson & Gustafson, 1996). Although acknowledging the challenges confronting families of children with chronic illness, other authors (Feetham, 1984; Wright & Leahey, 1990) point to the importance of recognizing family strengths as well as problems in meeting the challenges of childhood chronic illness. The enduring goal of health care providers has been to develop interventions that enhance child and family adaptation and quality of life.

Historical Perspectives on Children With Chronic Illness and Their Families

Children

Forty years ago children with chronic illnesses who survived were primarily cared for in hospitals and institutions, often for lengthy periods of time (Hobbs, Perrin, & Ireys, 1985). Children's care and support were the foci of nurses and physicians, with little attention paid to the children's families. Although maternal love and care were recognized as important, families were viewed as not having the skill or knowledge to care for their ill children, often employing poor child-rearing practices, being overprotective or overindulgent, and fostering dependence (Dixon, 1996; Young, 1992). Consequently, nurses perceived themselves as better able to provide the best care and often viewed themselves as mother substitutes. If the child was sent home, professional health care experts dictated how the family should behave and care for their child. In addition, the illness or disability of the child was assumed to put the child at risk for psychopathology, depression, and emotional and social retardation (Gortmaker, Walker, Weitzman, & Sobol, 1990).

There have been dramatic changes over the decades in how a child with a chronic illness is perceived and cared for by health care professionals. No longer are children viewed in isolation from their families. In fact, the term *family-centered* care has been used to indicate quality health care for children and families. Concepts, such as self-efficacy and self-care, have altered how families and health care professionals in-

teract with one another. The view of chronically ill children has shifted from perceiving them as isolated, incapable individuals needing constant support and protection to seeing them as individuals who are integral, accepted members of families and communities and capable of managing their own illnesses (Deatrick, Angst, & Madden, 1994).

Family

Prior to 1960, families of chronically ill children were rarely considered in planning the nursing care of children with chronic illness or a disability, and parents were often viewed as incompetent to provide adequate care for their seriously ill children. However, with the work of Bowlby (1969) and Robertson (1958) came recognition of the importance of maintaining family ties for the emotional and psychological well-being of the hospitalized child. As a result, there was a dramatic shift from perceiving the family as incapable of caring for an ill child to viewing the family as essential to the child's care (Rosenthal, Marshall, MacPherson, & French, 1980). This shift in perspective led to such innovations as open visiting hours, rooming-in, and family involvement in care (Dixon, 1996). New, more family-centered policies brought health care providers and family members into more frequent contact with one another. These increased contacts raised questions about appropriate roles for family members in the care of an ill or hospitalized child and led to a number of studies describing the kinds of relationships that develop between family members and health care providers (Kirschbaum & Knafl, 1996; Rosenthal et al., 1980; Thorne, 1993).

■ Domains of Research

In the past two decades, knowledge about chronically ill children and their families has expanded dramatically (Beck, 1988). Increasing numbers of better prepared nurse researchers have led to more sophisticated, better designed studies, with several authors documenting the growth and progress in child and family research (Austin, 1991; Beal & Betz, 1992; Beck, 1988; Burke & Roberts, 1990). The majority of the research can be categorized as focused on either the individual or family experience, or the interaction between the hospital and the family:

The overwhelming research focus of nurse investigators during the past 30 years has been on the levels of stress experienced by chronically ill children and their parents and how they coped and adapted. Whether viewing childhood chronic illness from a psychoanalytic, systems, developmental, or stress and coping framework, nurses have sought to capture this experience based on the assumption that nursing interventions would then be developed to reduce the stress and anxiety experienced by children and families. Initially, interventions focused on alleviating the stresses encountered in hospitals and included preparation for procedures and treatments, alleviation of pain, implementation of open visiting hours and rooming-in, and use of play and other projective techniques to reduce and master stress (Vessey, chap. 5 in this volume).

The Individual Experience

> If the parents reject a child's handicap, the child may think that he is not liked as a person. As parents may resent and reject the child, the nurse should make every effort to further good relationships between the child and his family. (Latham & Heckel, 1972, p. 326)

This section discusses research on the individual experience of chronic illness. Studies that address how children and adolescents respond to chronic illness initially and over time and those that address parental responses to childhood chronic illness are reviewed here. In the following section, studies that consider chronic illness from a family perspective are reviewed.

Children and Adolescents

Investigators have directed their attention to a number of topics related to how children and adolescents respond to chronic illness. This section considers studies that have focused on the period surrounding the initial diagnosis, ongoing stress and coping, functioning and adaptation, and self-care. Nurse researchers, in describing how children and adolescents have responded to the stress of having a chronic illness, have sought to identify the children's and adolescents' responses to the initial diagnosis, stresses and coping strategies, and individual functioning in the context of chronic illness. Chronic illness has been postulated to affect multiple areas of child/adolescent functioning, including body image, self-concept, social competence, and illness knowledge (Hobbs et al., 1985; LaVigne & Faier-Routman, 1993).

Initial Diagnosis

As Vessey (chap. 5 in this volume) has noted, nursing research conducted with chronically ill children in the 1970s focused on children's behaviors and responses to being hospitalized and their reactions to the illness, the hospital environment, and treatments. Parents and nurses, as opposed to the child or adolescent, typically were the source of data for these studies. Only recently have nurse investigators obtained data directly from children regarding their experiences of dealing with chronic illness or disability (Charron-Prochownik, Kovacs, Obrosky, & Ho, 1995; Dewis, 1989; Grey, Cameron, Lipman, & Thurber, 1994; Kieckhefer, 1988; Kyngas & Barlow, 1995; Ory & Kronenfeld, 1980). Much of this recent research points to the adaptability of children and adolescents in meeting the challenges of illness.

Dewis (1989) discussed the initial reactions of adolescents following spinal cord injury and found that they described feeling normal and actively worked to live what they viewed as a normal life. In a similar vein, Grey and colleagues' (1994) examination of initial responses to a diagnosis of diabetes, found no differences between newly diagnosed children and healthy children on the variables of depression, anxiety, adjustment, and self-perception. They reported that diabetic children were less withdrawn and more likely to cope by ventilating feelings than a comparison group of healthy children (Grey et al., 1994). Researchers are beginning to make progress in giving voice to those children who have chronic illnesses, and their efforts provide important insights for clinicians.

Ongoing Stress and Coping

In the earliest published descriptions of children's stress and coping responses, the clinical and single case studies published in *Maternal-Child Nursing Journal* documented young children's behaviors as they dealt with the illness experience, which included aggression, anger, and coping using play, language, and activity. Over 80 studies focusing on children's illness experiences were published between 1970 and 1990 (Faux & Deatrick, 1991), and they provide a rich source of information on this important topic. For example, Dittemore (1983) described the therapeutic use of play by a severely burned child and Carey (1976) described children's independence-seeking behaviors after a kidney transplant. These early studies, such as Woods's (1979) description of a deaf child's reaction to hospitalization and Scanlon's (1985) account of a toddler's response to multiple hospitalization, guided subsequent researchers' efforts to explore these phenomena with larger samples. Drawing on published case studies, Caty, Ellerton, and Ritchie (1984) developed a measure of stress

and coping for hospitalized chronically ill children. In a later study, they described the concerns and stressors of hospitalized chronically ill toddlers and preschoolers (Caty, Ritchie, & Ellerton, 1989).

The majority of stress and coping studies conducted over the past 20 years with children and adolescents focused primarily on school-age children and adolescents, with very little attention paid to infants, toddlers, and preschoolers. For example, sources of stress and coping behaviors were examined in school-age children and adolescents with asthma (Carrieri, Kieckhefer, Janson-Bjerklie, & Souza, 1991; Ryan-Wenger & Walsh, 1994; Walsh & Ryan-Wenger, 1992). These authors found that, overall, stress levels and coping strategies were comparable to healthy children, with the exception of girls with asthma who reported feeling sick more frequently and perceived themselves as more pressured by parents (Walsh & Ryan-Wenger, 1992).

Using Lazarus and Folkman's (1984) theory of stress and coping, Spitzer (1992b, 1992c, 1993) explored coping and appraisal patterns of school-age children with hemophilia. Spitzer identified two approaches to appraisal: amplifying when threats occurred and minimizing when few threats were noted. Knowledge and past experiences were used to manage anxiety and reduce fear, suggesting that, over time, children learn, affecting coping strategies.

One focus of the stress and coping research has been on exploring factors that contribute to children's resiliency in coping with the stresses of chronic illness. Burke (1980, 1986a, 1986b; Burke & Wiskin, 1984) developed a model of risk, vulnerability, resilience, and competence to describe children with chronic stress who handled stress with "extraordinary competence." In one of the rare studies of infants, Morrow (1995), who suggested that temperament is a stress mediator, found that infants with myelomingocele were rated by their mothers as less active but more approachable and adaptable than children in a control group of healthy infants. However, maternal evaluations were significantly related to mothers' age and education.

The interaction of environment with chronic illness continues to be explored with hospitalized children and adolescents (Hart & Bossert, 1994; Keller & Nicholls, 1990; Nuttall & Nicholls, 1992; Patton, Ventura, & Savedra, 1986; Pederson & Harbaugh, 1995; Stevens, 1986). Hart and Bossert (1994), using a tool developed by Broome and colleagues (Broome & Hellier, 1987; Broome, Hellier, Wilson, Dale, & Glenville, 1988), found that hospitalization led to intensification of chronically ill children's fears regarding their illness. Other researchers have found that adolescents who experience frequent hospitalizations, as a result of their chronic condition, view them as socially disruptive, with hospitalization itself associated with pain, anxiety, invasions of privacy, heightened awareness of knowledge deficits, and limited involvement in decision making (Nuttall & Nicholls, 1992; Pederson & Harbaugh, 1995; Stevens, 1986).

Child and Adolescent Functioning and Adaptation

Early nursing studies identified various negative outcomes for children and adolescents with chronic illness. Qualitative research, in particular, has contributed to understanding how children and adolescents adapt to illness and procedures, such as limb amputation and cancer. The earliest nursing report of children's responses to impairment was Stoll's (1969) description of the reactions of 3 girls to severe burns. In a subsequent grounded theory study, Kueffner (1975) observed 6 severely burned children throughout their hospitalizations and described distinct stages of recovery (i.e., agony, hope, and reorganization). Other early investigations documented a variety of responses

and outcomes of children and adolescents to chronic illness. Holaday (1974) found that children with a chronic illness exhibited lower achievement behaviors than did their healthy peers and that boys specifically avoided achievement situations. Garlinghouse and Sharp (1968) studied hemophiliac children and found positive correlations between frequency and duration of bleeding episodes and maternal stress levels. Researchers in the 1980s and 1990s continued to address the correlates of child and adolescent adaptation to illness, paying increased attention to the strengths that supported successful adaptation (Fulton & Moore, 1995; Haase, 1987; Hinds, 1984, 1988; Hinds & Martin, 1988).

An early longitudinal case study of a severely burned girl (Dittemore, 1983) equated disfigurement with distorted body image. However, other studies conducted since then have found little measurable impact of chronic illness on children's and adolescents' self-concept, when compared with healthy children (Macbriar, 1983; Saucier & Clark, 1994). Mobley, Harless, and Miller (1996) compared the self-portraits and self-competence scores of preschool children with spina bifida with those of healthy preschoolers. Those with spina bifida produced less sophisticated drawings, with fewer body parts (e.g., no legs or feet), and were considered less physically and cognitively competent than their peers. The researchers speculated that these differences were the result of the impaired children being aware that they are different (Mobley et al., 1996).

Social competence has been used as an indicator of child adaptation in two recent studies. Breitmayer, Gallo, Knafl, and Zoeller (1992) studied 66 children, ages 7–14 years, afflicted with a variety of chronic illnesses and found that mothers' perceptions of competence increased with maternal socioeconomic and educational status. However, both mothers and fathers felt that their children were at greater risk for social competence difficulties than did parents of children comprising a normative sample. Pless and colleagues (1994) also used social competence as the measure of chronically ill children's psychological health in a study to assess the effectiveness of a family nursing intervention. Nelms (1989) examined empathy, emotional responses, and depression with school-age diabetic and asthmatic children and reported no significant differences between the groups; however, the diabetic children were found to be the most aggressive.

In studying diabetic children, Grey and her colleagues (Grey et al., 1994; Grey, Cameron, & Thurber, 1991; Grey, Genet, & Tamborlane, 1980; Grey & Thurber, 1991) explored the relationship between psychosocial variables and physiological parameters in evaluating metabolic control among diabetic children. All of these studies found that moderate to severe adjustment problems related with poorer control, a finding consistent with that of other researchers (Lawler, Volk, Viviani, & Mengel, 1990).

Self-Care

Other investigators found that children often have a poor understanding of their illness. Such misunderstandings could compromise the child's ability to engage in competent self-care.

As chronically ill children mature and are capable of providing for their own needs, they become developmentally able to assume certain self-care responsibilities. In fact, a child's or adolescent's gradually increasing assumption of care is generally considered an indicator of positive adjustment to the illness or disability (Deatrick et al., 1994). Also, because providers seek to promote self-care, self-efficacy, self-regulation, and self-management in children with chronic illness, these concepts have been the focus of many studies. It has been found that younger adolescents with a chronic illness

exhibit better health care practices than older adolescents and that cognitive maturity, self-esteem, and perception of control over outcomes affect how children and adolescents implement self-care practices (Denyes, 1980; Frey & Denyes, 1989; Frey & Fox, 1990; Gaut & Kieckhefer, 1988; Heamon, 1995; Holaday, Turner-Henson, Harkins, & Swan, 1993; Kieckhefer, 1987; Monsen, 1992; Rew, 1987a, 1987b; Saucier, 1984). Children's involvement in decision making about medical and surgical treatments is another aspect of self-care that has been of interest to investigators. Older adolescents undergoing surgery tend to be included more frequently in care decisions by parents and health care professionals (Angst & Deatrick, 1996; Deatrick, 1984).

Based on Piaget's (1969) cognitive theory, children's knowledge of their illness and bodies has been examined and related to levels of stress and adjustment. Neff and Beardslee (1990), Gibbons (1985), and Spitzer (1992a) all found that children often have misconceptions of their illness and treatment regimens. For example, in a study of boys with hemophilia, Spitzer (1992a) found that children actively sought treatment and procedural information but often misunderstood how one contracted hemophilia and the purpose of therapy. Munet-Vilaro and Vessey (1990) demonstrated that chronically ill Hispanic children had minimal information about their illnesses, as their parents limited communication and discouraged the children's questions about their illness.

Other researchers have directed their attention to developing instruments to measure concepts related to children's and adolescents' self-care agency. Denyes's (1980) Self-Care Practice Instruments, Diabetes Self-Care Practice Instrument (Frey & Denyes, 1989; Frey & Fox, 1980), and Child and Adolescent Self-Care Practices Questionnaire (Moore, 1995) were developed to measure self-care among chronically ill children and adolescents. Instruments such as these are invaluable in furthering our understanding of children's and adolescents' responses and adaptation to illness.

Parents

Along with studying the individual child's or adolescent's response to chronic illness, nurse researchers have explored the response of other family members. The majority of studies have focused on how mothers reacted to the initial diagnosis or their responses to the ongoing stress of coping with their child's illness. Particular attention has been paid to the concept of chronic sorrow. Later investigators began to explore the experiences of fathers and siblings.

Initial Diagnosis

The emotions that parents live through when their child is diagnosed with a chronic illness/impairment have been thoroughly documented by researchers in both nursing and other disciplines (Austin, 1991; Hirose & Ueda, 1990; Hodges & Parker, 1987; McKeever, 1981). Across cultures, parents have been found to experience anger, guilt, disbelief, grief, and denial.

Parents' interactions with the health care professionals during the diagnostic period influence their initial responses to the illness. In a series of articles, Cohen (1993a, 1993b, 1995a, 1995b; Cohen & Martinson, 1988) described three stages characterizing the prediagnostic period (i.e., lay explanatory, legitimating, and medical diagnostic) as parents come to the realization their child is seriously ill. Using narrative techniques, Knafl, Ayers, Gallo, Zoeller, and Breitmayer (1995) analyzed data related to the diagnostic stories told by parents in 63 families and identified five distinct pathways to diagnosis: direct, delayed, detour,

quest, and ordeal. These studies provided insights into how parents' initial illness experiences influence their later adaptation and interactions with health care providers.

Ongoing Stress and Coping

The majority of the early family (maternal) studies were based on the belief that the child's illness was a significant source of maternal stress. Studies of parental attitudes toward children with diabetes (Watson, 1972), cardiac defects (Beck, 1973), or tracheostomies (Aradine, 1980; Aradine, Uman, & Shapiro, 1978) provided similar descriptions of maternal stresses and coping behaviors (Aradine, 1980; Aradine et al., 1978; Wills, 1983). Various authors explored correlates of maternal stress, linking it to such things as the relationship with the child and the seriousness of illness symptoms (Garlinghouse & Sharp, 1968).

Researchers have often used a stress and coping framework to describe family responses to childhood chronic illness. For example, Lewandowski (1980) examined the stress and coping styles of parents experiencing their child's open heart surgery. Mardiros (1982, 1987) described the stress of mothers of disabled children and provided a description of role alterations demanded by this situation. Clements, Copeland, and Loftus (1990) used a grounded theory approach to study 30 parents of children with cystic fibrosis or diabetes and described patterns of equilibrium and disequilibrium in family life over the course of the child's illness. They postulated that families encounter predictable critical times in their child's illness trajectory and offered health care professionals suggestions for providing interventions, such as anticipatory guidance, to diminish the stress (Copeland, 1993; Copeland & Clements, 1993).

In contrast to early research, later studies revealed that stress could lead to positive as well as negative outcomes. Gibson (1986) studied 56 parents of children with cystic fibrosis and found that they experienced strong social support and identified both positive and negative aspects of their situation. In a study of 100 parents of children with spina bifida, Van Cleve (1989) noted that the parents reported coping as being positively related to the strength of the marital relationship. Contrary to predicted relationships, in a study of one- and two-parent families of chronically disabled children, Keller and Nicholls (1990) found no differences between groups in family stress levels, although single parents reported more adaptability, fewer financial resources, and lower levels of coping.

More recently, nurse investigators have used interpretive methods to understand more fully the experiences of families and to identify themes that apply across diagnostic groups (Andersson-Segesten & Plos, 1989; Burkhardt, 1993; Christian, 1994; Cohen, Nehring, Malm, & Harris, 1995; Dashiff, 1993; Faulkner, 1996; Gibson, 1988, 1995; Hatton et al., 1995; MacDonald, 1995, 1996; Simon & Smith, 1992; Van Os, Clark, Turner, & Herbst, 1985).

Chronic Sorrow

The concept of chronic sorrow was first reported in the 1960s (Jackson & Vessey, 1996). Chronic sorrow has been shown to persist throughout the child's and parents' lives and is particularly intense at times when the child does not meet usual developmental milestones (Clubb, 1991; Damrosch & Perry, 1989; Fraley, 1986, 1990; Lawler, 1977; Phillips, 1991; Warda, 1992; Young, 1977). Damrosch and Perry (1989) noted differences in maternal and paternal patterns of adjustment, with mothers more frequently describing their adjustment in terms of chronic, periodic crises and fathers describing their adjustment as steady and gradual. Burke and colleagues (Burke, Hainsworth, Eakes & Lindgren, 1992; Eakes, 1995; Hainsworth, Burke, Lindgren, & Eakes, 1994; Lindgren, Burke, Hainsworth, & Eakes, 1992) explored this concept across the life span of persons with chronic disabilities and their families, lending support to the enduring nature of parental sorrow even in those families who have adapted well to the illness.

Fathers

As noted previously, both clinicians and researchers considered fathers peripheral to the chronic illness experience prior to 1980. An early study by McKeever (1981) found that fathers wanted information, described acute grief reactions at the time of the birth of a child with congenital anomalies, and viewed their primary priority as supporting their wives. They also felt that the presence of a chronically ill child in the family had decreased their career mobility and curtailed family social activities. In later studies, limited participation in care regimens by fathers continued to be noted (Anderson, 1990; Anderson & Elfert, 1989; Heamon, 1995; Holaday, Turner-Henson, & Swan, 1991; Mardiros, 1987). Increasingly researchers are including fathers as active participants in their studies. Dixon (1996) reviewed 16 qualitative studies of family response to childhood illness and found that fathers provided data in 13 of 16 studies. She identified this as an encouraging trend among researchers seeking to achieve a more comprehensive view of families' chronic illness experiences.

Siblings

The recognition of siblings as among the most potentially influential individuals in a chronically ill child's life and renewed focus on the potential impact of illness on well siblings are further evidence of nursing's growing interest in how the entire family responds to chronic illness. Early researchers documented the impact of chronic illness on well siblings' physical, emotional, and cognitive functioning. The first sibling study was done by Schwirian (1976) and examined the effect of increased caregiving responsibilities on siblings of hearing impaired preschoolers. Schwirian found that the oldest healthy female sibling performed more care activities than younger and/or male siblings. This same theme was apparent in research by Williams, Lorenzo, and Borja (1993), who studied siblings of children with neurological and cardiac impairments in the Philippines. They reported that the oldest female siblings were expected to assume considerable caretaking and household responsibilities and participated in fewer school and social activities than their peers (Williams et al., 1993).

During the past 15 years, numerous studies have been completed that either focused on or included siblings (Davies, 1993; Faux, 1991; Gallo, Breitmayer, Knafl, & Zoeller, 1991, 1992, 1993; Harder & Bowditch, 1982; Kiburz, 1994; Menke, 1987; Pinyerd, 1983; Taylor, 1980; Williams et al., 1993). These studies have drawn varying conclusion regarding the impact of childhood chronic illness on well siblings, with some authors reporting positive and some negative impacts.

■ The Family Experience

Not only does the child, but also the child's family, have to live with this condition and make friends with it. The emphasis should be on what the child can do rather than on what he cannot do. (Latham & Heckel, 1972, p. 393)

Long-term exposure to chronic stress has been postulated to have deleterious effects on the child and the family. Children with chronic illness have been assumed to be at high risk

for psychopathology, impaired personality, and poor social functioning. The family unit also has been viewed at risk for dysfunction and maladjustment. Although early research focused on the response of individual family members, in the past 15 years there has been a shift toward trying to illuminate how the family unit adjusts to having a chronically ill family member. In general, familial adaptation to the experience of having a chronically ill family member has been studied from two overarching perspectives: family functioning and family management. Recently, more attention has been paid to the influence of culture and environment on responses to chronic illness. Investigators also have continued to study more discrete aspects of the family's chronic illness experience, such as maternal attachment and parenting behaviors.

Family Functioning

Using varying conceptual frameworks and methodologies, researchers have studied how families respond to the experience of having a chronically ill child. Family adaptation studies have focused on both immediate and long-term adaptation to chronic stress and specifically on outcomes for individual family members. In early studies, Benoliel (1970, 1975, 1977, 1983) described the impact of childhood diabetes on family life. She identified four styles of parental functioning (protective, adaptive, manipulative, and abdication) and two patterns of family adaptation (stable and recurring crisis).

Feetham developed a measure of family functioning, the Feetham Family Functioning Survey (FFFS; Roberts & Feetham, 1982), to evaluate the impact of the chronically ill child on the family. This measure has been used by a number researchers to study family response to a variety of chronic illnesses. In a recent study using the FFFS, Sawyer (1992) found no significant differences between family functioning in families with and without children with cystic fibrosis.

By the mid-1980s, research programs on family adaptation to childhood chronic illness were firmly grounded in theoretical frameworks. The ABCX or Resiliency Model of Family Stress, Adjustment, and Adaptation (McCubbin & McCubbin, 1993) served as the basis for several studies. Austin, McBride, and Davis (1984) studied parents' beliefs about their child's epilepsy. In subsequent research, Austin and her colleagues used the Resiliency Model (McCubbin & McCubbin, 1993) to explore relationships between family characteristics and child attributes in families of children with asthma and epilepsy. Results indicated that families of children with epilepsy exhibited lower levels of adaptation and resources and that the children exhibited lower self-esteem and increased behavioral problems (Austin, 1988, 1989; Austin & McDermott, 1988; Austin, Risinger, & Beckett, 1992; Austin, Smith, Risinger, & McNelis, 1994).

McCubbin (1984, 1988, 1989) and McCubbin and Huang (1989) studied families of children with cystic fibrosis, cerebral palsy, and meningomyelocele, using family stress, resources, coping patterns, and family types to explain variation in the child's health status. They found that illness severity was significantly related to the child's health status and family variables.

Family system variables have been shown to contribute more to the health status of the child when the child was more severely impaired (Austin, 1991). Donnelly (1994) explored family hardiness, stressors, and functioning with 27 parents of asthmatic children and found that, in general, these families exhibited high hardiness and low stress. Youngblut, Brennan, and Swegart (1994), LoBiondo-

Wood, Bernier-Henn, and Williams (1992) and Stevens (1994) also have used the Resiliency Model (McCubbin & McCubbin, 1993) to examine family adjustment to having a child in the home who is medically fragile or dependent on technology. These studies found that families in these situations reported multiple stressors, including the persistent gravity of the situation, fear of incompetency, and inadequate respite care.

Using qualitative methods to facilitate understanding of the family adjustment and adaptation, Gagliardi (1991a, 1991b) and Wuest and Stern (1990a, 1990b, 1991) described how families learn to live with muscular dystrophy and chronic otitis media, respectively. The exploration of the process of family adaptation has been continued by other researchers (Christian, 1994; Copeland, 1993; Gibson, 1995; Jerrett, 1994; Lightburn, 1992; Perkins, 1993; Price, 1993; Turner, Tomlinson, & Harbaugh, 1992), who studied a wide variety of illnesses.

Family Management Style

Several studies addressed how families actively manage their child's chronic illness (Edwards-Beckett & Cedargen, 1995; Knafl, Breitmayer, Gallo, & Zoeller, 1996; Murphy, 1989, 1990; Wuest & Stern, 1991). These researchers were comparatively less interested in the impact of illness on family functioning and more interested in family participation in illness care. Wuest and Stern (1991) explored how families effectively managed their children's chronic otitis media and subsequently were empowered in their contacts with health care professionals. Using a grounded theory approach, Wuest and Stern found that parents progressed through four stages of managing their child's illness: acquiescing, helpless floundering, becoming an expert, and managing effectively. These stages were related to the child's response to disease, the amount of disruption to family life, and the family's relation to the health care system.

Knafl and Deatrick (1990) developed a conceptual model of family management style, which was based on a formal concept analysis. Family management style (FMS) was conceptualized by Knafl and Deatrick (Deatrick & Knafl, 1990; Knafl & Deatrick, 1990) as encompassing the components of each family member's definition of the situation, behaviors used to manage the chronic illness situation, and the sociocultural context that frames these definitions and behaviors. The FMS framework guided a number of other studies. Gallo (1990) used a case study approach to describe how a family with an 11-year-old boy with diabetes defined and managed his illness. Two other case studies illustrated the use of the FMS framework to understand family response to childhood illness (McCarthy & Gallo, 1992; Obrecht, Gallo, & Knafl, 1992).

In a similar vein, Murphy (1989, 1990) studied the responses of 20 mothers and 20 fathers to the birth of a high-risk infant and derived three management styles: disagreement on socially prescribed management styles, adoption of parallel styles, and negotiation of mutually interdependent management styles. More recently, Knafl and colleagues (Knafl, Breitmayer, Gallo, & Zoeller, 1994, 1996; Knafl, Gallo, Breitmayer, Zoeller, & Ayers, 1993) studied 63 families of chronically ill children to further develop the FMS framework and described five family management styles: thriving, accommodating, enduring, struggling, and floundering (Knafl et al., 1996). Using Knafl and Deatrick's (1990) conceptualization of family management style, Edwards-Beckett and Cedargren (1995) studied how families interacted, shared information, and obtained support in the sociocultural context of school, community, and health care environments.

Normalization has been identified as the preferred management style of many families, and many authors used the concept of normalization to understand how families respond to childhood chronic illness (Anderson, 1981; Anderson & Chung, 1982a, 1982b; Bossert, Holaday, Harkins, & Turner-Henson, 1990; Cohen, 1993a; Dashiff, 1993; Deatrick, Knafl, & Walsh, 1988; Gagliardi, 1991a, 1991b; Hatton et al., 1995; Jerrett, 1994; Knafl & Deatrick, 1986; Knafl, Deatrick, & Moore, 1996; Krulik, 1980; Ray & Ritchie, 1993; Robinson, 1987; Scharer & Dixon, 1989). Families who adopt a normalizing management style minimize the unusual, extraordinary aspects of their situation and work to develop strategies that support a normal family life.

Cultural and Environmental Influences

Family response and adaptation to the experience of having a chronically ill child always occurs within specific cultures and environments. However, few researchers have addressed this aspect of the family's illness experience. Those studies that incorporated a cultural perspective yielded extremely useful information for providing culturally sensitive care. Using ethnographic methods, Anderson and colleagues (Anderson, 1981; Anderson & Chung, 1982a, 1982b; Anderson, Elfert, & Lai, 1989; Elfert, Anderson, & Lai, 1991) examined how immigrant Chinese families experience chronic illness. In contrast to North American families, the Chinese families did not adopt normalization as a preferred management style. Similarly, Koizumi (1992) investigated how Japanese mothers described having a child with diabetes. Wuest (1991) looked at Native North American children with chronic otitis media and found that families de-emphasized illness control in favor of learning to live in harmony with the illness. Across different cultural groups, Munet-Vilaro and Vessey (1990) and Martinson and Yi-Hua (1992) found significant differences in children's knowledge of their illness and bodies and explored the implications of these differences for developing supportive nursing interventions.

Using Bronfenbrenner's (1979) model of ecology of human development, Holaday and colleagues (Holaday & Turner-Henson, 1987; Holaday, Turner-Henson, & Swan, 1994; Turner-Henson, 1993; Turner-Henson, Holaday, Corser, Ogletree, & Swan, 1994) conducted a longitudinal study of the experience of growing up chronically ill. Taken together, their work provides a view of the child with chronic illness as having few friends, not participating in school clubs or sports, and being excluded from certain school and developmental experiences.

Parenting the Chronically Ill Child

Nurse researchers have also focused on the challenges associated with parenting a chronically ill child. In particular, investigators have been concerned with how chronic illness affects usual patterns of interaction between parents and children in areas such as discipline and protectiveness. Much of the research in this area has addressed mother-infant interactions or parenting practices and concerns in the context of chronic illness.

Mother-Infant Interactions

The effects of stress on maternal-infant bonding have received limited attention by nurse researchers. Considerable research has focused on maternal-infant interactions after the birth of an infant with a defect (Hedrick, 1979; Mercer, 1974a; Waechter, 1977). Mercer (1974a) collected interview and observational data from 5 mother-infant dyads over a 3-month period. She found increased frequency and intensity of maternal appraisal and more maternal attachment than aversion responses. In contrast, Holaday (1981, 1982, 1987), Capuzzi (1989), Childs (1985), and Kikuchi (1986) found a negative impact of a child's impairment on the mother-infant relationship. Holaday (1982, 1987) discovered atypical interaction patterns among 6 mother-infant dyads.

Child-Rearing Concerns and Practices

In early studies, nurse researchers examined parents', primarily mothers', child-rearing concerns when they had a chronically impaired child (Crummette, 1979; D'Antonio, 1976; Gillon, 1972; Holaday, 1978; Meier, 1978). D'Antonio (1976) identified four parenting patterns in mothers of children with congenital heart defects: avoidance of conflict with the child; watchfulness; prevention of further harm; and restrictiveness. Mothers of children with asthma described altering their usual patterns of mothering in response to the illness (Crummette, 1979).

It has been postulated that differential parenting practices between the chronically ill child and well siblings within families leads to negative outcomes for both affected children and their healthy siblings (Schlomann, 1988). However, there has not been general support for this hypothesis (Faux, 1986; King, 1981; Khampalikit, 1983; Pinelli, 1981; Stullenbarger, Norris, Edgil, & Prosser, 1987; Williams, 1995).

With the move from institutional to home care, parents have increased needs for specific information and skills to care competently for their ill infant or child. A number of studies identified specific needs, such as managing emergencies, detecting changes in the child's condition, giving medications and treatments, providing a safe physical environment, and dealing with developmental issues (Aradine,

1980; Aradine et al., 1978; Crummette, 1979; Hymovich, 1976).

■ *The Family-Provider Interface*

> But the parents may be unwise in their treatment of the child. Perhaps they will consider present comfort and giving him what he wants of greater importance than what is for his best good. Or they might refuse to listen to the physician and nurse and follow nonprofessional advice. (Sellew, 1944, p. 3)

The third domain of understanding the experience of children with chronic illness and their families is that of the interface between families and the health care system. These interactions occur in the institution, home, and community. Investigators have explored the nature of relationships between family members and health care providers as well as interventions to support optimal family adjustment to the challenges of childhood chronic illness.

Central to families' abilities to adapt to their child's chronic illness are their relationships with health care professionals, which typically are long term and intense (Thorne, 1993). Relationships between families and health care providers are changing, with families no longer content to work within the paternalistic, authoritarian framework that has characterized these relationships for four decades. Increasingly, families are seeking to work collaboratively with professionals who understand how they view their situation (Faux & Knafl, 1996).

Thorne and Robinson (1988a, 1988b, 1989) developed a staged model of health care relationships derived from data collected from families of chronically ill children and adults. They proposed that, over time, families progress through three relationship phases—naive trust, disenchantment, and guarded alliance— and eventually establish positive relationships with health care professionals. Knafl, Breitmayer, Gallo, and Zoeller (1992) identified parents' views of the components of a positive working relationship with health care professionals to include information exchange, interactional style, establishing a relationship with the child, and fostering parental competence. In contrast, other researchers noted the difficulties encountered by parents as they attempt to negotiate roles and relations with home care providers (Patterson, Jernell, Leonard, & Titus, 1994; Ray & Ritchie, 1993; Scannell, Gillies, Biordi, & Child, 1993). Yet these researchers also identified the components of a positive working relationship. For example, Patterson and colleagues (1994) found that positive relationships were enhanced by parents' perceptions that providers were competent, genuinely cared for their child, and were respectful of parents and supportive of collaborative interaction with the family.

Parents' and health care professionals' perceptions of one another in hospital settings also have been studied. The illness trajectory of many chronic illnesses necessitated periodic hospitalization for acute illness episodes, surgery, or adjustments in medical regimens. Over time, as hospital policies changed and open visiting became the norm, attitudes of the nursing staff about parental participation were explored (Seidl, 1969; Seidl & Pilletteri, 1967). As recently as 1992, Young noted that the nursing staff still discouraged parental visits and participation in the care of their children. Numerous researchers explored the hospitalization experience of families with a chronically ill child (Burke, Costello, & Handley-Derry, 1989; Burke, Kauffmann, Costello, & Dillon, 1991; Callery & Smith, 1991; Hayes & Knox, 1984; Kruger, 1992; Ogilvie, 1990; Perkins, 1993; Robinson, 1984, 1985, 1987). These studies described the difficulties encountered by parents during their children's repeated hospitalizations as a result of discrepancies between parents' and nurses' expectations of one another.

Other studies sought to identify and explore selected aspects of parent-provider relationships, with considerable attention directed to the interaction that surrounds health decision making. Two recent studies addressed parental decision making in the context of childhood illness to explore how parents and providers interact. Drawing on a secondary analysis of two qualitative data sets, Kirschbaum and Knafl (1996) described three patterns of decision making between parents and health care providers: dependent, independent, and collaborative. Higgins and Kayser-Jones (1996) recently explored parental decision making in accepting a cardiac transplant. They identified two styles of parental decision making, spontaneous and logical, and found that the major factor influencing decision making was family beliefs related to the quality of the family's and the child's life. Physician endorsement of a treatment option with which the parents disagreed led to parents changing their decision in only 2 of the 15 families studied (Higgins & Kayser-Jones, 1996). Based on her review of 16 qualitative studies in which there was a child with a chronic illness, Dixon (1996) identified four meta-themes that shaped the parents' relationships with health care providers: trust, information gathering, participation in care, and decision making.

■ *Trends in Child and Family Research*

Since 1980 there has been a surge in nursing research dealing with children with chronic illness and their families. The use of interpretive methods (grounded theory, ethnography, and phenomenology) was the dominant feature of these studies (Deatrick, Faux, & Moore, 1993; Dixon, 1996; Faux & Deatrick, 1991). The recent focus on families reverses an earlier trend of research concentrating on the child's experiences and adjustment.

Perhaps the greatest change in child and family research related to the experience of chronic illness has been the shift away from a deficit view of how families respond to chronic illness. Forty years ago, the experience was described as totally negative for the child and mother. However, as research increasingly shows that the majority of children and their families adapt well to the illness experience, researchers are examining family strengths to understand how they may be fostered and supported (Burke, 1980, 1986a, 1986b; Knafl et al., 1994).

Nonetheless, most studies failed to incorporate a well-articulated conceptual framework. Batey (1977) and Barnard and Neal (1977) noted that studies done in the 1960s and 1970s were inadequately conceptualized and incorporated few conceptual or theoretical frameworks. In a review study of the care of chronically ill and disabled children, Burke and Roberts (1990) found that only 22% of the 50 studies they reviewed used a conceptual model to guide the study design and interpretation of findings. Certainly, few nursing models have been used or tested in pediatric nursing. Betz and Beal (1993) found that only 17 (9%) of the studies they reviewed incorporated nursing frameworks. In spite of these shortcomings, there is some evidence of greater attention being directed to specifying conceptual frameworks as an integral part of the research design, primarily stress and coping, developmental, systems, crisis, and attachment theories. Feminism is another lens that researchers are beginning to incorporate when framing their studies and interpreting results (Anderson, 1990; Anderson et al., 1989; Wuest & Stern, 1991). Both McBride (1994) and Ganong (1995) predict that this trend will increase in the future as caregiving and chronicity disproportionately affect women's lives.

Several authors completed major reviews of the research related to family response to childhood chronic illness. These reviews provided useful insights into the relative strengths and weaknesses of various study designs. Burke and Roberts (1990) classified 75% of the studies conducted in the 1980s with chronically ill children as descriptive and exploratory, with Beck (1988) noting that only 3% of reviewed studies employed experimental or quasi-experimental designs. Austin (1991) estimated that 80% of the family studies examined were descriptive and correlational, with the remaining 20% incorporating comparison groups. Similarly, in their sample of 319 studies, Beal and Betz (1992) noted that only 17% tested nursing interventions; the majority of these were informal program evaluations.

In the 20 years between 1970 and 1990, designs were primarily descriptive, cross-sectional, and often employed qualitative approaches. Although the use of qualitative designs continues, by the mid-1980s, these studies were better designed and more rigorous, often using specific approaches (grounded theory, ethnography, or phenomenology) to guide data collection and analysis (Deatrick et al., 1993) and frequently triangulating qualitative and quantitative methods (Austin et al., 1994; Holaday et al., 1994; Knafl, Breitmayer, et al., 1996).

In examining children and adolescents and their families' responses to chronic illness, researchers have continued to use developmental stages as a basis for sample selection. To date,

the overwhelming predominance of samples of school-age children is a significant limitation to building an understanding of the effects of chronic illness on the full developmental range of children.

Moreover, convenience samples with small numbers of subjects continue to predominate. Although Turner-Henson, Holaday, and O'Sullivan (1992) described strategies to obtain larger samples, few studies have been conducted based on large samples. On the other hand, there has been a trend to include multiple family members in this research, therein contributing to a more comprehensive view of family response to chronic illness.

During the past four decades, nurse researchers have made great strides in the scope and rigor of their studies in describing how children and families live with chronic illness. At the same time, relatively little effort has been directed toward the systematic development of interventions that would support optimal family adaptation (Bell, 1996), with the exception of Wright and Leahey (1994a) and Robinson (1994) who have developed innovative models for working with families experiencing difficulty dealing with a member's illness.

Several groups of investigators have proposed typologies of family interventions that may guide future studies (Craft & Willadsen, 1992; Nolan, Keady, & Grant, 1995). Certainly, the many theoretical models that have guided various groups of investigators have the potential to support interventions as well (Deatrick, in this volume; Hymovich, 1976; Hymovich & Hagopian, 1992; McCubbin & Huang, 1989; Wright & Leahey, 1990, 1994a). Further, the research programs of several researchers exhibit great potential for creating innovative interventions that can enhance the quality of life of children with chronic illness and their families. In particular, the Resiliency Model (McCubbin & McCubbin, 1993), which guided McCubbin's and Austin's research, may lead future investigators to develop interventions that foster coping and family hardiness.

Ganong (1995) predicted that future family research will employ multidisciplinary teams, using multiple approaches, emphasizing cultural and feminist contexts to further understand how families experience chronic illness. It is imperative that pediatric and family nursing research (a) determine what needs to be further explored, (b) develop and test appropriate interventions, and (c) prepare nurses who can interact and care appropriately and effectively for this high-risk population.

10

■

INTEGRATIVE REVIEW OF ASSESSMENT MODELS FOR EXAMINING CHILDREN'S AND FAMILIES' RESPONSES TO CHRONIC ILLNESS

■ *Joan K. Austin and Sharon L. Sims*

In recent decades, the number of chronically ill children has increased (Gortmaker, 1985). Many nurse researchers have been studying these children and their families with the goals of improving their nursing care and enhancing quality of life. To advance the science in this area, it is essential that these nurse researchers use the best assessment models and instruments available. This chapter reviews the nursing research literature related to children's and families' responses to chronic childhood illness. Our purposes are to (a) describe the major child and family domains assessed, (b) evaluate the status of assessment models and instruments measuring these domains, and (c) make recommendations for future development of assessment methods. Following a description of the search process and an overview of the articles selected, we present our major findings.

■ Selection of Articles

Two major computerized databases (Cumulative Index to Nursing and Allied Health Literature and MEDLINE) were searched using the key words *children* and *chronic illness* to identify relevant nursing literature from 1989 to 1994, and a hand search was conducted to locate relevant research articles in the key pediatric and nursing research journals. For the purpose of this review, chronic

AUTHORS' NOTE: Work on this chapter was supported in part by Grant No. NS22416 to Joan K. Austin from the National Institute of Neurological Disorders and Stroke. The authors acknowledge the assistance of Judy Williams in conducting the literature search.

illness refers to a primarily physical disease or disorder in an otherwise healthy child. Reports focusing exclusively on mental illness, substance abuse, and mental retardation were excluded. The age of the chronically ill children studied ranged from 1 month to 18 years. Articles were selected for review if they reported results from a study related to chronic childhood illness or if they reported on the development of an instrument for use with this population. All relevant articles in nursing journals were included; those in interdisciplinary journals were included only if at least one of the authors was a nurse.

Overview of Selected Articles

Of the 38 articles selected for review (see appendix), 30 (79%) were in nursing journals, and most of these were concentrated in three pediatric journals: *Journal of Pediatric Nursing, Maternal-Child Nursing Journal,* and *Pediatric Nursing.* As noted in an earlier review (Austin, 1991), the literature was almost evenly divided between those using a more inductive approach, with primarily qualitative methods, and those using a more deductive approach, with more quantitative methods. A few authors combined qualitative and quantitative methods. With the exception of 6 articles, which focused primarily on instrument development, all were reports of completed research studies. For ease of reporting findings, the articles that describe development of an instrument are presented separately. Moreover, the 32 articles describing completed research studies were separated into two groups based on primary assessment method (quantitative or qualitative) and reviewed separately. Four reports of completed studies where both qualitative and quantitative methods were used (Breitmayer, Gallo, Knafl, & Zoeller, 1992; Gallo, Breitmayer, Knafl, & Zoeller, 1993; Loebig, 1990; Ray & Ritchie, 1993) are reviewed in both sections.

Our major findings are presented under three major headings: instruments developed, quantitative assessment methods, and qualitative assessment methods. These findings are followed by conclusions and recommendations.

■ Instruments Developed

Four groups of authors developed scales that could be used in the area of chronic childhood illness and reported the development and psychometric properties of these scales in 6 articles. Three of the 6 instruments were developed by Austin and colleagues (Austin & Huberty, 1989, 1993; Austin, Patterson, & Huberty, 1991) for use with school-age children with either epilepsy or asthma. A fourth scale, previously developed by Ryan-Wenger (Ryan, 1989; Ryan-Wenger, 1990) to measure coping in general population schoolagers, was further tested by the author in a sample of children with asthma. Punnett and Thurber's (1994) scale is a revision of an existing scale to make it relevant for evaluation of a camping experience for children with asthma. The final scale was developed by Dragone (1990) to measure primary health care needs of chronically ill adolescents. Each of these instruments is described below.

Revised Family APGAR

The original Family APGAR is a 5-item scale for adults and adolescents that measures satisfaction with five aspects of family functioning: adaptation, partnership, growth, affection, and resolve (Smilkstein, 1978). Austin and Huberty (1989) found that children under 10 years of age had trouble completing the scale independently, and so they revised each of the 5 items to be understandable for children as young as 8 years of age. For example, the item "I am satisfied with the way my family expresses affection and responds to my emotions, such as anger, sorrow, or love" was revised to read "I like what my family does when I feel mad, happy, or loving." Children respond using a 5-point scale of *Never, Hardly, Some of the time, Almost always,* and *Always.* To obtain information on internal consistency and test-retest reliability, Austin and Huberty (1989, 1993) carried out two studies. The revised version was found to have good test-retest reliability ($r = .73$) and good internal consistency reliability (alpha coefficients = .68 to .71). Support for validity was found when the scores from administrations of the original and revised versions 2 weeks apart were correlated with each other ($r = .79$ and .74).

Child Attitude Toward Illness Scale (CATIS)

The CATIS was developed to assess attitudes or how children feel (e.g., happy/sad, good/bad) about having a health condition (Austin & Huberty, 1993). The summated rating scale was developed so that any health condition could be measured in children at least 8 years old. Sample items include "How good or bad do you feel it is that you have (asthma/seizures)?" and "How often do you feel sad about being sick?" Children rate the items on 5-point scales (e.g., *Very good, A little good, Not sure, A little bad,* and *Very bad*; or *Never, Not often, Sometimes, Often,* and *Very often*). Following support for content validity, two studies were carried out to examine reliability and validity. Test-retest reliability was supported when the scores from two administrations of the scale 2 weeks apart were found to be correlated ($r = .80$). Confirmatory factor and coefficient alpha analysis indicated that the CATIS is a unidimensional instrument with good internal consistency reliability (coefficient alpha = .80).

Moreover, support for validity was found when the score was positively correlated with self-concept ratings ($r = .48$) and negatively correlated with parents' ratings of behavior problems ($rs = -.22$ to $-.43$; Austin & Huberty, 1993).

Coping Health Inventory for Children (CHIC)

CHIC (Austin et al., 1991) was developed for parents to report on their school-age children's coping behavior. This 45-item scale, which was developed for episodic illnesses such as epilepsy and asthma, provides scores for five different coping patterns: develops competence and optimism; feels different and withdraws; is irritable, moody, and acts out; complies with treatment; and seeks support. Parents report on their children's observed behavior on 5-point scales reflecting frequency (*Never* to *Almost always*). Two studies were carried out to obtain information on reliability and validity. Confirmatory factor analysis provided support for the 5-factor solution. Internal consistency reliability was strong for each of the five factors (i.e., coefficient alpha ranged between .72 to .86). Validity was also supported when coping patterns were significantly and appropriately correlated with child self-concept, attitude, and behavior problems. Support for test-retest reliability was found when coping pattern scores were correlated with each other ($rs = .68$ to .91 for mother sample) over two administrations.

Schoolagers' Coping Strategies Inventory (SCSI)

SCSI was developed on a general population sample (Ryan, 1989; Ryan-Wenger, 1990) and was selected for review here because of its use with children with asthma by the nurse developer (Ryan-Wenger & Walsh, 1994). SCSI is a self-report scale where children, ages 8–13 years, rate 26 coping strategies on 3-point scales for both frequency (*Never* to *Most of the time*) and effectiveness (*Never do it* to *Helps a lot*). Even though SCSI was developed using samples of primarily Caucasian children, it was found to have good reliability (alpha coefficients were .80 for frequency and .73 for effectiveness) with a sample of African American children from low-income families (Ryan-Wenger & Copeland, 1994). Support for validity was found in that study when scores discriminated between groups of children with different levels of stress-related problems. The scale was also found to be reliable for measuring frequency and effectiveness of coping strategies when addressing a problem with asthma at an asthma camp (Ryan-Wenger & Walsh, 1994). The alpha coefficients for the asthma sample were .85 and .89 for frequency and effectiveness, respectively. No specific information was provided on validity with the asthma sample.

Revision of Child Evaluation Inventory (CEI)

Punnett and Thurber (1994) reported on a revision of CEI (Kazdin, Esveldt-Dawson, French, & Unis, 1987), a scale developed originally to assess the outcomes of individual psychotherapy in children with mental illness. Punnett and Thurber revised the scale to be applicable to evaluating satisfaction with an asthma camping experience. For example, "camp" was substituted for "psychotherapy" and "asthma" for "behavior." The 21-item unidimensional scale asks children to rate different aspects of camp on 5-point scales ranging from *Unfavorable* to *Favorable*. For example, one item was "Please rate how you felt about your nurse." The scale was found to have good internal consistency reliability (coefficient alpha

= .91). Validity was not addressed by the authors, but they did suggest that the inventory could be easily adapted for evaluation of camping experiences for children with other chronic conditions.

Primary Health Care Needs Assessment (PHCNA)

Dragone (1990) reported on both the development of an instrument and a completed research study using the newly developed scale. PHCNA is a 60-item scale designed to identify the primary health care needs of adolescents with a variety of chronic illnesses. Dragon developed the scale based on her personal experience and reports in the literature describing health care needs of both healthy and chronically ill adolescents. Items focus on issues related to development, management of the illness, and health promotion. Sample items are "had a toothache," "gotten drunk," "had a skin rash," and "been anxious a lot." Adolescents respond by checking each event that has happened to them in the past year and by identifying the 5 items they are most concerned about. Parents are also asked to complete the scale, based on their knowledge of their child. Content validity was established by review from experts. Test-retest reliability was supported when, over a 2-week period, 88% of the adolescents and 85% of the parents agreed with their initial responses to 10 randomly selected items. In a sample of 24 chronically ill adolescents, Dragone (1990) found that the health concerns that were both most frequent and important were boredom, concern about how illness would affect their future, inability to do things friends did, worry about health, headaches, concern about ability to have children, depression, and concerns about school progress.

In summary, this overview of newly developed or revised instruments indicates a moderate amount of activity by nurse authors, who, for the most part, appear to be knowledgeable about how to revise old or develop new instruments that possess good psychometric properties. Although none of the three newly developed scales is widely used, Revised Family APGAR and CATIS appear to meet the criteria for moderately established scales (i.e., ongoing development of psychometric properties, and use in published research other than the instrument development studies) set forth by Sawin and Harrigan (1995). Following their development, Revised Family APGAR and CATIS were used in studies whose results have been published (Austin, Smith, Risinger, & McNelis, 1994). The other newly developed scales would be considered newly established because they have some psychometric properties but no or limited use in published studies. SCSI, which was originally developed for the general population and used in this sample, would also meet the criteria for moderately established.

■ Quantitative Assessment Methods

The 18 completed research studies using quantitative methods were analyzed to identify the individual assessments made. At least one assessment of an attribute of the chronically ill child was made in 16 of the articles, and at least one assessment of a family or family member attribute was made in 13 articles. With few exceptions, most of the researchers were using previously developed instruments. For ease of presentation, the assessments were divided into two groups: attributes of the chronically ill child and attributes of the family or family members. For each of these groups, we present the domains assessed, the different instruments used, and an overview of results.

Attributes of the Chronically Ill Child

As would be expected in research focused exclusively on chronic childhood illness, characteristics of the chronic condition or health behaviors were the most frequently described child attributes. The next most commonly assessed attribute was child psychosocial adjustment. Other attributes commonly measured were the child's perceptions of self, coping and social support, and affect. An overview of assessments made in each child attribute area follows.

Characteristics and Health

An assessment of the severity of the child's chronic condition was made in almost all studies describing the illness. The majority of the authors developed their own questions to measure illness characteristics and symptoms. Information on the psychometric properties of these author-developed scales was rarely reported. Only one group of researchers (Breitmayer et al., 1992; Gallo, Breitmayer, Knafl, & Zoeller, 1992) included a previously developed scale. They asked mothers to use a 7-item version of Stein and Jessop's (1982) Functional Status Measure (FSM) to rate their child's ability to perform age-appropriate activities. FSM has been found to have good content validity and satisfactory internal consistency reliabilities, with alpha coefficients ranging between .62 and .83 (Stein & Jessop, 1982). Moreover, the scale could discriminate between groups of children with differing levels of functioning. Two studies (Austin et al., 1994; Nelms, 1989) included school absences in assessing the severity of the condition. Two others (Grey, Cameron, & Thurber, 1991; Lawler, Volk, Viviani, & Mengel, 1990) used a physiological variable to reflect health status, and both of these measured glycosylated hemoglobin to reflect diabetic control.

TABLE 10.1 Instruments Assessing Child Adjustment

Domain	*Instrument(s)*
Behavior problems	Child Behavior Checklist; behavior problem scores (Achenbach, 1991a) Child Behavior Checklist–Teacher's Report Form; behavior problem scores (Achenbach, 1991b)
Social competence	Child Behavior Checklist; social competence items (Achenbach, 1991a) Child and Adolescent Adjustment Profile (Ellsworth, 1981)
Adjustment within the Family	Kinetic Family Drawing–Revised (Spinetta, McLaren, Fox, & Sparta, 1981) Emotion Triangulation Scale (Lawler, Volk, Viviani, & Mengel, 1990)
Anxiety	State-Trait Anxiety Inventory for Children (Spielberger, 1973)
Depression	Children's Depression Inventory (Kovacs, 1985) Beck Depression Inventory (Beck, Ward, Mendelson, Mock, & Erbaugh, 1961)
Aggression	Feshbach Aggression Measure (Feshbach, 1956)
Self-concept	Piers-Harris Self-Concept Scale (Piers, 1984) Self-Perception Scale for Children (Harter, 1985) Sears Self-Concept Inventory (Sears, 1964) Coopersmith Self-Esteem Inventory (Coopersmith, 1967)
Ego development	Objective Measure of Ego Identity Status (Adams, Bennion, & Huh, 1989)

Health behaviors related to the chronic condition were assessed in studies by Grey and colleagues (1991) and Ray and Ritchie (1993). Grey and colleagues (1991) assessed self-care activities related to the chronic condition, using Self-Care Questionnaire (SCQ; Saucier, 1984), a previously developed 15-item instrument measuring self-care behaviors related to diabetes. Content validity has been supported for SCQ, and internal consistency reliabilities, as measured by coefficient alpha, ranged between .63 and .85. In their study of children needing home health care, Ray and Ritchie (1993) measured parents' reports of their children's illness care using Clinician's Overall Burden Index (COBI; Stein & Jessop, 1982), a scale developed for clinicians that measures differences in care for an ill child and a healthy child. Support for the validity of the scale was found when scores on the scale were highly correlated ($r = .82$) with a clinician's independent rating of burden involved in providing the child's care (Stein & Jessop, 1982).

In summary, there were many different approaches to measurement of illness variables, with most studies using author-developed instruments. Factors influencing this diversity of measurement approaches include the vast differences in illness symptoms, impact of the chronic illness on the child and the family, and the purpose of the research study. It could be argued that a uniform scale to describe all chronic illnesses would allow comparison of illness severity across studies, but the development of such a scale would be most difficult because of the need to address diversity in illness symptoms, illness impact (e.g., physical, social, and cognitive), and child developmental levels. A scale that was general enough to address all illnesses most likely would not only be lengthy but lack sufficient specificity to examine differences within a given illness sample. For example, global physical functioning scales do not differentiate among children with seizure conditions and no other physical problems.

Psychosocial Adjustment

An assessment of psychological adjustment of the chronically ill child was made in 8 studies. Most of these authors used previously developed scales with strong reliability and validity and, in some cases, norms for the general population. Table 10.1 lists the previously developed child adjustment rating scales and sources of the scales. It is important to note that all adjustment scales were developed for general population children and do not specifically measure child adjustment related to chronic physical illness. Some authors used more than one instrument or more than one source to assess psychological status. For example, Grey and colleagues (1991) measured adolescents' anxiety, depression, adjustment, and self-perceptions. Austin and colleagues (1994) measured several aspects of adjustment in the measurement of quality of life, including mothers', teachers', and children's ratings of psychological and social adjustment.

The most commonly used scale to measure child psychological adjustment is Child Behavior Checklist (CBCL; Achenbach, 1991a), which was used by two different groups of investigators (Austin, Risinger, & Beckett, 1992; Austin et al., 1994; Breitmayer et al., 1992; Gallo et al., 1992). CBCL is a 138-item scale that measures behavior problems and social competence. Behavior problems are measured on 3-point scales, with higher scores reflecting more problems. Scores are provided for total behavior problems as well as for higher-order factor scores of internalizing and externalizing. Social competence has three subscales: Social Activities, Social Relationships, and School Activities and Performance. Internal consistency reliability for the total score and major factors are excellent, with coefficient alpha ranging between .89 and .96 for total behavior score, and .57 and .64 for social competence. Test-retest reliability over a 1-week period has also been found to be excellent, with a mean of .89 for behavior problems and .87 for social competence. Norms are available based on age and gender (Achenbach, 1991a). Besides the CBCL form that parents complete, there are forms available for teachers and youths. Results from studies using the instrument indicated that children with epilepsy had more behavior problems than children with asthma (Austin et al., 1994). Moreover, children with chronic illness were found to be less socially competent than general population norms (Breitmayer et al., 1992); their healthy siblings, however, were not found to be different from population norms (Gallo et al., 1992).

A second scale used by more than one group is Children's Depression Inventory (CDI; Kovacs, 1980-1981), a 27-item scale that measures overt symptoms of childhood depression. Children respond to each item with a rating of 0 to 2 in the direction of increasing psychopathology. The scale has been found to have strong reliability (coefficient alpha = .86; Kovacs, 1980-1981) and concurrent validity (Kovacs, 1985). Using CDI, Nelms (1989) found that children with asthma or diabetes were more depressed than well children, and Grey and colleagues (1991) found that older adolescents were significantly more depressed than younger pre-adolescents.

The final scale used by more than one group is Kinetic Family Drawings–Revised (KFD–R; Spinetta, McLaren, Fox, & Sparta, 1981), which makes use of a projective technique to assess children's adjustment within the family context. KFD–R uses a family picture drawn by the child to assess the child's communication, self-image, and emotional tone within the family context. Recurring objects and themes in the pictures are scored in the three areas. Bossert and Martinson (1990) reported on studies in the literature supporting the reliability (alpha coefficient = .72) and validity (correlated with a family adjustment scale) of the use of this assessment technique with families of chronically ill children. Mullis, Mullis, and Kerchoff (1992) found that children with leukemia reported more problems than healthy children with emotional tone using this scale.

Only one author-developed measure of adjustment was used: Lawler and colleagues' (1990) Emotion Triangulation Scale, which measures adolescents' emotional boundaries and behaviors when there are problems in their parents' marital relationship. The authors found the internal consistency reliability using

Cronbach's alpha to be .72. No information on validity was reported. In that study, only 1 of the 16 adolescents with diabetes was experiencing more than minimal triangulation in the parents' marital relationship.

Four different authors measured child self-concept or self-perceptions. Each used a different scale, and all scales were well developed by researchers in other disciplines. Piers-Harris Self-Concept Scale (Piers, 1984) is an 80-item scale on which children respond with *Yes* or *No* to statements about self. Estimates of internal consistency reliability for the total score ranged from .89 to .93; test-retest reliabilities ranged from .42 to .96 (Piers, 1984). Self-Perception Scale for Children (Harter, 1985) is a 36-item scale on which children select one of four options that most describes how they perceive themselves. The scale and its six subscales have coefficient alphas ranging from .71 to .85. Sears Self-Concept Scale (Sears, 1964) is a 20-item scale on which children compare themselves to other children the same age on aspects of self. Coefficient alpha for the total scale was .88. The final scale, the school form of Coopersmith Self-Esteem Inventory (SEI; Coopersmith, 1967), is a 58-item scale on which school-age children respond with *Like Me* or *Unlike Me.* The scale has been found to have strong test-retest reliability ($r = .70$) and internal consistency reliability, with coefficient alphas ranging from .80 to .86. Results from the use of these self-perception scales indicated some differences between chronically ill samples and well samples. For example, Mullis and colleagues (1992) found that children with leukemia had more negative self-concepts only in the area of school academics, and Nelms (1989) found that children with asthma had lower self-concept scores than children with diabetes or well children.

Only one study focused on ego identity development. Lawler and colleagues (1990) measured level of ego identity development using the extended version of Objective Measure

of Ego Identity Status Instrument (EOMEIS; Adams, Bennion, & Huh, 1989), a 64-item self-report scale that categorizes adolescents on four levels of identity status. Internal consistency reliability using coefficient alpha ranged from .70 to .86 (Lawler et al., 1990). Ego identity was not found to be related to any family or adolescent adjustment variables in adolescents with diabetes.

In summary, psychosocial adjustment of chronically ill children was assessed with scales designed to measure adjustment in general population children. With the exception of CBCL (Achenbach, 1991a) and Teacher's Report Form (Achenbach, 1991b), where parents or teachers rate the children's behavior, children complete the adjustment scales. It should be noted that even though children spend a large amount of time at school, only one group of researchers (Austin et al., 1994) included an assessment of the child's behavior at school in the assessment of adjustment. In that study, Austin and colleagues (1994) found children with asthma to have fewer problems at school than children with epilepsy. When adjustment differences were found between chronically ill and healthy children, they were in the direction that chronically ill children were faring worse. Moreover, comparisons between chronically ill children showing differences between illness groups lend support for investigating differences between groups of chronically ill children.

Coping and Social Support

Coping and social support were combined for review because coping scales frequently include behaviors of seeking and using social support. Along with the two newly developed coping scales described previously, 3 studies (Grey et al., 1991; Keller & Nicolls, 1990; Lawler et al., 1990) used instruments measuring aspects of coping and social support. Two of the scales were developed specifically for adolescents. Adolescent Coping Orientation for Problem Experiences (ACOPE; Patterson & McCubbin, 1991) is a 54-item self-report questionnaire that assesses 10 categories of coping behaviors found helpful in managing problems or difficult situations. The scale has been found to have good reliability, with coefficient alphas ranging from .67 to .78 (Grey et al., 1991). In their study, Grey and colleagues (1991) found differences in coping strategies based on developmental stage, with ventilating feelings being used more by younger adolescents, and avoidance and relaxation behaviors being used more by older adolescents. Moreover, poorer adjustment was found to be related to coping strategies of ventilating feelings and avoidance.

Young Adult Social Support Inventory (Patterson, McCubbin, & Grochowski, 1991), used by Lawler and colleagues (1990), is a 60-item scale that measures five areas of social support—emotion, esteem, network, appraisal, and altruistism—from several different sources. Internal consistency reliability for the total score using coefficient alpha was .89 (Lawler et al., 1990). Lawler and colleagues found that adolescents with diabetes received minimal social support from others.

Keller and Nicolls (1990) used a scale initially developed for adults, Jaloweic Coping Scale (JCS; Jaloweic, Murphy, & Powers, 1984), to measure coping in adolescents. JCS is a 40-item scale that asks subjects to rate how often they have used different coping strategies and how helpful they found the strategy to be. While support for reliability and validity has been found with adults with hypertension (Jaloweic et al., 1984), no information was reported on the reliability and validity with an adolescent sample. Keller and Nicolls (1990) found that chronically ill adolescents used more emotive coping strategies than their parents.

In summary, only 3 studies assessed coping or social support. Moreover, all studied adolescents, and all used different scales. The significant relationships found between coping strategies and adjustment by Grey and colleagues (1991) suggest that more research should focus on coping strategies.

Affect

Children's affect or feelings were measured in three different studies. Austin and colleagues (1994) measured children's feelings about having their chronic condition using the previously described Child Attitude Toward Illness Scale (Austin & Huberty, 1993) and found that children with epilepsy had more negative attitudes than children with asthma. Fleming, Holmes, Barton, and Osbahr (1993) assessed children's perceptions via color preferences using the Luscher Color Test (Luscher, 1969). Although validity data were not reported on the Luscher Color Test, the authors did report that reproducibility of the choice of favorite color selected first or second was 64%. The differences in color preference found that were based on the child's health state led the authors to propose that color preference could be used to assess the child's affective state. For example, physically disabled children selected the color blue more than acutely ill children did.

Nelms (1989) asked children to complete questionnaires and respond to videotapes and audiotaped vignettes, developed by Feshbach (1982), to measure empathy and emotional responsiveness. Using Feshbach Audiovisual Empathy Measure, children reported their own feelings after viewing videotapes of real children expressing five different emotions. Using Feshbach Emotional Responsiveness Measure, children listened to audiotaped vignettes and reported their level of emotional intensity. Results indicated that children with either asthma or diabetes did not differ from each other but scored higher than well children on emotion.

In summary, few studies used measures of affect. Moreover, authors were diverse in their approaches to the measurement of affect, with

TABLE 10.2 Previously Developed Family Assessment Instruments

Domain	*Instrument(s)*
Family stress	Family Inventory of Life Events and Changes (McCubbin, Patterson, & Wilson, 1991e)
	Adolescent-Family Inventory of Life Events and Changes (McCubbin, Patterson, Beuman, & Harris, 1991d)
Family resources	Family Inventory of Resources for Management (McCubbin, Comeau, & Harkins, 1991a)
	Family Hardiness Index (McCubbin, McCubbin, & Thompson, 1991c)
Family functioning	Revised Family APGAR (Austin & Huberty, 1989)
	Impact on Family Scale (Stein & Riessman, 1980)[a]
	Family Adaptability and Cohesion Evaluation (Olson, Portner, & Lavee, 1985)
	Family of Origin Scale (Hovestadt, Anderson, Piercy, Cochran, & Fine, 1985)
	Feetham Family Functioning Survey (Roberts & Feetham, 1982)
Family coping	Coping Health Inventory for Parents (McCubbin, McCubbin, Nevin, & Cauble, 1991b)[a]
	Chronicity Impact and Coping Instrument (Hymovich, 1984)[a]

a. These scales were developed for chronic childhood illness.

self-report, observation, and projective techniques being represented. Differences in affect found between and within samples suggest that more research on chronically ill children should include measures of affect.

Development

Assessment of developmental status other than age was rare. Only one study focused on physical development. Grey and colleagues (1991) used five Tanner stages (Morris & Udry, 1980) to measure sexual maturation. Adolescents were shown pictures of stages of physical development for pubic hair and genitalia; this method has been found to have correlations above .70 with ratings by physicians (Grey et al., 1991). Differences were found between three groups based on these stages, with older adolescents reporting more anxiety, worse peer relations, and less self-competence than younger children.

Attributes of Family or Family Members

A content analysis of family assessments in the 13 studies led to the following categories:

family stressors, family functioning, family resources and coping, and family member involvement and adjustment. In the assessment of family variables, most authors used scales previously developed for the general population and were consistent in reporting psychometric information on them. These scales and sources are listed in Table 10.2, and many are described in Sawin and Harrigan (1995). As noted in this table, only three previously developed family scales focused on parents of chronically ill children. Author-developed scales were used in 3 studies (Grey et al., 1991; Nagy & Ungerer, 1990; Williams, Lorenzo, & Borja, 1993).

Many authors assessed different aspects of the family in the same study. For example, Lawler and colleagues (1990) administered four scales to measure different aspects of the family. Although most of the authors collected data on the family only from parents, a few collected information from youths. For example, Austin and colleagues (1994) had children with epilepsy and asthma complete Revised Family APGAR (Austin & Huberty, 1989) as part of their assessment of quality of life of children with asthma and epilepsy, and Lawler and colleagues (1990) had adolescents with diabetes complete several family scales in their measurement of family stress, functioning, and emotional health. An overview of assessments made in each attribute category follows.

Family Stress

Family stress was assessed in 6 studies. The assessment model used in 4 studies asked respondents to identify which stressful events had occurred in a past time period using a self-report format. Three studies (Austin et al., 1992; Donnelly, 1994; Lawler et al., 1990) used Family Inventory of Life Events and Changes (FILE; McCubbin, Patterson, & Wilson, 1991e), or a shorter version of this scale. FILE is a 71-item self-report instrument that provides information on strains and life changes in nine areas relevant to family. The scale has been found to have good reliability (coefficient alpha = .72, and test-retest reliability between .72 and .77) and validity through predicted relationships with other family measures (McCubbin & Patterson, 1991). Reliabilities were reported for the study sample in only two studies. Austin and colleagues (1992) reported a coefficient alpha of .82 for the 71-item version, and Donnelly (1994) reported a coefficient alpha of .43 for the 10-item version. In the study by Austin and colleagues (1994), family stress was found to be a significant predictor of behavior problems in children with epilepsy. Lawler and colleagues (1990) found no significant relationships between stress and other family variables.

In the final study where parents reported on stress, Ray and Ritchie (1993) used a 1-item unsegmented visual analog scale to measure parental perceived stress. No reliability or validity data were reported. The authors, however, did find that the stress score was significantly related to caregiving burden and the coping strategy of maintaining family integration.

Adolescents reported on stressors in two studies. Lawler and colleagues (1990) used the adolescent version of FILE (AFILE; McCubbin et al., 1991e) and did not report reliability

results from their sample. Grey and colleagues (1991) developed a 57-item Life Event Scale using items from three other child and adolescent life event scales. The internal consistency reliability using Cronbach's alpha was .86 for this new scale. Stress was not found to be significantly related to physical development, child coping, child adjustment, or self-concept. The correlation between stress and parent coping, however, was −.29.

Only the study by Nagy and Ungerer (1990) measured sources of stress that were related specifically to rearing the child with cystic fibrosis. They used a semistructured interview to assess sources of stress in the areas of child health and treatment, cost, impact of illness on family, and school problems. Parents were asked to report how much they worried about potential problems related to the child's illness. No reliability or validity data were provided. In that study, no differences in stress were found between mothers and fathers.

In summary, the concept of family stress was commonly assessed and most frequently operationalized by the number of stressful events in the past year. Relationships between family stress and other child and family variables have been inconsistent, with some authors finding a relationship with child outcomes (Austin et al., 1992) and others not (Grey et al., 1991). Relationships between stress and other family variables also have not been consistent, with some groups supporting relationships (Grey et al., 1991; Ray & Ritchie, 1993) and one group (Lawler et al., 1990) not doing so.

Family Functioning

Assessments of family functioning were made primarily using scales previously developed for use with the general population (see Table 10.2). Revised Family APGAR (Austin & Huberty, 1989) is the shortest, with only 5 items and one dimension measuring satisfaction with family relationships. Using this scale, Austin and colleagues (1994) found that children with epilepsy rated family functioning more negatively than children with asthma did.

Family Adaptability and Cohesion Evaluation Scale (FACES; Olson, Portner, & Lavee, 1985) was used in two studies (Donnelly, 1994; Lawler et al., 1990). The most recent version (20-items) of FACES has two independent factors that measure family adaptability and cohesion. Coefficient alpha reliability was .76 for cohesion and .58 for adaptability (L'Abate & Bagarozzi, 1993). Using this scale, Lawler et al. (1990) found that adolescents with diabetes rated their families as more rigid and less emotionally healthy than norms. Donnelly (1994) used the score to create a family type score and found it to be significantly related to family hardiness.

Family of Origin Scale (Hovestadt, Anderson, Piercy, Cochran, & Fine, 1985) was used in the study by Lawler and colleagues (1990) on adolescents with diabetes. The self-report instrument is a 40-item scale that measures autonomy and intimacy perceived in one's family of origin. The scale is relatively new, and only data on content validity and test-retest reliability ($r = .97$) have been reported (L'Abate & Bagarozzi, 1993). Results indicated that 15 of 16 adolescents with diabetes rated their families as less healthy than norms for college students.

Feetham Family Functioning Scale (FFFS; Roberts & Feetham, 1982) was used in the study by Sawyer (1992) to compare functioning families of children with cystic fibrosis with a general population sample. The scale was developed by nurses to measure family functioning in three areas: relationships between family and larger social elements, relationships related to roles within the family, and interpersonal relationships within the family. Parents respond to 21-items three times to measure how much of the attribute is there now, how much of the attribute is desired, and how

important the attribute is. Estimates of internal consistency reliability ranged from .66 to .84, and test-retest reliability was .85 in past research (Roberts & Feetham, 1982; Sawin & Harrigan, 1995). In Sawyer's (1992) study, no differences in functioning were found between families with a child with cystic fibrosis and general population families.

A scale measuring family functioning (Impact on Family Scale), developed by Stein and Riessman (1980) specifically for families of chronically ill children, was used by Loebig (1990) to study families of children with spina bifida. This 24-item scale reflects both positive and negative changes in the family as a result of the chronic illness. The scale has four subscales, Financial Impact, Social/Familial Impact, Personal Strain, and Mastery, and also assesses effects on siblings. Estimates of reliability resulted in coefficient alpha ranging from .60 to .88. No differences were found between the sample of children with spina bifida compared to the reference sample, but differences were found within the sample based on demographic variables. For example, mothers with more than one child were found to score higher on the Financial Impact subscale than mothers with only one child.

In summary, with one exception, assessment of family functioning was made with scales developed for the general population. Results comparing differences in family functioning were mixed, with the study by Sawyer (1992) showing no differences in functioning between general population families and those with a child with cystic fibrosis, whereas in the study by Lawler and colleagues (1990) that had adolescents with diabetes rate their families, functioning was rated less favorably than norms. There also were differences in family functioning between different illness groups, with children with epilepsy reporting less satisfaction with their families' functioning than did children with asthma in the study by Austin and colleagues (1994).

Family Resources and Coping

Three studies measured family resources or strengths (Austin et al., 1992; Donnelly, 1994; Nagy & Ungerer, 1990). Two scales—Family Inventory of Resources for Management (FIRM; McCubbin, Comeau, & Harkins, 1991a) and Family Hardiness Index (FHI; McCubbin, McCubbin, & Thompson, 1991c)—are self-report questionnaires completed by parents. FIRM is a 69-item scale with four subscales: Esteem and Communication, Mastery and Health, Financial Well-Being, and Extended Family Social Support. Estimates of internal consistency reliability were adequate, with coefficient alpha ranging from .62 to .85. Validity was supported when FIRM scores were correlated with results from other family scales (McCubbin et al., 1991a). Austin and colleagues (1992) found that two FIRM subscales—Mastery and Health and Extended Family Social Support—are significant predictors of behavior problems in children with epilepsy. FHI (McCubbin, McCubbin & Thompson, 1991c) is a 20-item scale with four subscales: Co-oriented Commitment, Confidence, Challenge, and External Control. Coefficient alpha for the total scale was .82 (McCubbin et al., 1991c). FHI was used in the study by Donnelly (1994) and was found to be related to family type but not family stress.

In the third study, Nagy and Ungerer (1990) used a semistructured interview to assess sources and types of social support. No information was provided on reliability and validity of the interview schedule. Results from this study showed that mothers received significantly more instrumental support and social support from friends than did fathers.

Parental coping was measured in 3 studies (Grey et al., 1991; Keller & Nicolls, 1990; Ray & Ritchie, 1993) using two scales that were both developed specifically for parents coping with a chronically ill child. Two studies used Coping Health Inventory for Parents (CHIP;

McCubbin, McCubbin, Nevin, & Cauble, 1991b), a 45-item scale with three subscales: Maintaining Family Integration, Maintaining Resources, and Medical Consultation. Past research found the scale to be valid, based on predicted relationships with other family variables, and coefficient alpha for the subscales were .79, .79, and .71, respectively. Grey and colleagues (1991) found that parental coping was moderately correlated ($r = -.25$) with depression in children with diabetes. Ray and Ritchie (1993), in their study of parents of chronically ill children, found that parental coping was inversely related to the level of burden.

The third study, by Keller and Nicolls (1990), used Chronicity Impact and Coping Instrument (Hymovich, 1984), a 167-item scale with seven subscales: Help, Self-Concern, Help Wanted, Self-Coping Strategies, Spouse Coping Strategies, Sibling Communication, and Beliefs. Reliability estimates using coefficient alpha ranged from .43 to .95 for the subscales (Hymovich & Baker, 1985). Keller and Nicolls (1990) found that mothers of adolescents with chronic illness used more emotive coping strategies than did their fathers.

In summary, family resources were measured using only scales developed for the general population. Results from studies measuring resources found that family resources were significantly related to child outcomes. In contrast, family coping strategies were measured using scales developed specifically for coping with a chronically ill child. Results indicated that parental coping was related to both child outcomes and parental burden.

Family Member Involvement and Adjustment

Only 2 studies measured aspects of parental involvement in child-rearing and caregiving activities; both were developed by the authors for their specific studies. Nagy and Ungerer (1990) used a semistructured interview, with an unspecified number of items, asking parents to estimate the amount of time in the past week spent in activities such as caring for the chronically ill child, completing household tasks, meeting children's physical needs, and managing family finances. No information was provided on the reliability or validity of the interview protocol. The authors found that mothers were more involved than fathers in rearing the child with cystic fibrosis. Williams and colleagues (1993) used a 31-item structured interview to measure maternal behavior related to caretaking and housekeeping as well as behavior in the provider role, social activities, and marriage-role-related activities. The authors reported that the interview protocol was found to have good content validity and to be sensitive to change in pilot testing. Results indicated that mothers decreased their caregiving to well siblings, housekeeping, job, and social activities prior to and after the illness onset.

Parental adjustment was directly assessed in only Nagy and Ungerer's (1990) study, in which two instruments—Mental Health Inventory (MHI; Veit & Ware, 1983) and State-Trait Anxiety Inventory (STAI; Spielberger, Gorusch, Lushene, Vagg, & Jacobs, 1983)—were administered to parents of children with cystic fibrosis. MHI is a 38-item self-report instrument with five subscales: Anxiety, Depression, Behavioral/Emotional Control, Positive Affect, and Emotional Ties. Support has been found for validity when subscales were related to other mental and physical health factors. Coefficient alpha in the Nagy and Ungerer (1990) sample of children with cystic fibrosis ranged from .52 to .95. STAI is a 20-item scale that measures immediate feelings reflecting anxiety. It is a well-developed scale with strong reliability coefficients (e.g., alpha = .91) in a general population sample (Spielberger, 1973). Nagy and Ungerer (1990) found that mothers had more anxiety and poorer mental health than normative samples and less emotional and behavior control than their husbands.

Sibling adjustment was assessed in 2 studies (Gallo et al., 1992, 1993; Williams et al., 1993). Gallo and colleagues (1992, 1993) used the previously described CBCL problem and social competence scores and found that siblings' adjustment did not differ significantly from the normative sample. They did find relationships with birth order, however, with siblings younger than the ill child displaying poorer adjustment than siblings older than the ill child. In Williams and colleagues' (1993) study, mothers were asked open-ended questions to determine any changes in siblings' response to their ill sibling. No information was provided on exact number of items, reliability, or validity. Results showed that siblings' household activities increased and their school and social activities decreased after onset of their sibling's chronic illness.

In summary, measurement of other family members focused on involvement or adjustment. In general, results indicated that mothers were most affected by the child's chronic illness. Mothers were more involved in caregiving (Nagy & Ungerer, 1990) and less involved in other activities (Williams et al., 1993). Moreover, they also appeared to have more symptoms of emotional distress (Nagy & Ungerer, 1990). Although siblings as a group did not appear to experience adjustment problems, Gallo and colleagues (1992, 1993) found differences based on birth order in relationship to the chronically ill sibling.

■ *Qualitative Assessment Methods*

The 18 research articles using qualitative methods were analyzed to identify major models or themes relevant to the assessment of children's and families' responses to chronic illness. As with the studies using quantitative methods, these studies focused on attributes of the chronically ill child or on attributes of the family or on both. One major difference, of course, is that these studies were generally not concerned with the measurement of attributes. Often, the purpose of the studies was to describe processes used by families in the management of childhood chronic illness. Samples in 17 of the 18 studies were composed of children and their families; the remaining study included a subset of children and families in a larger sample that ranged from infants to elderly persons.

In this group, 14 authors relied solely on qualitative methods and data, including interviews, case analysis, or projective techniques. Four used some combination of quantitative and qualitative methods/data. Five identified a specific methodology, such as grounded theory or phenomenology. Seven of the reports were generated from a single, large grounded theory study. A summary of study purposes, methods, and major themes from the analyses is presented in Table 10.3.

Assessment Themes

Family Management Style. Seven studies were reported in the development and explication of this model. All data in these articles were generated from a single, large grounded theory study of 63 families with a chronically ill school-age child. Knafl and Deatrick (1990) presented the original concept analysis of Family Management Style (FMS), illustrated with interview data from two of the families. Two reports (Gallo, 1990; McCarthy & Gallo, 1992) used a case study analysis of one family over time to further develop the FMS theme. They illustrated three features of FMS: definition of the situation, management behaviors, and sociocultural context. Deatrick and Knafl (1990) used a case analysis to describe elements of the management behav-

iors component of the model: target behaviors, goal, dimension, focus, and implementation of management behavior. Gallo, Breitmayer, Knafl, and Zoeller (1991) and Gallo (1990) analyzed interviews with parents and healthy siblings to explore the theme of sibling perception of stigma of illness and sibling adjustment to chronic illness.

Breitmayer and colleagues (1992) examined child social competence using interview data as well as quantitative measures, which are reported in the quantitative section of this chapter. This group also examined sibling psychosocial adjustment to chronic illness in a wholly quantitative report of data from the same study (Gallo et al., 1992). Even though it is evident that a variety of family and child attributes were studied by this group, the conceptual model of FMS was central to all.

Child Attributes

An assessment of child coping was made in 2 of the studies reviewed. Spitzer (1992) assessed children's perceptions of, and coping with, illness and treatment. The main themes of this study were illness (hemophilia) and treatment constraints or hardships and their meaning to children. Types of coping (emotion-focused and problem-focused) were described. Breitmayer and colleagues (1992) investigated the social competence of chronically ill children, differentiating this concept from the incidence of behavior problems. Major themes in the attainment of social competence centered on the roles of parents and children in managing illness.

In general, developmental differences among children in these studies were not addressed. Only the one conducted by Clements, Copeland, and Loftus (1990) identified developmental concerns as a central focus of the research. Gallo and colleagues (1991), McCarthy and Gallo (1992), and Gallo (1990) reported some data about school issues, but none specifically assessed school performance as a feature of adjustment to chronic illness.

Family Attributes

Assessment of family attributes constituted the main focus of the rest of the qualitative studies. Phillips (1991) described the concept of chronic sorrow in mothers caring for chronically ill children at home, noting that hopelessness and uncertainty were important elements in the development of this emotional state.

Loebig (1990) and Dashiff (1993) studied the impact of chronic illness on the family system. Loebig (1990) reported mothers' assessments of the impact of a child with spina bifida on the family, including concerns about the child's social development, rehabilitation prospects, and future independence. Dashiff (1993) studied the impact of diabetes on families, focusing on parents' perceptions of their adolescent daughters with diabetes. The daughters' illness was perceived to have a positive impact on family closeness and yet present a challenge to the spousal relationship. Families concentrated on minimizing the negative impact of the illness and on managing emotional distress.

Cohen (1993, 1995a, 1995b) generated a grounded theory of family behavior under conditions of sustained uncertainty due to having a child with a chronic illness. She described the prediagnostic period in chronic illness with its attendant intensification of uncertainty; the triggers of increased uncertainty in families; the chronic illness trajectory as experienced by families; and six dimensions of living with uncertainty: namely, managing (a) time, (b) awareness, (c) environment, (d) information, (e) the illness, and (f) social interaction.

Clements and colleagues (1990) described critical times in childhood chronic illness that result in disequilibrium in family interactions and function: initial impact, parent absence, developmental changes, relocation of the child, and increasing physical symptoms.

Burkhardt (1993), using a thematic analysis, studied health perceptions of mothers caring for chronically ill children. Major themes in mothers' perceptions of their own, and their children's, health were acceptance, relationships, coping, uncertainty, time perspective, hope, normalization, and heightened awareness of the illness.

Sims, Boland, and O'Neill (1992) studied family decision making roles in caring for persons with chronic illness, including a subset of families caring for chronically ill children at home. They described a process of taking control that allowed families to reassert their decision-making authority in the caregiving process.

Ray and Ritchie (1993) described both the coping strategies used by parents in managing their child's care and the factors that influenced parents' appraisal of stress and choice of coping strategies. The major themes presented in this study were parental coping, coping strategies, appraisal, burden, and situational and personal factors in coping.

It is difficult in such a reductionistic presentation of results to adequately situate findings in an appropriate context. The reader is reminded that in qualitative research the circumstances and stories of each family are inseparable from the findings. Nonetheless, this brief review of qualitative studies demonstrates the wide range of themes and concepts that have emerged from the study of families and children with chronic illness.

■ Summary, Conclusions, and Recommendations

Our summary comments address five broad areas: focus of assessments, source of information, validity issues, developmental issues, and knowledge development. Recommendations for future development of

(text continued on p. 216)

TABLE 10.3 Overview of Studies Using Qualitative Assessment Methods and Findings

Author(s) and Date	Purpose	Method(s)	Themes or Concepts
Knafl and Deatrick (1990)	Concept analysis of Family Management Style in families with chronically ill child	Concept construction Case analysis Case illustration	Family Management Style How family as a unit responds to child's chronic illness Definition of situation Management behaviors Sociocultural context
Gallo (1990)	Illustrate three interactive components of Family Management Style model	Case analysis	Family Management Style Definition of situation Management behaviors Sociocultural context Categories of definition: seriousness of illness, illness management philosophy, parental philosophy, and consequences of illness
McCarthy and Gallo (1992)	Describe how a family defines and manages diabetes; compare responses of family members on two occasions	Case analysis	Family Management Style Definition of situation Management behaviors Sociocultural context
Gallo, Breitmayer, Knafl, and Zoeller (1991)	Describe how well siblings view potential stigma in childhood chronic illness	Content analysis of sibling interviews	Stigma in chronic illness Responses to ill child Impact of illness on sibling's daily life Decision making about revealing or not revealing the illness to others

Author (year)	Purpose	Methods	Concepts
Breitmayer, Gallo, Knafl, and Zoeller (1992)	Explore relations between families' management of child's chronic illness and measures of individual and family functioning; illustrate contrasting styles of family management and child coping	Case vignettes Quantitative measures (reported previously)	Social competence Roles of parents and children in treatment regimens Responsibility in illness management
Gallo, Breitmayer, Knafl, and Zoeller (1993)	Examine variations in sibling behavioral adjustment in relation to mothers' perceptions of illness experience and family life	Interviews Quantitative measures (reported previously)	Sibling adjustment to illness Family response to illness Illness management Impact of illness Parenting philosophy Stressors Social support
Deatrick and Knafl (1990)	Elaborate management behaviors component of Family Management Style model	Concept illustration Case analysis	Family Management Style Management behaviors Daily adjustments to child's special needs
Loebig (1990)	Describe mothers' assessments of impact of child with spina bifida on the family	Interviews Content analysis Quantitative measures (reported previously)	Impact of illness on family system Mothers' concerns about child: social development, rehabilitation, and independence
Phillips (1991)	Concept development: Chronic sorrow in mothers caring for chronically ill child at home	Interviews Content analysis	Chronic sorrow Denial Hopelessness Uncertainty
Ray and Ritchie (1993)	Describe coping strategies of parents in managing child's care and the factors influencing parents' appraisal and coping strategies	Interviews Quantitative measures (reported previously)	Parent Coping Coping strategies Appraisal Burden Situational and personal factors in coping

TABLE 10.3 *Continued*

Author(s) and Date	Purpose	Method(s)	Themes or Concepts
Spitzer (1992)	Document type of illness constraints and their meaning for school-age children with hemophilia Document relationships between coping strategies used by children and illness constraints encountered	Projective technique/interview Constant comparative analysis	Child coping Physical and psychosocial illness constraints Identity development/differentness Illness and treatment concerns
Burkhart (1993)	Identify health perceptions as described by mothers of children with chronic illness	Interviews Thematic analysis	Health perceptions of mothers: personal health and child's health Acceptance Coping Uncertainty Hope Normalization Heightened awareness
Dashiff (1993)	Description of parental perceptions of diabetes in daughters Impact on family during adolescence	Interviews Content analysis	Impact of diabetes on family unit, marital dyad, and child with illness Closeness of family unit Minimizing negative impact of illness Managing emotional distress
Clements, Copeland, and Loftus (1990)	Describe parents' perceptions of specific periods viewed as difficult while caring for chronically ill child	Grounded theory Interviews	Critical times in chronic illness, resulting in disequilibrium in family interactions and support: Initial impact Parent absence Developmental changes Relocation of child Increase in physical symptoms

Source	Purpose	Method	Concepts

Cohen (1993)	Generate theory of family behavior under conditions of sustained uncertainty due to diagnosis of chronic, life-threatening illness of a child	Grounded theory	Uncertainty in illness
			Diagnostic closure and the spread of uncertainty
			Living with sustained uncertainty
			Six dimensions of daily life:
			  Managing time
			  Managing awareness
			  Managing environment
			  Managing information
			  Managing the illness
			  Managing social interaction

Cohen (1995a)	Explicate theory of family behavior under conditions of uncertainty due to child with chronic illness	Grounded theory	Stages of prediagnostic period in chronic illness of child Intensification of uncertainty Parental response to diagnosis
Cohen (1995b)	Explicate theory of family behavior under conditions of uncertainty due to child with chronic illness	Grounded theory	Triggers of increased uncertainty Chronic illness trajectory framework
Sims, Boland, and O'Neill (1992)	Describe experiences of families caring for chronically ill child at home (sample included subset of families caring for children)	Grounded theory Interviews	Decision making in home health care Family decision-making roles Problem framing Taking control

assessment methods are presented in each of these areas.

Focus of Assessments

Even though authors rarely referred to a theory that guided their focus of assessment, it was apparent that family stress theory was a guiding paradigm in most of the studies. As a result, the focus of many of the assessments of child and family attributes was on stressors, resources, coping strategies, and family functioning. A major focus of assessment was on adjustment—either on the chronically ill child or on the family. Very often in the quantitative studies, the focus of assessment was on general psychosocial adjustment of the chronically ill child and not specifically on the child's adjustment to illness. Authors conducting qualitative studies tended to focus their assessments more on adjustment to illness.

A trend was also found for measurement of child adjustment to focus on maladjustment, even though the majority of children with chronic conditions were found to be doing well. For example, CBCL (Achenbach, 1991a) focuses primarily on problem behaviors. It is surprising that nursing's focus would be on general psychosocial adjustment rather than on the adjustment of the child or the family specifically to an illness, especially because it is the illness that leads to contact with the nurse. More important, nurses are the ones with responsibility to intervene to help families adjust to the illness. One could hypothesize that adjustment to the illness would be reflected in an assessment of general adjustment, but without measuring it specifically it is difficult to know why and how illness affects psychosocial adjustment. For example, five different children could be maladjusted for five different reasons. Nursing assessments need to focus on factors that are within the purview of the nurse's target of intervention. It could be ar-

gued that for the pediatric nurse, interventions should focus on factors that are related to adjustment to illness rather than on general psychosocial dysfunction.

A related theme was the limited focus of assessment on process, especially in the quantitative studies. As noted in a previous review by Austin (1991), time since onset was rarely included as a variable, so it was not known if the processes of adjustment changed over time. Authors using qualitative methods more frequently focused on process. Neither group of researchers, however, studied the process of nursing care and how it was related to outcomes. The target of assessment for the researchers using qualitative methods was more on how the family managed or responded rather than on the interface between the family and nursing care. It can be safely assumed that quality of nursing care should influence adjustment to illness. Moreover, considering that nursing is an applied profession and research should have as a major goal the development of interventions to improve nursing care, it is surprising that nursing care attributes were rarely a focus of assessment.

If assessment methods are to provide a stronger foundation for nursing interventions, assessment tools must be developed that discriminate between patients needing different types of nursing care. It is essential that assessment instruments not only be more narrowly focused but, more important, address nursing care behaviors. With the trend for individually tailored interventions, it is especially important that assessment tools be developed that provide for the identification of individual attributes amenable to nursing interventions. For example, Austin and colleagues (1992) found family resources of mastery and health and extended family social support to be positively related to child adjustment. Before appropriate interventions can be designed, however, it will be necessary to identify the specific nature and timing of these family resources that lead to successful child adaptation to the chronic illness (Austin, 1991; Feetham, 1984).

Source and Type of Assessment Data

Self-report was the major method used to collect data in these studies. Authors using quantitative methods predominately used paper-and-pencil questionnaires. Face-to-face interview was the primary method used by authors employing chiefly qualitative methods. Only a few studies made use of other techniques such as child drawings and response to vignettes. Noticeably absent was the use of observational methods where systematic procedures were used to watch and record behavior. This lack of using observational methods was surprising in light of its relevancy for family research and its increasing use to study families in other disciplines (Miller, 1986).

As noted previously by Feetham (1984), there was a trend for data to be collected only from one source. With few exceptions, data on child adaptation were collected from only one family member, usually the mother or the child. Authors using qualitative methods generally gathered data primarily from parents and rarely from children. Teachers' ratings of the child were also rare, even though children spend a great deal of time at school. Furthermore, school is a context where many chronically ill children experience problems. The reliance on data from one source can lead to problems with method variance bias, a condition where the magnitude of the relationship between two variables varies based on the source of the data (Lorenz & Melby, 1994). The use of multiple sources and multiple methods for the measurement of the same concept is one strategy for addressing method variance bias (Lorenz & Melby, 1994). This strategy is being used by researchers in other disciplines to study chronic childhood illness. For example, Pianta and

Lothman (1994) used observation of mother-child interaction, mothers' ratings of the child's behavior, teachers' ratings of the child's behavior, and questionnaires in their research on childhood epilepsy.

Validity Issues

Many of the authors employing quantitative methods used instruments developed specifically for the general population. These scales, however, may not be valid measures of adjustment in children with chronic health conditions. For example, symptoms of depression or behavior problems may be caused by characteristics of the chronic condition and not be representative of maladjustment. CBCL (Achenbach, 1991a) and CDI (Kovacs, 1985) both contain items (e.g., appetite, fatigue, sleep) that could be caused by the chronic condition. As a result, these children could receive inflated scores if scoring procedures do not take into account illness characteristics (Perrin, Stein, & Drotar, 1991). Bennett (1994) suggested that it is important to analyze data with and without these items to determine if their inclusion is inflating scores. To advance the field, nurse researchers might need to revise general population scales to make them more valid for children with chronic illness.

Authors using primarily quantitative methods consistently reported in the methods section the reliability and validity of scales. In contrast, data on how valid the measurement instrument was for their samples of chronically ill children or how well the results discriminated among families needing different treatments were rarely mentioned. If nurse researchers would be more systematic in their reporting of results from using scales, we could accumulate information on how well these scales fared with samples of chronically ill children. As noted by La Greca (1994), it is also very important that samples are thoroughly described and the results (e.g., means, standard deviations, range, reliabilities) systematically reported. When problems with instruments are found or any changes are made to make a scale more valid for chronic illness, these should be thoroughly described in the report of the research. It is also important that assessment instruments not only meet the customary standards for reliability and validity but render scores that discriminate among patients needing different levels of care (Keith & Lipsey, 1993).

Developmental Issues

A related concern is the lack of attention to issues related to the developmental level of the child. With very few exceptions, age was the only developmental variable measured, and little was mentioned about how cognitive level might affect adjustment. Deatrick, Faux, and Moore (1993) pointed out that child developmental level also influences the validity of assessment methods. Developmental issues are especially important because wide age ranges are often needed to obtain appropriate samples in the area of chronic illness (Austin, 1991). Even though age is certainly related to psychological and neurobehavioral maturation, and all three are embedded in cognitive development, it is not accurate to assume that age alone will substitute for cognitive development. It appears that more attention to developmental differences is needed in nursing assessment. In measurement studies, cognitive development could be a variable addressed in sample selection and study design. In interpretive studies, differences in cognitive development could be accounted for in the theory generated or in the descriptive findings.

Related to this concern is the application of family stress theory without considering the vast developmental differences among family members. Midence's (1994) criticism, that re-searchers studying childhood chronic illness tend to apply adult models of stress and coping to children, appears to be supported in this review. It is recommended that nurse researchers include assessment of developmental variables so it can be determined if theories and assessment methods are valid across developmental levels.

Knowledge Development

As the use of interpretive methodologies and qualitative methods increases in nursing, the debate about how best to use the knowledge generated from these approaches becomes more important. This debate is no longer focused on the position of interpretive research relative to other kinds of research. Currently, we are more interested in understanding how we might use interpretive knowledge in the development of theory or nursing interventions.

One possibility is that knowledge gained from interpretive work gives us better contextual assessment of families and children with chronic illness. Because of its (generally) more holistic approach, it may allow us to better assess families as units versus as sets of individual responses adding up to a family. This issue is specifically addressed in Knafl and Deatrick (1990). Also, methodologies such as grounded theory were designed to examine process in a less time-bound way than is possible with quantitative instruments.

Experimental and measurement design seems firmly fixed in the repertoire of nursing science. As with interpretive research, few are naive enough to engage in circular debates about their worth in the development of nursing knowledge. As can be seen in this review, quantitative methods have their own points of vulnerability that must be addressed. For example, the validity of using adult-focused measures with children has been questioned.

Overall, the knowledge generated by the studies reviewed for this chapter is still in a fragmentary state. It is a good reflection of knowledge development in nursing generally. The next step appears to be finding ways to integrate knowledge gained from a variety of study designs into useful applications for the practice of nursing. These studies indicate that we could be using triangulation where it counts the most: at the conceptual and theoretical levels of knowledge development in the assessment of family responses to chronic childhood illness.

APPENDIX

■ *Articles Reviewed*

Austin, J. K., & Huberty, T. J. (1989). Revision of the Family APGAR for use by 8-year-olds. *Family Systems Medicine, 7,* 323-327.

Austin, J. K., & Huberty, T. J. (1993). Development of the Child Attitude Toward Illness Scale. *Journal of Pediatric Psychology, 18,* 467-480.

Austin, J. K., Patterson, J. M., & Huberty, T. J. (1991). Development of the Coping Health Inventory for Children. *Journal of Pediatric Nursing, 6,* 166-174.

Austin, J. K., Risinger, M. W., & Beckett, L. A. (1992). Correlates of behavior problems in children with epilepsy. *Epilepsia, 33,* 1115-1122.

Austin, J. K., Smith, M. S., Risinger, M. W., & McNelis, A. M. (1994). Childhood epilepsy and asthma: Comparison of quality of life. *Epilepsia, 35,* 608-615.

Bossert, E., & Martinson, I. M. (1990). Kinetic Family Drawings–Revised: A method of determining the impact of cancer on the family as perceived by the child with cancer. *Journal of Pediatric Nursing, 5,* 204-213.

Breitmayer, B. J., Gallo, A. M., Knafl, K. A., & Zoeller, L. H. (1992). Social competence of school-age children with chronic illness. *Journal of Pediatric Nursing, 7,* 181-188.

Burkhart, P. V. (1993). Health perceptions of mothers of children with chronic conditions. *Maternal-Child Nursing Journal, 21,* 122-129.

Clements, D. B., Copeland, L. G., & Loftus, M. (1990). Critical times for families with a chronically ill child. *Pediatric Nursing, 16,* 157-161.

Cohen, M. H. (1993). The unknown and the unknowable—managing sustained uncertainty. *Western Journal of Nursing Research, 15,* 77-96.

Cohen, M. H. (1995a). The stages of the prediagnostic period in chronic, life-threatening childhood illness: A process analysis. *Research in Nursing and Health, 18,* 39-48.

Cohen, M. H. (1995b). The triggers of heightened parental uncertainty in chronic, life-threatening childhood illness. *Qualitative Health Research, 5,* 63-77.

Dashiff, C. J. (1993). Parents' perceptions on diabetes in adolescent daughters and its impact on the family. *Journal of Pediatric Nursing, 8,* 361-369.

Deatrick, J. A., & Knafl, K. A. (1990). Management behaviors: Day-to-day adjustments to childhood chronic condition. *Journal of Pediatric Nursing, 5,* 15-22.

Donnelly, E. (1994). Parents of children with asthma: An examination of family hardiness, family stressors, and family functioning. *Journal of Pediatric Nursing, 9,* 398-408.

Dragone, M. A. (1990). Perspectives of chronically ill adolescents and parents on health care needs. *Pediatric Nursing, 16,* 45-50.

Fleming, J. W., Holmes, S., Barton, L., & Osbahr, B. (1993). Differences in color preferences of well school-age children and those in varying stages of illness. *Maternal-Child Nursing Journal, 21,* 130-142.

Gallo, A. M. (1990). Family management style in juvenile diabetes: A case illustration. *Journal of Pediatric Nursing, 5,* 23-32.

Gallo, A. M., Breitmayer, B. J., Knafl, K. A., & Zoeller, L. H. (1991). Stigma in childhood chronic illness: A well sibling perspective. *Pediatric Nursing, 17,* 21-25.

Gallo, A. M., Breitmayer, B. J., Knafl, K. A., & Zoeller, L. H. (1992). Well siblings of children with chronic illness: Parents' reports of their psychologic adjustment. *Pediatric Nursing, 18,* 23-27.

Gallo, A. M., Breitmayer, B. J., Knafl, K. A., & Zoeller, L. H. (1993). Mothers' perceptions of sibling adjustment and family life in childhood chronic illness. *Journal of Pediatric Nursing, 8,* 318-324.

Grey, M., Cameron, M. E., & Thurber, F. W. (1991). Coping and adaptation in children with diabetes. *Nursing Research, 40,* 144-149.

Keller, C., & Nicolls, R. (1990). Coping strategies of chronically ill adolescents and their parents. *Issues in Comprehensive Pediatric Nursing, 13,* 73-80.

Knafl, K. A., & Deatrick, J. A. (1990). Family management style: Concept analysis and development. *Journal of Pediatric Nursing, 5,* 4-14.

Lawler, M. K., Volk, R., Viviani, N., & Mengel, M. B. (1990). Individual and family factors impacting diabetic control in the adolescent: A preliminary study. *Maternal-Child Nursing Journal, 19,* 331-345.

Loebig, M. (1990). Mothers' assessments of the impact of children with spina bifida on the family. *Maternal-Child Nursing Journal, 19,* 251-264.

McCarthy, S. M., & Gallo, A. M. (1992). A case illustration of Family Management Style. *Journal of Pediatric Nursing, 7,* 395-402.

Mullis, R. L., Mullis, A. K., & Kerchoff, N. F. (1992). The effect of leukemia and its treatment on self-esteem of school-age children. *Maternal-Child Nursing Journal, 20,* 155-165.

Nagy, S., & Ungerer, J. A. (1990). The adaptation of mothers and fathers to children with cystic fibrosis: A comparison. *Children's Health Care, 19,* 147-154.

Nelms, B. C. (1989). Emotional behaviors in chronically ill children. *Journal of Abnormal Child Psychology, 17,* 657-668.

Phillips, M. (1991). Chronic sorrow in mothers of chronically ill and disabled children. *Issues in Comprehensive Pediatric Nursing, 14,* 111-120.

Punnett, A. F., & Thurber, S. (1994). The Child Evaluation Inventory: An adaptation for asthma camp. *Children's Health Care, 23,* 69-74.

Ray, L. D., & Ritchie, J. A. (1993). Caring for chronically ill children at home: Factors that influence parents' coping. *Journal of Pediatric Nursing, 8,* 217-225.

Ryan-Wenger, N. M., & Walsh, M. (1994). Children's perspectives on coping with asthma. *Pediatric Nursing, 20,* 224-228.

Sawyer, E. H. (1992). Family functioning when children have cystic fibrosis. *Journal of Pediatric Nursing, 7,* 304-311.

Sims, S., Boland, D. L., & O'Neill, C. A. (1992). Decision making in home health care. *Western Journal of Nursing Research, 14,* 186-200.

Spitzer, A. (1992). Coping processes of school-age children with hemophilia. *Western Journal of Nursing Research, 14,* 157-169.

Williams, P. D., Lorenzo, F. D., & Borja, M. (1993). Pediatric chronic illness: Effects on siblings and mothers. *Maternal-Child Nursing Journal, 21,* 111-121.

11
■

INTEGRATIVE REVIEW OF INTERVENTION RESEARCH WITH CHILDREN WHO HAVE CHRONIC CONDITIONS AND THEIR FAMILIES

■ *Janet A. Deatrick*

Intervention research tests blueprints for assisting children with chronic conditions and their families. The scientific literature is replete with suggestions to use the results of descriptive studies to design interventions. Testing these interventions in experimental studies then contributes evidence regarding their effectiveness.

Experimental and quasi-experimental studies constituted 5% of published pediatric nursing research between 1980 and 1987 (Burke & Roberts, 1990) and approximately 10% between 1968 and 1992 (Hester, 1992). Today, these studies still constitute only a small portion of research done in the discipline; however, they can provide guidance for future care of vulnerable children and their families.

The characteristics of effective as well as ineffective interventions can be identified across existing studies so as to design the most pro-

ductive approaches to use with chronically ill children and their families. Such efforts are consistent with today's increased attention to developing cost-effective models of care that link patient care problems with interventions and outcomes. This chapter provides an integrative review (Broome, 1993; Lee, Picard, & Blain, 1994) of studies that tested interventions with children who have chronic conditions and their families in order to make recommendations for clinical research. The review was designed to answer the following research questions:

- What intervention strategies have been effectively used with children who have chronic conditions and their families?
- What interventions have not been successful?
- What is the methodological adequacy of these studies?
- What are the reported psychometric properties of the outcome measures?

- What were the substantive findings of these studies?

This analysis complements and further develops knowledge gained from previous reviews concerning intervention studies focused on children and their families (Beal & Betz, 1992; Brennan, 1994; Olson, Heater, & Becker, 1990), current initiatives regarding guidelines for early intervention practice (Magyary, Brandt, Fleming, Kieckhefer, & Padgett, 1993), and the classification of nursing interventions and functions related to the family (Craft & Willadsen, 1992; Grobe, 1990; Martin, Scheet, & Stegman, 1993; McCloskey & Bulechek, 1994; Saba, 1992; Verran, 1986).

The working definition of *intervention* used in this analysis is based on Feetham's (1992) description of practitioner-family interventions: "the direct activities by the practitioner to affect family function and/or structure through work with the individual family members and/or the family system. The intervention can result in a short-term or a long-term effect" (p. 105). A conceptualization of practitioner-child-family interventions ideally considers characteristics of each (Knafl, 1992) and the interrelationships between the psycho-biological-spiritual structure of the child and the family (Wright & Leahey, 1994a; Wright & Levac, 1992) and the practitioner. Therefore, interventions are considered in the context of characteristics of the practitioner, child, and family.

Interventions typically occur on cognitive, affective, or behavioral levels (Wright & Leahey, 1994a) with effects or outcomes that can be attributed to the same level or possibly to others. That is, cognitive interventions can result in affective changes (e.g., preoperative instruction will reduce preoperative anxiety). Less is known about how changes in the cognitive domain will affect actual behaviors (Gilliss & Davis, 1992).

■ Past Research

A number of past studies and research programs set the stage for recent intervention research. The research of Kathryn Barnard, Ida Martinson, Mary Lauer, Mary Ann Lewis, and their colleagues in the 1970s and 1980s formed the foundation for today's understanding concerning the efficacy of nursing interventions with children who have serious, chronic conditions and their families. In particular, these early studies revealed the critical elements of nursing interventions. In a recent review of parent-infant nursing science, Walker (1992) analyzed the key components in Barnard's program of research regarding supportive interventions for parents and infants. Timing is crucial. She concluded, with Barnard, that the prenatal period is the optimal time to begin interventions with parents who are socially at risk. Moreover, the types of interventions must be shaped to the characteristics of the caregivers. For example, Barnard found that a mental health intervention emphasizing the development of a therapeutic relationship was more effective for mothers with lower IQ scores, whereas an intervention emphasizing information and resources (IR) was more effective for mothers with higher IQ scores, who together with their children had significantly better outcomes from the IR intervention (Barnard, Snyder, & Spietz, 1991).

Martinson and colleagues (1978) and Lauer, Mulhern, Wallskog, and Camitta (1983) sensitized nursing to the importance of the setting and nature of care regarding terminally ill childrens who were dying in the home and hospital. In their pioneering work, they identified the social, psychological, and economic outcomes of their interventions. Again, the differences among families' responses to treatment were emphasized, which were attributed to the intervention as well as to unknown factors.

Over the past 20 years, Lewis and Lewis have participated in the design, implementation, and evaluation of research intent on empowering children to participate in their own well-child care and illness-related care. Two reviews of that work (Lewis & Lewis, 1989, 1990) concluded that children are competent to self-select into programs where they learn decision-making skills and how to apply them in clearly defined situations. However, resistance to diffusion and implementation of these programs derives from the health care system, children, and families. Deeply rooted patterns of behavior are unlikely to change without strong inducements. Lewis and Lewis concluded that successful programs must involve the providers and families themselves and not just the children.

The U.S. General Accounting Office (GAO; 1990) reviewed home visiting in the United States and Europe in order to describe its effectiveness as an early intervention strategy. Included in this analysis was Brooten and colleagues' (1986) comprehensive program of discharge planning and home follow-up care with low-birth-weight infants and their families, which employs advanced practice nurses. Also included was Olds, Henderson, Tatelbaum, and Chamberlin's (1986) nurse home visitation program with socially disadvantaged primiparous women. Although the programs included in the GAO (1990) review were not all nursing studies, home visiting was found to be an important ingredient in nursing interventions with high-risk populations. Home visiting across provider groups was associated with improved outcomes for participants, including improved birth outcomes, better child health, improved child welfare, and improved development, when compared to individuals who did not receive the interventions tied to home visits. The GAO study concluded that critical components of home visiting programs include clear objectives that are used to manage the problem, matching the home visitor's skills and abilities to the services being provided, working through an agency with the capacity to deliver or access a wide range of services, and developing secure funding over time. Projects that did not achieve desired outcomes failed to (a) use objectives to guide the program and its services, (b) design and structure services, (c) sufficiently train and supervise home visitors, and (d) provide access to a range of services. Home visits remain a central element to much community-based nursing care, and the results of the GAO review are applicable to nursing interventions.

Recently, Burke, Kauffman, Wiskin, and Harrison (1995) proposed the following characteristics for successful interventions with children who had chronic conditions: parent-focused, multifaceted, organized around periods of potential or actual parent or child distress, and professionally delivered by individuals especially trained concerning the intervention. Successful interventions also vary (a) in response to parents' needs over time, (b) by nurses' experience and skill, and (c) by availability of health care services. Less successful interventions deal with a wide range of issues, are provided by individuals without training specific to the intervention, and require contacts that are not necessarily linked to specific client problems.

Lee and colleagues (1994) suggested issues that are especially relevant for the methodological critique of intervention studies: (a) relevancy of the demographic data to the experience of chronic illness, (b) qualifications of the individual performing the intervention, (c) integrity of the design, (d) characteristics of the treatment, (e) source of assessment data, and (f) appropriateness of statistical analysis.

This past research forms the foundation for the critique and synthesis of the studies identified

TABLE 11.1 Summary of Critical Methodological Elements in the 9 Articles

Methodological Element	No. Occurring (no. applicable)
Relevancy of demographic data	
Age	8(9)
Diagnosis or disabilities	7(8)
Duration of condition	2(5)
Parents' education/occupation	4(4)
Gender	7(9)
Race/ethnicity	5(9)
Social history	3(7)
Social economic status	3(9)
Attrition noted	5(9)
Sample size or statistical power defended	0(9)
Characteristics of treatments	
Skills/qualifications of providers	
Background	7(9)
Gender	1(9)
Program training	7(9)
Number of providers	6(9)
Conceptual basis	4(9)
Interventions[a]	
Objectives	9(9)
Timing	0(9)
Length of contact	7(9)
Type and number of contacts	6(9)
Nature	9(9)
Family/maternal context	6(9)
Community linkages	2(9)
Future funding support	0(0)
Measurement and analyses	
Analyses	
Demographics	7(9)
Univariate statistics	8(8)
Inferential statistics	7(7)
Themes	2(2)
Psychometrics	
Reliability	7(19)
Validity	10(19)

a. Also see Table 11.3 for a description of the interventions.

for this review as they provide critical information for shaping interventions that have the desired outcome. These critical elements are summarized in Table 11.1 in terms of the relevancy of demographic data, characteristics of the treatment, measurement, and analysis. Numbers in the table reflect the presence of these elements in articles sampled in this review.

■ *Method*

The literature search had three components: (a) a manual search of 16 peer-reviewed nursing research and practice-based journals from 1966 to 1995; (b) a computerized literature search using the keywords *intervention, children, adolescents,* and *families*; and (c) examination of the reference lists of articles to identify articles not located in the other two components of the search process (see Table 11.2). To be included in the review, articles had to meet the following criteria: a full research report, one or more authors was a nurse, and a focus on infants (older than 1 month), children, and/or adolescents with chronic conditions, with one of the following also needed: comparison or control group, single group design with pre- and postintervention assessment, or random assignment of participants to groups for posttest assessment only. Interventions could be directed at the family unit or at individual family members.

Each article was summarized and critiqued using three organizing grids. First, critical

TABLE 11.2 Journals Used in Manual Search[a]

Advances in Nursing Science
Applied Nursing Research
Children's Health Care
Family Relations
Image
Issues in Comprehensive Pediatric Nursing
Journal of Advanced Nursing
Journal of Pediatric Health Care
Journal of Pediatric Nursing
Maternal-Child Nursing Journal
MCN: American Journal of Maternal-Child Nursing
Nursing Research
Pediatric Nursing
Research in Nursing and Health
Scholarly Inquiry for Nursing Practice
Western Journal of Nursing Research

a. MEDLINE and CINAHL searched from 1966 to the present.

methodological elements were assessed (see Table 11.1) in terms of the number of times and number of applicable instances that each issue was addressed. A rating of over 60% was considered typical when describing the sample as a whole. The sample, design, and interventions for each article were described (see Table 11.3). Substantive findings were organized according to their focus, target constructs, and outcomes (see Table 11.4). Other issues such as ethical concerns (Lewis, Rachelefsky, Lewis, & Richards, 1994) and analyses of cultural competence (Villarruel, 1995) were beyond the scope of this review. For clarity, the term *children* in this review refers to individuals of all ages affected with a chronic condition, and the term *siblings* refers to their brothers and sisters.

■ Results

Numerous articles described interventions, but few tested them. Nine articles, representing 8 different studies, were identified that met the criteria for inclusion in the review. One project had two publications of pertinent results. Lewis, Salas, de la Sota, Chiofalo, and Leake (1990) described the intervention outcomes for children, and Lewis, Hatton, Salas, Leake, and Chiofalo (1991) described the outcomes for parents. In all studies, authors used a pretest-posttest approach to data collection. Random assignment of study participants to groups was done in only a few articles (Black et al., 1994; Lewis et al., 1991; Lewis et al., 1990; Pless et al., 1994). Four studies had no control groups (Brandt & Magyary, 1993; Craft, Lakin, Oppliger, Clancy, & Vanderlinden, 1990; Hills & Lutkenhoff, 1993; Smith et al., 1991). Of the 5 that had a control group, 1 used a no-treatment control group (Heiney, Goon-Johnson, Ettinger, & Ettinger, 1990) and 4 used a routine care control group

(Black et al., 1994; Lewis et al., 1991; Lewis et al., 1990; Pless et al., 1994).

Black and colleagues (1994) implemented an intervention with 60 pregnant, drug-abusing women to provide maternal support and promote child development, parenting, and utilization of informal and formal resources. Brandt and Magyary (1993) implemented an intervention with 17 diabetic children and 1 of their parents to increase the children's diabetes knowledge, skills, and feelings of competency and parents' supportive network. Craft and colleagues (1990) used an intervention to increase independence in 15 children with cerebral palsy through their siblings (*n* = 31). Heiney and colleagues (1990) worked with 14 siblings of children with cancer to increase the siblings' social adjustment. Hills and Lutkenhoff (1993) designed an intervention to increase the social skills of children with chronic conditions and tested it with 12 children with myelomeningocele. Lewis and colleagues (1990, 1991) studied 236 children with epilepsy and their parents to increase the knowledge of both children and parents, decrease the parents' anxiety, and strengthen the children's self-perception, disclosure, and coping/adaptation. Pless and colleagues' (1994) study of 332 children with various chronic conditions and their families sought to optimize family and parental functioning and increase the children's psychosocial adjustment. Smith, Schreiner, Brouhard, and Travis (1991) designed a stress management intervention for children with chronic conditions and tested its effectiveness with 108 diabetic children.

■ Critical Methodological Elements

Each study was critiqued in terms of the methodological elements that were important in past intervention studies. The results of

(text continued on p. 230)

TABLE 11.3 Summary of Studies

Reference	Sample/Design	Intervention
Black, Nair, Knight, Wachtel, Roby, and Schuler (1994)	60 pregnant women who were abusing drugs (40% HIV positive) Randomized clinical trial; routine care control group	Two prenatal home visits and biweekly postnatal visits for 18 months; structured curriculum on child development and parenting taught by community health nurses; women encouraged to enroll in drug rehabilitation program
Brandt and Magyary (1993)	17 children, ages 8–13 years, with diabetes and one of their parents One group, pretest/posttest design; (note: 3-month follow-up scores reflect change from the posttest scores)	5-day program with 11 sessions of 50 minutes each; 3 to 5 children and one of their parents in each group; focus of the groups was on diabetes knowledge and skills, children's feelings of competency, and parents' supportive network
Craft, Lakin, Oppliger, Clancy, and Vanderlinden (1990)	31 siblings, ages 4–17 years, of 15 children, ages 4–19 years, with cerebral palsy One group, pretest/posttest design	4-month intervention by Ph.D.-prepared nurse; four developmentally tailored classes for the siblings focused on knowledge of cerebral palsy and how to motivate their brother or sister to be more independent; home visits (number not specified) and sibling meetings (twice a month) focused on learning reinforcement
Heiney, Goon-Johnson, Ettinger, and Ettinger (1990)	14 siblings, ages 9–15 years Nonequivalent, control group design (comparisons possible on social adjustment only)	7 sessions of group therapy using the Yalom framework and co-led by fellow in child psychiatry and a pediatric oncology nurse practitioner; goal was to increase social adjustment of siblings of children with cancer
Hills and Lutenhoff (1993)	12 children, average age 11.6 years, with myelomeningocele One group, pretest/posttest design	18 sessions of 3 hours' duration; social skills group; Erikson developmental framework; focused on awareness, mastery, and social interaction; also went on outings
Lewis, Hatton, Salas, Leake, and Chiofalo (1991)	365 parents of children with epilepsy See below	See below

226

Source	Sample and Design	Intervention
Lewis, Salas, de la Sota, Chiofalo, and Leake (1990)	236 children, ages 7–14 years, with epilepsy Randomized clinical trial (note: posttest results are 5 months after the program); routine care control group	4 sessions of 90 minutes each in Chile, each taught by elementary school teachers and social worker; family-focused, child-centered educational program concerning epilepsy, medications, disclosure, coping/adaptation, and working as a family control group had 3 sessions of 2 hours each that were traditional lectures
Pless, Feeley, Gottlieb, Rowat, Dougherty, and Willard (1994)	332 children, ages 4–16 years, with various chronic conditions Randomized clinical trial	Telephone, home, and/or office/clinic visits with BSN-prepared nurse; minimum of 12 contacts over 1 year; based on McGill Model of Nursing; goals were to optimize family and parent functioning to increase psychosocial adjustment of children with chronic illness
Smith, Schreiner, Brouhard, and Travis (1991)	108 campers, average age 14.5 years, with diabetes One group, pretest/posttest design	7-day camp; life skills curriculum taught by a trained college-educated young adult in small groups; included specific topics; used variety of techniques to teach them, including stress management

227

TABLE 11.4 Outcomes From 9 Intervention Studies With Children Who Have Chronic Conditions and Their Families

Constructs	*Outcome*
Child-Focused Interventions	
Child ratings	
Coping strategies (Ways of Coping Checklist–Revised; Smith, Schreiner, Brouhard, & Travis, 1991)	Increased problem-focused strategies ($p < .03$) Decreased detachment strategies ($p < .001$)
Effect of program on knowledge perceptions (Hills & Lutkenhoff, 1993)	Qualitative reports of and improvement in self-concept, mastery, social interaction, awareness
Sibling ratings	
Self-Care Abilities Scale (Craft & Willadsen, 1992)	No significant differences pretest to posttest
Parent ratings	
Self-Care Abilities Scale (Craft & Willadsen, 1992)	No significant differences pretest to posttest
Therapist ratings	
Self-Care Abilities Scale (Craft & Willadsen, 1992)	No significant differences pretest to posttest
Range of motion (Functional Status Scale; Craft & Willadsen, 1992)	Increased range of motion in shoulder, elbow, and wrist ($p < .05$); no significant changes in lower body
Sibling-Focused Interventions	
Child rating	
Effect of program on knowledge and perceptions (Heiney, Goon-Johnson, Ettinger, & Ettinger, 1990)	Qualitative reports of trust, sadness, anger, and uncertainty; therapeutic indicators included universality, interpersonal learning, catharsis, cohesiveness, and imparting of information; satisfaction with group
Social Adjustment Scale (Heiney, Goon-Johnson, Ettinger, & Ettinger, 1990)	No significant differences pretest to posttest
Parent rating	
none	none
Family-Focused Interventions	
Child ratings	
Effect of program on knowledge and perceptions (Lewis, Salas, de la Sota, Chiofalo, & Leake, 1990)	More general knowledge ($p < .01$); more knowledgeable about seizure management ($p < .05$) and unnecessary restrictions to social and play activities ($p < .05$); increased participation in normal activities ($p < .03$) and gains in skills ($p < .02$); no impact on disclosure to friends and others or on self-care
Self-concept (Harter Self-Perception Profile; Brandt & Magyary, 1993)	Increased cognitive competence ($p = .037$; posttest) but no significant differences at 3-month follow-up
Lewis, Salas, de la Sota, Chiofalo, and Leake (1990)	Better social interactions and skills ($p < .05$) and better behaved ($p < .002$)
Pless, Feeley, Gottlieb, Rowat, Dougherty, and Willard (1994)	Increased scholastic competence ($p < .05$), behavior ($p < .01$), and global self-worth ($p < .01$) for older children
Knowledge and problem solving (Brandt & Magyary, 1993)	More knowledgeable at posttest ($p = .003$) and 3-month follow-up ($p = .008$); increased problem solving at posttest ($p = .002$) but no significant differences at 3-month follow-up

TABLE 11.4 *Continued*

Constructs	Outcome
Sibling ratings	
Taylor Manifest Anxiety Scale (Lewis, Hatton, Salas, Leake, & Chiofalo, 1991)	Reduced anxiety in experimental group ($p < .01$)
Child Abuse Potential Inventory (Black, Nair, Knight, Wachtel, Roby, & Schuler, 1994)	No significant difference
Child adjustment (Personal Adjustment and Role Skills; Pless, Feeley, Gottlieb, Rowat, Dougherty, & Willard, 1994)	Decreased children's anxiety and depression ($p = .001$)
Child psychopathology	
(Achenbach Child Behavior Checklist; Pless, Feeley, Gottlieb, Rowat, Dougherty, & Willard, 1994)	No significant differences
Drug abuse (Black, Nair, Knight, Wachtel, Roby, & Schuler, 1994)	Marginally more drug free ($p = .059$); women who had more home visits more likely to be drug free ($p = .002$)
Effect of program on knowledge and perceptions (Lewis, Hatton, Salas, Leake, & Chiofalo, 1991)	No significant differences in knowledge; experimental group perceived that they were significantly more knowledgeable ($p < .05$) and had a better understanding regarding the importance of medications ($p < .01$)
Knowledge and problem solving (Brandt & Magyary, 1993)	More knowledgeable at posttest ($p = .008$) but no significant differences at 3-month follow-up; increased problem solving at posttest ($p = .002$) but no significant differences at 3-month follow-up
Maternal social support (Brandt & Magyary, 1993)	No significant differences
Parenting Stress Index (Black, Nair, Knight, Wachtel, Roby, & Schuler, 1994)	No significant differences
Therapist ratings	
Child development (Bayley Scale of Infant Development; Black, Nair, Knight, Wachtel, Roby, & Schuler, 1994)	No significant differences
Compliance (Black, Nair, Knight, Wachtel, Roby, & Schuler, 1994)	Marginally more compliant ($p = .069$); women who had more home visits were more compliant ($p = .016$)
Home Environment Scale (Black, Nair, Knight, Wachtel, Roby, & Schuler, 1994)	Marginally more likely to live in a child-centered home ($p = .061$), being more emotionally and verbally responsive ($p = .033$) and having more opportunities for variety in stimulation ($p = .065$)
Self-care (Brandt & Magyary, 1993)	Increased children's skills with insulin injections at posttest ($p = .003$) but no significant differences at 3-month follow-up; no significant differences for parents with insulin injections or children with chemstrips

this critique are summarized in Table 11.1, which lists the criteria used to judge each study, the number of times the criteria were met, and the number of times they were applicable; that is, if a study was solely child focused, reporting a parent's occupation would not be applicable.

Relevancy of Demographic Data

Demographic data typically included the age of the child and sibling(s), the child's diagnosis, education of the parents, and the gender of the child, sibling(s), and parents. Less attention was paid to parents' age, duration of the child's condition, and the race, socioeconomic status, or social history of the children, sibling(s), or parents. Both the data typically included and those less often reported are all vital in studies with chronically ill children and their families and important to consider in all intervention studies as both modifying and mediating variables.

Sample attrition rates were typically not described. This is especially serious in that none of the articles contained a justification for the number of participants comprising their samples. These deficiencies raise questions, as they would in any intervention study, about the power of statistical tests used in the studies to differentiate an effective intervention from one that is ineffective with these particular samples.

Characteristics of Treatments

Skills/Qualifications of Providers

The qualifications of the providers, as well as the number of providers, were usually described in terms of background and intervention-specific training. However, their gender was not usually described. The gender of the providers is critical data to consider due to the possible role that gender may play in communication and interpersonal relationships.

Conceptual Basis

The conceptual/theoretical perspectives of the studies were typically not identified. Two of the studies that did so were consistent with an ecological/systems framework (Black et al., 1994; Pless et al., 1994). Two other studies used social-psychological theories (Heiney et al., 1990; Hill & Lutkenhoff, 1993). Each framework was consistent with the purposes of its respective study. However, it should be noted that successful interventions consider a wide range of influences and services, as is consistent with frameworks, such as those with an ecological perspective.

Interventions

The following aspects of the interventions were evaluated: objectives, timing, length of contact, type and number of contacts, nature, family/maternal contexts, community linkages, and future funding support.

Objectives. All studies had clear objectives. Explicitly identifying, from a conceptual and clinical perspective, if the interventions denote child-focused, sibling-focused, and/or family-focused interventions and if they are cognitive, affective, and/or behavioral is suggested (Wright & Leahey, 1994a). Although such an analysis can create artificial dichotomies (Robinson, 1995a), used judiciously it can be invaluable in terms of adding clarity to the study.

Timing. None of the studies gave a rationale for the timing of the interventions (Walker, 1992). To justify future expenditure of resources, plan effectively, and replicate interventions, this rationale is imperative.

Length of contact: Type and number of contacts. Most studies, however, did stipulate the length or duration of the intervention, as well as the type and number of the contacts involved in the intervention. Of special importance were the studies that specified a minimum number of contacts and then further explained how many contacts were needed to meet the specific needs of the individual and/or family (Pless et al., 1994). Black and colleagues (1994) had no minimum number of contacts and stipulated that the study's underlying assumption was based on the intention to provide any intervention. Therefore, individuals were retained in the study if they consented, even though they refused certain types of contacts. The number of contacts per individual/family ranged from none to 75 (home visits and telephone calls), with an average of 25 and a standard deviation of 19.

Nature. Not surprisingly, given the focus of these studies, the nature of the interventions was described. Child-, sibling-, and family-focused interventions were used and are described in detail in Table 11.3. Child-focused interventions were designed for children, ages 4–19 years. The format of the child-focused interventions ranged from 1 hour (Smith et al., 1991) to 3 hours each (Hills & Lutkenhoff, 1993) for 7 days (Smith et al., 1991) to an unknown number of total contacts over 4 months (Craft et al., 1990). Content focused variously on emotions and perceptions of self, on social interactions, stress management, problem solving and decision making, motivation, and knowledge.

A sibling-focused intervention was conducted by Heiney and colleagues (1990) for 9- to 15-year-olds. The seven 1-hour sessions were oriented toward group processes to increase the siblings' social adjustment.

Family-focused interventions were conducted during three 2-hour sessions (Lewis et al., 1991; Lewis et al., 1990) or five 50-minute sessions (Brandt & Magyary, 1993) and home visits were made over a period of 1 year (Pless et al., 1994) to 18 months (Black et al., 1994). Family-focused interventions attempted to intervene with the parent(s) and affected children.

The duration of the interventions may have affected their effectiveness (Connell, Turner, & Mason, 1985). Results of the School Health Evaluation project found that stable effects on knowledge, attitudes, and behavior occur only after 50 classroom hours, with relatively more hours required to produce significant attitude change than either knowledge or behavior. This project involved more than 30,000 children in Grades 4 through 7 in 1,071 classrooms across 20 states. Although the transferability of these results to the situations of these families may be questioned, perhaps some of the interventions should have been of a longer duration.

Family-focused interventions appeared more successful than child-focused interventions. Content addressed child behavior, child development, compliance with primary care, drug abuse, emotions and perceptions of self, family relationships, knowledge, parenting, problem solving, school performance, socialization, and skills (see Table 11.3). However, inclusion or exclusion of family issues such as communication patterns, problem-solving ability, and communication style was not addressed when describing the interventions. Deatrick, Feetham, Hayman, and Perkins (1993) specified that interventions with children who have chronic conditions and their families should consider (a) the way that the family and its members define their situation and (b) how they manage the daily work directly related to the child's condition. In fact, Wright and Leahey (1994a) and Robinson (1994) underscored the centrality of the definition or meaning that families and their members ascribe to their situation in making therapeutic change. In future work, assumptions about the contribution of family issues need to be recognized, even if they are not directly studied.

Traditional assumptions about how to effect change in individuals with chronic conditions and their families include a singular perception of the reality of their situation and a belief that a linear relationship exists between aspects of the situation (i.e., family functioning) and the response of the individual family member (i.e., adherence to treatment). Nontraditional perspectives call for recognition of the multiple realities that may be present in a situation and the systemic nature of processes within individuals and families (Robinson, 1994).

Moreover, these intervention studies typically did not use advanced practice nurses, who can function beyond a standardized protocol and shape specific interventions to the characteristics of family members and family units. It is crucial to include the use of advanced practice nurses in the design of future studies, as they have been used successfully with maternal-infant, oncology, and geriatric populations (Brooten et al., 1986; Brooten & Naylor, 1995; McCorkle et al., 1989; Naylor et al., 1994).

Family/maternal context. Although most studies did give some implicit descriptions of the family and/or maternal context for the intervention, more explicit details of the context of care could strengthen future intervention studies by providing useful information on how to individualize interventions to be appropriate in varying contexts. From these data, the relative risk of the family and the parental subsystem can be ascertained. For instance, has the pregnant woman had inadequate or no prenatal care in the past?

Community linkages. Other available client services were seldom addressed and were rarely included as a project objective. For instance, if a project focuses on teaching related to diet, the intervention may need to include provision for access to food stamps for eligible clients. Because access to a wide variety of client services/community linkages has been found to be important in the long term outcomes of studies involving families with multiple problems, both referrals for existing problems and helping families and their members learn to advocate for needed services could be crucial components of successful interventions.

Future funding support. No study mentioned whether or not additional funding was being procured or had been procured to extend or continue the work of the project. Discussions of barriers to continued funding and any creative solutions to these problems are needed to sensitize consumers, policymakers, and other researchers to the ongoing needs of families.

Measurement and Analyses

Analyses. Demographic characteristics were analyzed in most articles. Studies appropriately used both univariate and inferential statistics. However, in the absence of power estimations, the statistical results are in question because it is not possible to determine if the statistical tests had the power to ascertain if the interventions made any true difference.

Qualitative descriptive themes were identified in 2 of the studies. A rationale for the manner in which themes are identified can strengthen further research by providing a basis for further developing the themes and evaluating their credibility.

Psychometrics. Neither reliability nor validity of the instruments was typically described. If an instrument has strong reliability and validity, support for the efficiency of the intervention is strengthened. However, if the instruments' reliability and validity are in question, the results must be interpreted with caution. Of special concern is the lack of psychometric data on instruments used with children who have chronic conditions.

■ Outcomes

Measures

Most assessments were self-assessments; that is, children, siblings, and parents rated themselves. Black and colleagues (1994; parent and observer), Brandt and Magyary (1993; parent, child, and observer), and Craft and colleagues (1990; parent, child, and sibling) all gathered data from more than one source. Craft and colleagues (1990) were the only investigators to measure the same concept, functional status, from the perspective of different individuals and use different instruments to measure the same concept. Self-concept and self-perception were most often used as outcome measures (Brandt & Magyary, 1993; Lewis et al., 1990; Pless et al., 1994). Few studies followed up their posttests with additional measures over time.

Of the 19 instruments used across the studies, the only standardized one that was used in more than one study was Harter Self-Perception Profile (Brandt & Magyary, 1993; Lewis et al., 1990; Pless et al., 1994). Three studies used varying forms of a program evaluation instrument designed for the study to measure the effect of the program on knowledge and perceptions (Heiney et al., 1990; Hills & Lutkenhoff, 1993; Lewis et al., 1990).

Most studies used either quantitative or qualitative approaches to measure outcomes related to the objectives, but not both. However, a combination of well-accepted quantitative and qualitative methods may be needed to enhance nurses' understanding about the effectiveness and efficiency of intervention outcomes over time. For instance, although Heiney and colleagues (1990) did not achieve significant results with quantitative instrumentation, qualitative results were important in understanding the results of the intervention.

■ Results

As noted in Table 11.4, areas of improvement were identified for child and parent variables. Statistically significant results were obtained for Black and colleagues' (1994) family-focused intervention in terms of maternal emotional and verbal responsivity, with numerous areas of marginal, but not statistically significant improvement, including having a child-centered and stimulating home environment. No significant differences between the control and experimental groups were noted for the developmental parameters of the infants, the parents' overall stress, or the parents' child abuse potential. Women who had more home visits (beyond the minimum specified in the protocol) were more likely to be drug free and compliant regarding health care.

Brandt and Magyary (1993) significantly improved selected posttest results for children and mothers concerning diabetes knowledge and problem solving. The children's insulin injection skills and cognitive self-perception also significantly improved. Children's social, physical, and general self-perception and their chemstrip ability did not improve. The social support network of the mothers remained unchanged. The children's gains were not maintained at 3 months postintervention.

Craft and colleagues (1990) obtained a significant change in the range of motion of the shoulder, elbow, and wrist for the children with cerebral palsy. However, there was no significant change in the children's hip, knee, or ankle range of motion or in the children's self-care abilities.

As previously explained, Heiney and colleagues (1990) did not obtain a significant change in social adjustment for siblings of children with cancer. However, qualitative results documented changes in mood state and indicators of therapeutic effects. Qualitative results for Hills and Lutkenhoff (1993) indicated improved social skills for the group members, but no quantitative measures were used. Lewis and colleagues (1990, 1991) significantly improved children's knowledge about epilepsy and seizure management but did not improve their parents' knowledge. The children's self-perception significantly improved, yet their self-care, disclosure, and behavior remained the same. The parents' manifest anxiety significantly decreased.

Pless and colleagues (1994) detected significant differences between the control and experimental groups related to personal adjustment, role skills, and self-perception. Behavior and social adjustment did not significantly change. Smith and colleagues (1991) found that the intervention significantly increased problem-focused strategies and significantly decreased detachment strategies.

Because the exact length and number of intervention contacts was often omitted from these articles, it is not possible to analyze the outcomes in regard to the relative strength of the intervention. The basis for each of the interventions was typically lacking, including the theoretical, research, and clinical rationale. Therefore, it is difficult to understand the rationale for the outcome measures that were chosen and possible reasons why the interventions may or may not have been successful.

Although researchers did not choose to measure family-level outcomes, such as family functioning, significant quantitative outcomes were obtained in discrete areas of individual family-member functioning or dyadic functioning. Examples of these variables are (a) certain aspects of the home environment that were measured by parents' report of their parenting behavior (emotional and verbal responsivity, as well as stimulation); (b) children's anxiety, depression, knowledge, play, scholastic competence, global self-worth, and socialization; and (c) parents' anxiety, perceptions of knowledge, and understanding.

■ Discussion

This integrative review has synthesized studies that employed interventions with children who have chronic conditions and their families. The scope and purpose for past reviews of intervention studies with children and their families differed from the scope and purpose of this review. Previous authors reviewed studies across health care conditions and situations (Beal & Betz, 1992; Olson et al., 1990) and during procedures (Brennan, 1994) and reported on studies whether or not they tested the intervention (Beal & Betz, 1992; Brennan, 1994). Recommendations were consistent with this review in terms of increasing the quantity and quality of intervention studies to guide the practice of pediatric nursing and underscoring the importance of reviews that synthesize results of studies.

The results of this review are consistent with the work of practicing nurses who are formulating research-based protocols, guidelines, and critical pathways for care. These all attempt to synthesize what is known about phenomena so as to improve care outcomes. For instance, Magyary and colleagues (1993) published such guidelines for nursing specialty practice with children in need of early intervention.

Finally, the results of this review are consistent with the work of individuals classifying nursing functions and interventions. It is most closely aligned with McCloskey and Bulechek (1994) and Craft and Willadsen (1992) due to their concentration on interventions related to the family (Craft & Willadsen, 1992) that were developed through consensus of experts and through a review of the literature. Evidence for the efficacy of 8 of the 9 family interventions identified by Craft and Willadsen was found in these studies: family support, family process maintenance, family integrity promotion, family involvement, family mobilization, caregiver support, sibling support, and parent education. Whereas Craft and Willadsen's parent education was confined to adolescent children, this review highlighted educational interventions with parents who had infants, children, and adolescents. No studies were reviewed that used family therapy.

Although the scope of this review is limited to studies with nurse authors, some recommendations can be made for clinical research. First, the review should be extended to include other disciplines. Discipline- or paradigm-specific reviews exist, but there are none that effectively integrate findings across disciplines. For instance, Finney and Bonner (1992) synthesized the results of behavioral family interventions with children who have chronic conditions. Their conclusions are similar to those stated in this review but are enriched through considering how to balance the needs of the child and the family.

Second, use of the criteria developed for this review should be refined and used to guide other reviews. These criteria would be helpful in ongoing integrative reviews of intervention research, in planning projects, and in reviewing individual projects. If future reviews done in nursing and other disciplines refine and use these criteria, the results could be compared and contrasted. When planning future intervention projects and reviewing proposals for possible implementation, these criteria can serve as a gauge on the completeness and scientific merit of proposals in light of what is currently understood about children with chronic conditions and their families.

Third, the results of past qualitative and quantitative studies need to be systematically

integrated into designing future proposals. Even though the results of past research were considered in these research designs, the literature tended to be discipline and paradigm specific. For instance, no evidence was found that qualitative research findings were used to design the content of interventions. The systematic understandings gained from qualitative studies can be very helpful in determining how to approach complex issues like those that one inevitably confronts when designing family interventions (Deatrick & Knafl, 1988).

Fourth, nursing theories and models consistent with the family/ecological perspective need to be examined for use in future studies. Characteristics of the practitioner, child, and family were critical to the planning, implementation, and testing of interventions in this review. However, many studies do not consider these characteristics. Theories that describe the characteristics of the practitioner(s), whether they are nurses, physicians, social workers, psychologists, or individuals from other disciplines or professions, need to be incorporated in the conceptualization of intervention studies. Models that describe the child and family may include concepts from various, albeit consistent, perspectives but should be broad rather than narrow. The family and community need to be considered when trying to influence children with chronic conditions and measure the outcome of those influences, which speaks to the appropriateness of ecological models.

Feetham (1992) noted, "Interventions with family members and families are complex and multifaceted. This complexity, coupled with the complexity of health care delivery, makes it imperative that the interventions to be studied are focused and linked conceptually and in time to the outcomes measured" (p. 103). Although much is known about these issues, much more needs to be learned. Use of these guidelines and lessons learned through past research can help shape the journey.

12
■

MEETING THE CHALLENGES OF CHRONIC ILLNESS FOR CHILDREN AND FAMILIES

Research Implications and Future Directions

■ *Kathleen A. Knafl*

The experience of chronic illness presents families and their individual members with multiple challenges that change over time in their nature and intensity. Making sense of the illness in terms of its meaning for the person's life, mastering treatment regimens, adapting the family routine and budget to the demands of the illness, creating a "normal" life for the child and family in spite of the illness, and negotiating with health care and school professionals are challenges typically cited in the literature. At the same time, the challenges presented by chronic illness for nurses are distinctly different from those for families. For nurses, the challenge and ultimate goal are to identify and implement interventions that contribute to the family's success in adapting to and managing the illness, with researchers, clinicians, and educators making unique contributions to achieve this goal.

A recent book on home and community care for chronically ill children noted that the "goal of policies and programs should be to maximize the strengths and abilities of families to care for and nurture their children" (Perrin, Shayne, & Bloom, 1993, p. 25). In short, the challenge to professionals is to work with families and help them respond to chronic illness in a way that promotes individual and family adaptation and growth. Although the nursing profession has a long history of striving to meet this challenge, the scientific basis for developing and implementing effective interventions for helping families and their individual members meet the challenges of chronic illness is poorly developed, a fact clearly demonstrated in the previous chapter (Deatrick, chap. 11).

Leff and Walizer (1992), in their book *Building the Healing Partnership,* noted that maximizing family strengths requires providers to adopt a care rather than a cure treatment model by "caring for the child and parents as they struggle to create a healthy family life despite the unrelenting demands of chronic illness/disability" (p. 38). Adopting such a caring model, although entirely consistent with nursing's goals and values, raises numerous questions about what we need to learn about families, about the chronic illness experience, and about parent-professional relationships to work effectively with families to meet the challenge of chronic illness. Austin and Sims (chap. 10 in this volume) identify the tremendous progress that has been made in this area. Their review supports the conclusion that a great deal is known about the subjective experience of chronic illness, its impact on family and individual functioning, and those factors that contribute to adaptation difficulties in ill children and their families.

Changes over the past several decades in family roles and prevailing family structures have fueled debate over the ability of the American family to fulfill its traditional functions and the relative merit of divergent family forms and values (Coontz, 1992; Gilliss, 1996; Popenoe, 1993; Whitehead, 1993). In spite of ongoing debate about the capabilities of the American family, another considerable body of literature supports the greater involvement of families in the care of their ill members. In contrast to past discussions of family involvement in care, current literature addresses the cost-effectiveness of such involvement as well as the benefits, both objective and subjective, for patients and their families. Notably, there is considerable evidence that most families with a child who has a chronic illness or disability, even a severe one, believe that home care is better for both the child and the family (Perrin et al., 1993). As a nation, we are not waiting to resolve the debate about the capabilities of the American family to encourage, and increasingly require, greater family involvement in health care.

If nothing else, contemporary discussions about the American family have increased professional awareness of the diversity of family forms, situations, and capabilities that pediatric nurses are likely to encounter. As Jessop and Stein (1989) maintained, each of these family forms has its own unique challenges and state: "Superimpose on these demanding relationships and styles of life a child's chronic illness and the situations may become overwhelming" (p. 63). Yet in spite of this concern that families may be overwhelmed by the demands imposed by a child's chronic illness, both firsthand accounts (Mullins, 1987) and current research (Austin, 1991) confirm the ability of many families to adapt well and even thrive in the context of childhood chronic illness. The tremendous variation in child and family response to chronic illness underscores the complexity of the challenges facing pediatric nurses and raises two fundamental questions that the authors of chapters in this section sought to address. First, how can nurses best meet the needs of diverse families confronting diverse chronic illness situations? Second, how can nurse researchers, clinicians, and educators work together to integrate clinical and academic expertise with regard to families and chronic illness to help families meet illness-specific demands while still sustaining their ongoing family life?

In venturing to synthesize what is known about child and family response to chronic illness, the contributors in this section were guided by a shared vision. Individual chapters were developed to provide a critical review of current research focusing on assessment and intervention and to ground contemporary efforts in a broader historical context. From the outset, our shared hope was that, through integration and critical review, the individual chapters, when viewed collectively, would reveal new insights about child and family response to chronic illness and provide definitive direction for future researchers, clinicians, and educators.

As authors, we have had our ups and downs along the way. In some areas, we were overwhelmed by the volume of literature; in other areas, we were dismayed by the paucity. All the section contributors were equally challenged by the task of bringing order to a widely disparate and often unwieldy body of literature. This chapter takes a more holistic look at child and family response to chronic illness by identifying issues and themes that characterize contemporary assessment and intervention research and considers the extent to which current efforts build on one another as well as on past research. In particular, the chapter identifies major substantive and theoretical advances in the field and discusses methodological positions and issues that have both facilitated and hindered knowledge development related to children with chronic illness and their families. Implications for future research and the translation of research findings into practice are offered.

■ *Common Themes and Distinguishing Issues*

The preceding chapters in this section, when viewed collectively, point to both shared and divergent themes in the assessment and intervention research with regard to substantive focus, theoretical base, and methodological emphasis. These themes are indicative of investigators' judgments about the specific critical aspects of the chronic illness experience that must be assessed and understood if nurses are to develop and implement effective interventions. They also reflect the discipline's collective wisdom about what theoretical positions and methodological strategies are best for advancing knowledge development in the field of pediatric chronic illness. Certain themes have characterized research on the

chronic illness experience in children and families over time; others reflect contemporary trends and issues.

Assessment Themes and Issues

In examining the research on assessment, one is struck by the methodological balance across quantitative and qualitative approaches and the substantive disparity of the research using each approach. Austin and Sims's review (chap. 10 in this volume) ascertains that underlying the methodological differences in assessment research are divergent substantive interests, with quantitative researchers more interested in the domains of illness impact and qualitative researchers more interested in the process of illness management.

Although concerned with a variety of topics related to children's adaptation to chronic illness (e.g., illness characteristics, psychosocial adjustment, coping, and social support), quantitative researchers have concentrated their efforts on assessing the child's adjustment to illness and exploring variables, especially demographic and illness characteristics, linked to different levels of adaptation. With regard to the family's experience of chronic illness, quantitative researchers typically have viewed chronic illness through a stress and coping lens and have focused their research on exploring the nature and extent of the stresses associated with chronic illness and the quality of family functioning when a child has a chronic illness.

In contrast, qualitative researchers have directed their efforts at describing family life in the context of chronic illness and conceptualizing how families and their individual members manage the challenges presented by the illness. They also continue to develop and refine a number of inductively derived concepts such as chronic sorrow, critical times, and normalization, that capture important aspects of the child's and the family's illness experience.

These differing emphases in quantitative and qualitative research are long-standing, as indicated by Faux (chap. 9) and Austin and Sims (chap. 10) in this volume and in other reviews (Austin, 1991). The differences are at least in part a function of the relative strengths and weaknesses of the two methodological approaches in addressing distinct research purposes and questions.

The assessment chapter (Austin & Sims, chap. 10) also revealed considerable variation in the measures used to study individual and family adaptation to chronic illness. With the exception of Child Behavior Checklist (Achenbach & Edelbrock, 1983), there are few shared measures across the quantitative studies in spite of the overall emphasis on child adjustment. For example, each of the four studies cited in the chapter that assesses child self-concept uses a different measure. Similarly, in spite of an interest in illness variables that is addressed in both the quantitative and qualitative studies, there is considerable variation in what illness-related variables are assessed and a general reliance on investigator-designed measures—a situation that contributes to fragmentary knowledge development. However, in discussing the possibility of developing a uniform scale to describe all chronic illnesses, Austin and Sims (chap. 10 in this volume) argue that it would be both unrealistic and not particularly useful to develop a scale that was general enough to address all illnesses. Although their point regarding objective measures is well taken, there still could be value in developing a single measure for tapping family members' subjective perceptions of common aspects of chronic illness, such as perceived severity, visibility, and uncertainty. Such a measure, when combined with more illness-specific objective measures of severity, would facilitate comparisons across samples and studies, contribute to the identification of aspects of the illness that children and their families find especially difficult to manage, and

have the potential to incorporate distinctive aspects of the illness experience into a standardized measure.

There is also evidence in the Austin and Sims assessment chapter that nurse researchers are making considerable progress in developing not only measures that address unique aspects of individual adjustment and family functioning when a child has a chronic illness but instruments that give voice to multiple family members. Four of the six newly developed instruments target the chronic illness experience as opposed to general adaptation, and five target the child or adolescent. Moreover, there is clear acknowledgment of the importance of considering more than chronological age when assessing the child's developmental level. Although Austin and Sims appropriately criticize nurse researchers for their overreliance on age as an indicator of development, it is interesting to note that this is a shortcoming we share with our colleagues in, surprisingly enough, developmental psychology. In reviewing the research on pediatric chronic illness for a special issue of *Journal of Pediatric Psychology,* Wallander (1993) concluded that

unfortunately, pediatric psychology research has not been exemplary in generally recognizing the notion that children are developing beings. In an attempt to be developmental in our research we incorporate chronological age as a variable. However, age is only a marker for developmental psychological processes, which have to be studied in their own right to understand truly how children behave. (p. 8)

Nurse researchers also need to consider the underlying developmental processes that shape child adaptation to chronic illness.

In other areas, evidence of progress in developing useful assessment techniques is less apparent. Austin and Sims reported no instances of qualitatively derived concepts being translated into standardized assessment tools even though the development of such instruments would be a useful endeavor that would contribute to the assessment of aspects of the chronic illness experience identified by family members as especially salient.

The importance of specifying and developing the theoretical underpinnings of assessment instruments is emphasized by Austin and Sims and supported by other family researchers. Grotevant (1989), arguing that there is no such thing as an atheoretical assessment, states that "theories should provide the guide for separating elements that are worthy of attention from those that are not" (pp. 108-109). He goes on to identify the following principles that underlie the link between theory and assessment: (a) "Theory should specify the domain of family functioning that is being investigated so that the full relevant domain can be sampled" (p. 109); (b) "Theory should lead to clear definitions of constructs and variables" (p. 109); (c) "Theory should drive decisions about assessment strategies" (p. 110); and (d) "Theory should provide guidance for the level of analysis" (p. 111). These principles can serve as a useful guide for nurse researchers as they continue to develop and refine increasingly sophisticated assessment tools.

Clearly, considerable progress has been made in the area of assessing the chronic illness experience of children and families. Quantitative researchers have expanded the focus of their research to include multiple family members, and qualitative researchers increasingly have focused their attention on concept and theory development as opposed to description. However, there needs to be more effort directed to linking the insights that come from both quantitative and qualitative assessment approaches. A full understanding of the chronic illness experience requires knowledge of both the processes by which children and families manage the experience and the outcomes associated with different subjective perceptions and management approaches.

Another variable that merits further attention is gender. Ganong (1995) identified an overall inattention to gender issues as a major shortcoming of family nursing research and his conclusion is supported by Austin and Sims's review (chap. 10 in this volume). At this point, it is unclear how important gender issues are in family adaptation to chronic illness and how gender varies in its importance across different cultural and socioeconomic groups. Also notably missing from both past and current research efforts are studies that focus on the link between the family and the health care system. This is a neglected area of study by family researchers in other disciplines too. For example, in her review of family and health research conducted during the 1980s, Patterson (1990) found that only 5% of the 86 studies reviewed focused on family-provider relationships. Yet a recent review by Dixon (1996) that focused on parent-provider relationships identified 16 articles and uncovered the following common themes that characterized and shaped these relationships: trust, information exchange, participation, and decision making. The identification of these themes provides needed direction for this important area of inquiry. More than anything else, inattention to the family-health care interface has detracted from the potential of current assessment-focused research to provide a basis for subsequent intervention research. The consequences of this shortcoming are reflected in the number and nature of current intervention studies.

Intervention Themes and Issues

It is difficult to discuss dominant themes in intervention studies that focus on children with chronic illness and their families. In spite of Deatrick's liberal inclusion criteria, the scarcity of intervention studies is startling. This shortage of intervention studies was underscored in a recent editorial in *Journal of Family*

Nursing titled "Wanted: Family Nursing Interventions" (Bell, 1995). In that editorial, Bell asked, "Where are the rich descriptions of practice? In-depth descriptions of the nursing of families or research about family nursing practice have comprised less than 20% of the 62 submitted manuscripts and a mere 18% of the 17 articles published in this first volume" (pp. 355-356).

The variations in both topic and design used in the handful of studies identified by Deatrick (chap. 11 in this volume) makes comparison among them difficult. In spite of considerable pressure from both funding agencies and influential nurse researchers to undertake intervention research in the realm of childhood chronic illness (U.S. Department of Health and Human Services, 1992), only a few adventuresome investigators have risen to the challenge.

Current intervention studies appear to target the child and to a lesser extent other family members, usually the parent. Although Deatrick describes some of the studies she reviewed as family focused (Black et al., 1994; Brandt & Magyary, 1993; Lewis et al., 1991; Lewis & Lewis, 1990), these studies actually target individual family members rather than the family unit. In her classic discussion of family nursing research, Feetham (1984) emphasized the importance of differentiating between family-related and true family research, defining family research as that which focuses on contributing to our understanding of the family unit as a whole as opposed to the roles of individual family members. Subsequent work by Feetham (1990) further elaborated these distinctions and continued to stress their importance. Recently, Robinson (1995b) identified other distinguishing aspects of family research based on the investigator's focus of attention, area of interest, and type of data. However, despite considerable efforts to identify the defining characteristics of family research, most of the intervention studies identified by Deatrick (chap. 11 in this volume),

including those that claimed to be family focused, were directed to the individual.

The individual focus of the intervention studies was especially apparent in the investigators' outcome measures. Most often these studies measured child outcomes related to adjustment. Unfortunately, those in which an intervention was directed at the family unit (Lewis et al., 1991; Pless et al., 1994) did not include a family unit outcome measure.

As a group, investigators engaged in intervention research related to child and family response to chronic illness have undertaken varied projects with regard to both the target and focus of their interventions. Although Deatrick identifies shortcomings of these projects, she also provides a comprehensive framework for critically reviewing intervention research and for planning future studies. Her discussion of conceptual and methodological issues provides much needed direction for both clinicians and educators as they develop, implement, and evaluate new interventions and highlights the importance of taking into account and reporting information on a fuller range of child, family, and provider variables. Deatrick also challenges those devising new interventions and studies to consider how the results of qualitative studies that have identified key elements of the child's and family's chronic illness experience might be used to shape future interventions.

Stewart and Archbold's (1992, 1993) work on nursing intervention research provides further guidance for nurse scientists. Addressing the importance of selecting appropriate outcome measures, they offer recommendations for addressing questions that arise in seven critical areas: (a) the conceptual link between the intervention and the outcome, (b) the extent to which the outcome variable is amenable to change, (c) the adequacy of the outcome variable for detecting change, (d) the construct validity of the outcome measures, (e) the distribution of scores, (f) the appropriateness of the reliability assessment, and (g) the interpretation of the stability of the outcome scores.

Bell (1995) too reminds us of the importance of also taking into account the processes underlying the outcomes of interventions. She argues that by focusing on the process as well as the outcome of interventions, nurse researchers will move toward identifying a common language for describing, evaluating, and communicating interventions. Robinson's (1996) work offers some intriguing insights in this regard. Based on her research with families who identified themselves as experiencing difficulties in managing a member's chronic illness, Robinson found that "from the families' perspectives, interventions that made a significant difference were primarily those that promoted and enhanced particular kinds of relationships: among family members and between the family and the nurse" (p. 153). Her work further supports the importance of understanding the processes underlying intervention outcomes, and recognizing that the human relationships that develop in the context of working with ill individuals and their families can influence the effectiveness of interventions.

The work of the Nursing Intervention Classification (NIC) project (McCloskey & Bulechek, 1994) has also influenced the advancement of intervention research. These investigators focused on identifying interventions currently in use by nurses, including those directed to the family unit, and their findings need to be taken into account when developing and implementing interventions directed at children with chronic illness and their families.

Deatrick (chap. 11 in this volume) also points to the need for ongoing discussion of the defining characteristics of family interventions. Although she concluded that family-focused interventions were more successful, these were typically directed to family members rather than the family as a unit. Clearly, there needs to be more effort in clarifying what is meant by a family intervention and exploring the appropriateness and relative merits of interventions directed to the family unit as opposed to individual family members.

Based on a review of the nursing literature on families, chronic illness, and interventions, Robinson (1994) identified three distinct orientations to nursing interventions with families (traditional, transitional, and nontraditional) and described how these orientations varied in regard to their perspective on objectivity and the merits of a systemic orientation. Her work raises important questions about the beliefs and assumptions that underlie different intervention approaches that target desirable family responses to chronic illness and appropriate family and health care provider roles. Also, it is important to keep in mind that family versus individual interventions are typically grounded in different theoretical positions and that ongoing discussion and research therefore must take into account broader issues about the relative merits of conceptualizing responses to chronic illness as an individual or family unit experience.

Deatrick also highlights an almost paradoxical quality of research in this area, revealing a tension between the need to individualize interventions to meet client needs and the need to standardize interventions to conform to generally accepted criteria of a well-conceived research design. Recognizing the importance of individualizing family interventions that are directed at helping the family cope with a disabled child, Gallagher (1990) argued that the most appropriate research design may be the case study approach with replication as "it allows for the careful analysis of interactive factors in a given situation" (p. 556). Deatrick has suggested that from a clinical perspective it is important to "use advanced practice nurses, who can function beyond a standardized protocol and shape specific interventions to the characteristics of family members and family units" (p. 232). Her conclusion is consistent with that of Dixon (1996), who noted, "The interventions that were most successful in changing the health care experience for parents were those in which the nurse used herself to build trust, openly shared information, and let family members tell their stories to someone who would listen" (p. 128). As discussed further in the following section, more effective linking of assessment and intervention research will not only contribute to more appropriate individualization of interventions but also establish the scientific merit of individualized intervention protocols.

Linking Assessment and Intervention Research

In looking across the assessment and intervention research, there is evidence of considerable parallel play. Although researchers in both areas have tended to focus on the child's psychosocial adjustment to chronic illness, few linkages are being made between the two areas. With the exception of Child Behavior Checklist and Harter Self-Perception Scale, the measures of child adjustment used in assessment studies are different from those used in intervention studies. Whereas assessment researchers have tended to focus on both the child and the family, intervention studies have focused more exclusively on child adjustment, especially as an outcome measure.

In comparing the assessment and intervention chapters in this volume there is no evidence of programs of research that encompasses both these domains. The investigators cited in the assessment chapter do not reappear in the intervention chapter, suggesting that investigators to date have been inclined to focus their efforts in one realm or the other. This conclusion is supported by Ganong (1995) in his critical review of the state of family nursing research, which noted a lack of well-developed programs of research focusing on the family.

Taking a somewhat different approach to linking assessment, intervention, and outcome research are scientists from the University of Iowa who are developing taxonomies related to nursing diagnoses, interventions, and outcomes (McCloskey & Bulechek, 1994). From its inception, this research team has been interested in both individual- and family-level response to illness. However, unlike most of the research cited in the chapters in this section of the volume, the Iowa group (McCloskey & Bulechek, 1994) has built its taxonomies based on nurses' reports of their practice rather than the responses of individuals and families experiencing chronic illness. However, given the growing recognition of the importance of the relationship between the family and the nurse as a key determinant of the effectiveness of the intervention, it is important to take both the family and professional perspectives into account when developing and evaluating interventions. The work of the Iowa group makes an important contribution to understanding the nursing perspective.

Nursing intervention studies related to child and family response to chronic illness appeared only recently in the literature. The few brave souls undertaking such studies are doing so while the discipline is still very much in the throes of developing sophisticated assessments and resolving theoretical issues about suitable intervention targets and appropriate outcome measures. The situation in nursing mirrors that in other fields. For example, psychologists Finney and Bonner (1992) cite numerous examples from both psychology and family therapy that point to the infancy of family intervention research. Their own review of family intervention research directed to families with children with juvenile rheumatoid arthritis, cancer, or insulin dependent diabetes mellitus concluded that "the literature has produced more questions than answers and the findings are tenuous at best" (p. 167). Their conclusion suggests that Ganong's (1995) assertion that family nursing research is lagging behind that of other disciplines in this area is overstated; investigators and clinicians across varied disciplines are struggling with having to develop and determine the effectiveness of family interventions.

Although one might argue that intervention studies should await resolution of ongoing methodological and theoretical debates, there are pressures from both clinicians and funding agencies to engage in intervention studies that are clearly linked to shaping practice and make evident the contribution of nursing care to patient outcomes. From the viewpoint of having a fully developed database from which to proceed, the resources for undertaking intervention research are scarce. Thus, it is even more critical that intervention researchers make efficient and effective use of the knowledge base available to them by building on the strengths of prior research rather than lamenting its weaknesses.

As a scientific discipline, nursing has appropriately honed its critical skills. However, we must not be overly dismissive of the current body of knowledge and recognize that even imperfect studies can reveal important results and insights that can inform practice and contribute to the design of future research. Similarly, the historical debate over the relative merits of quantitative and qualitative methodologies has not served us well. Although, in recent years researchers from both traditions have been more willing to acknowledge their respective contributions to the advance of nursing science, there still is relatively little building on one another's efforts. Perhaps the issue is that reasearchers are too inclined to link their research programs to their methodologies rather than to overarching conceptual and substantive interests. Whether interested in individual or family adaptation to illness or both, investigators need to be guided by their ultimate purpose, understanding and fostering child and family adaptation to chronic illness, rather than by the methodological means to achieve this

goal. In an environment of scare resources for developing intervention studies, it is important that all those available resources, in the form of previous studies, be considered as potential building blocks for future research endeavors.

Assessment-focused studies are beginning to address a combination of illness, child, and family variables. As such, considerable progress is being made in identifying and developing measures that evaluate the impact of chronic illness on children and families, as well as the coping processes in which they engage. Other assessment efforts, usually relying on qualitative designs, have revealed explanatory insights into how families manage chronic illness and the kinds of interventions that support or detract from their coping efforts. Clearly, both kinds of data are useful in developing intervention studies. Whereas data from qualitative studies provide useful information for developing and individualizing interventions, more standardized assessment efforts provide useful information on salient family and individual outcomes that are amenable to nursing interventions.

Although the chapters in this section have focused on assessment and intervention research, important insights on child and family response to chronic illness also come from creative practice initiatives like the Family Nursing Unit (FNU) of the University of Calgary (Wright & Leahey, 1994a, 1994b; Wright, Watson, & Bell, 1990). Grounded in an integrated service, research, and teaching mission, the FNU uses an advanced practice nursing model to offer assistance to families who present themselves as having difficulty managing a member's chronic illness. Nursing efforts focus on working with families to help them develop beliefs about the illness situation that support their ability to manage effectively. The research and systematic clinical observations that accompany nursing practice on the FNU have revealed useful data about the nature and development of effective working relationships between nurses and families. In particular, the individuals associated with the FNU have done an especially fine job of articulating the clinical implications of the theoretical premises on which their practice is based (Leahey & Harper-Jacques, 1996). The FNU is an excellent example of a practice initiative that is shaping research through the ongoing dissemination efforts of it originators.

The emphasis of this section has been on intrafamilial responses to childhood chronic illness. It is, nonetheless, important to take into account broader cultural and sociopolitical issues that influence how families respond to chronic illness and the resources available to them. Within nursing, Anderson has done an especially good job of linking family response to these larger issues. Anderson (1990) reminds nurses that "health care management is enmeshed within broader sociopolitical and economic structures and is not simply based on decisions made by health care professionals" (p. 80). For example, the qualities that nurses view as desirable in families may change as a result of contemporary social trends. As noted in the Faux's chapter (chap. 9 in this volume), the nurse's view of the ideal parent has changed considerably over the past 30 years. Whereas dependence used to be encouraged, today it is viewed as a threat to appropriate parental involvement in illness management. Macrolevel trends and issues such as this also need to be considered when deciding on the focus of assessment efforts and interventions.

Over 6 years ago, I wrote that family research was a field "for those with a pioneering spirit, a tenacious mind set, and a high tolerance for ambiguity!" (Knafl, 1992, p. 100). That conclusion holds today. However, I would add that it is a field uniquely suited to the strengths of nurse researchers who can meld their methodological and theoretical sophistication with their clinical grounding to identify and pursue research questions that address the concerns and needs of families in which there is a child with a chronic illness.

PART IV

CHILDREN AND FAMILIES AND THE HEALTH CARE SYSTEM

■ *Suzanne L. Feetham, Editor*

■ *Overview*

Strong, efficient care delivery systems are critically necessary to provide the highest quality of care for children and families and to assure an environment for the conduct and utilization of research. As identified in the chapters of this book there is breadth and depth to the knowledge from the research of children and their families to inform care by nurses and other health professionals. This section is unique as each of its chapters addresses content (historical, health services research and health policy research) and contexts (systems-health centers and community) not traditionally examined by pediatric clinicians and nurse researchers. Also, the interdependence of the in-

fluence of social and health policy on the care of children and families is analyzed from historical and current research to define strategies for action.

Of significance are the areas where research is the most limited: those related to the health systems for children and their families and the relationships between these health systems and the social, cultural, economic, and political environments. In this time of dramatic change in the financing and distribution of care, this paucity of research is a significant challenge to the ability to sustain or improve health services for children and their families.

In this section, the authors address many of the limitations through systematic reviews of relevant articles and analyses of both integrated reviews and reports of policy analyses. They use exemplars to demonstrate the potential of historical, health services, and health policy research to improve the systems for services for children and their families.

As noted by these authors, there are significant influences on the distribution of resources for the health and health care of children and their families. Although programs of research of children are affected by many of the same influences, there are additional factors to be addressed related to the systems of care. One of these is the lack of proactive, comprehensive health policies resulting in the lack of initiatives to improve the health of children and their families. The second is the adult orientation of our society. The third is the failure to conduct practice and research with attention to the broader system contexts. The authors address these influences from the contexts of history, acute care systems, and community-based systems.

Each chapter in this section documents the relevancy of the challenges and provides direction to clinicians and researchers to correct the paucity of nursing research in health services and health policy related to systems for the care of children and their families. Frameworks such as benchmarking are used to relate the concepts of health services research to the practice of clinicians.

In each chapter, the need for clinicians and researchers to extend their traditional lens of personal health (individual child and family) to the aggregate or the public health view is discussed. To document the outcomes of care, nurses need to reframe their clinical knowledge across two dimensions: first, to move from a clinical perspective of individual children and their families to recognizing the influence of broader system factors on the care of the child, and second, to consider how knowledge of the care and outcomes of individual children and families can be used to inform unit, institutional and health policy decisions. The authors have delineated factors that influence nurses'

ability to transfer their significant clinical knowledge to and from the perspective of the clinical unit where they work, to the organization, and to state and national policy.

In the chapters on care systems, Meister and Feetham and Frink describe the processes and linkages from the personal health (individual child) data to the need in systems for aggregate data. As the operations of health systems become more integrated, the need for nursing data is a significant challenge. The direction of health care is toward data/information systems that are integrated within and across systems The authors describe how nursing can contribute data and note that nurses bring a critical dimension to the discussion in the development of these integrated information systems.

The authors in this section stress that it is critical that clinicians and researchers clearly differentiate the health and service delivery needs of children from adults. The relationship of the inability to differentiate the needs of children, the effects on the allocation of health services for children and their families, and the lack of comprehensive health policy for children are emphasized.

Comprehensive policy directed to the health of children and families is not a historical tradition in the United States. Policy for children and families tends to be directed to specific conditions or circumstances such as pediatric AIDS or Head Start. This categorical approach often results in short-term attention to and resources allotted to child and family issues. Besides the lack of policy, a confounding factor is that the limited health services and systems research that does exist is rarely applied to inform health and social policy to improve the health of children and families. The authors identify the beginning changes of increased attention to the health and education of U.S. children emanating from the president and some members of Congress. Such attention provides a window for nurses and other health professionals to frame their clinical knowledge and research to inform policymakers of their contributions to improve the health of children and families.

In summary, the factors affecting the progress of research of health systems for children and families are analyzed in this section. These factors include (a) the need for knowledge from research to differentiate the care needs of children from those of adults, (b) the limited measures of quality and outcomes in research of children and families, (c) the need for integrated data/information systems for health care systems and research of children and families, (d) the limited efforts by nurses and other health professional to examine practice and conduct research within the contexts of the broader systems affecting care, and (e) the need to frame knowledge from research of children and families to inform policy. The analyses presented in each chapter provide specific direction to increase nursing's ability to improve the health of children and families at both the individual and the aggregate level.

13

■

HISTORICAL OVERVIEW OF HEALTH CARE DELIVERY MODELS FOR CHILDREN AND THEIR FAMILIES

■ *Doris J. Biester and Barbara Velsor-Friedrich*

Within the context of our current health care model, children occupy a small but important segment. Although most of the children in the United States are healthy and have lower per capita health care costs than adults, a small minority have chronic conditions or multiple complex health problems and hence an ongoing need for access to comprehensive physical and mental health care (Anthony, 1995). Children have special needs that must be met by the health care delivery system within a family context.

This chapter focuses on types of health care delivery models that have played a central role in child health care in the 19th and 20th centuries. The discussion covers such topics as the initial lack of societal differentiation of children and the eventual recognition of children within the societal context. The history of hospitals and other complementary models of care for children are presented as are the govern-ment forces that have impacted the development and maintenance of these models. A new delivery system, integrated systems of care, is then reviewed.

■ Lack of Societal Differentiation of Children

Public responsibility for the health and welfare of children was an idea that developed slowly in the United States. Historically, American values included a belief that children were the property of their parents, and therefore, intervention from outside the family was not tolerated. Laws prohibiting cruelty to animals existed long before laws prohibiting cruelty to children. It was not until 1876 that the New York legislature passed a law that created the Society for the Prevention of Cruelty to Children (Abt, 1923).

Prior to the 19th century, care for children was not differentiated from adults based on development. Children were viewed as miniature, incomplete adults who grew into maturity through parental care and guidance. Early child health care services did not consider that anatomy, physiology, cognition, growth, and development of children differed significantly from that of adults. Children received the same remedies and treatments as adults in the same facilities.

In the early phases of the delivery of health and welfare services for children, foundling homes were established. Although for centuries, these institutions were the only places where children could receive care, they had little impact on improving children's health status. The advent of hospitals did not initially improve the status of children's health as they were excluded from hospital care. Women with young children were also barred from admission because the hospital did not want the responsibility of caring for their children, and hospital managers did not want their patients disturbed by the noise of children (Radbill, 1955; Rosenberg, 1987). Children's early health care services were thus minimal and reflected society's lack of value given its children.

■ Recognition of Children Within a Societal Context

Government influences have had a significant impact on the development and implementation of child health and welfare services. Since the early 1900s, the level of federal support for child health issues has varied, with support often tied to crisis-related issues such as war and poverty. Child health issues were given national attention when the first White House Conference on Children was convened by President Theodore Roosevelt in 1910. Subsequent White House conferences focused on issues such as child health

and welfare standards. Although these conferences dealt with important issues, they were criticized for their overall lack of action and limited outcomes. The last White House Conference on Children was held in 1970. Since then, child- and family-related conferences have been held sporadically (King, 1993).

As a result of the first White House Conference on Children, the Children's Bureau was created in 1912. The purpose of this government-sponsored institution was to investigate the problems associated with high infant mortality, orphanages, juvenile courts, desertions, dangerous occupations, accidents, diseases of children, and employment legislation affecting children in several states and territories. Specialists with expertise in all these fields were called on to help stimulate plans of action to improve the overall health and welfare of children (Hutchins, 1994).

The Children's Bureau was housed in the Department of Labor and included, as an initial responsibility, the administration of the child labor laws passed in 1916 (Rudolph, 1991). Later, this bureau provided grants for the development of diagnostic clinics for the mentally retarded. The Children's Bureau existed until 1969 and was eventually subsumed under the Office of Child Development in the Department of Health and Human Services.

In 1921, the Sheppard-Towner Act authorized $1.2 million to improve health services for all classes of children and their families. Its passage marked the first direct federal grant-in-aid program to any group for health services. The major functions of the Act were the following:

- Federal financial aid to the states
- Application of grants-in-aid for the problem of reducing maternal and infant mortality
- Vesting states with the authority to initiate and administer the plan, subject to the approval by the Federal Board of Maternity and Infant Hygiene

Over an 8-year period, this Act was responsible for the registration of all births, the establishment of well-baby clinics, and the creation of maternal child health programs in state and local health departments (Rudolph, 1991). These programs ceased to function in 1929, due to strong opposition from the American Medical Association (AMA) against what was seen as an early form of socialized medicine (Baker, 1994; Cone, 1979b).

Between 1929 and 1935, there was limited activity related to federally sponsored programs for children and their mothers. In 1935, Title V of the Social Security Act was passed. The majority of programs under this title were directed to address the integration of health services for poor children and their mothers and for crippled children. These services were to be directed through official state health agencies (Rudolph, 1991).

Aid to Families With Dependent Children (AFDC) originated under Title V. The overall concept of AFDC was to provide assistance to the working poor and to those unable to work. Initially, the program provided various levels of cash grants for the support of eligible children and their families. In 1967, the focus of AFDC was enlarged to provide economic rehabilitation for eligible heads of households through job placement services (Grotberg, 1976).

During the late 1930s and early 1940s, programs for children experienced several cutbacks. These cutbacks reflected, in part, a lack of society's sense of responsibility toward women and children. However, during a recognized crisis such as war, the government supported child health care. For example, in 1943 Congress supported the Federal Emergency Maternal and Infant Care Program (EMIR), which provided federal funds for states to purchase medical and hospital care for servicemen's wives and children. This was the largest public medical program in the United States and was administered through state health departments. The program ended in 1947 after it had cared for 1.25 million mothers and their infants (Sinai & Anderson, 1948).

Unfortunately, no plan existed for the continued care of women and children after the war ended. For the most part, new initiatives/programs were freestanding and not designed to fit into the infrastructure of the existing health care delivery system. Over the years, a costly pattern developed of terminating preventive maternal-child health (MCH) services instead of transitioning them into existing programs. This has been one of the critical flaws in the government's attempt to develop, implement, and evaluate maternal child health and welfare services.

In 1965, during the "War on Poverty," Medicaid (Title XIX of the Social Security Act) was passed by Congress and signed by President Lyndon Johnson. The original goal of this legislation was to reduce or eliminate differentials regarding the availability of and access to quality medical care by race, socioeconomic standing, and financial barriers for families. This goal was to be achieved through statewide, unified medical assistance programs for individuals eligible to receive federally aided money payments from public assistance programs. The passage of Medicaid was considered a breakthrough, as earlier programs for the medically needy applied only to those age 65 and older. Poor pregnant women, children, and adolescents were now also eligible for health care services.

Medicaid is the largest public medical care program for children in this country. This program has been shown to substantially improve access for economically disadvantaged children in poor health. However, not all eligible poor children receive its benefits. Children in low-income families make up 50% of the beneficiaries, although they account for only 15% of Medicaid expenditures. The elderly and disabled account for the largest percentage (59%)

of spending, related to intensive use of acute- and long-term care services (Kaiser Commission on the Future of Medicaid, 1995).

The Office of Economic Opportunity opened in 1965 and housed Head Start, an important program developed for preschool children of poverty-level families and based on the premise that early social and intellectual stimulation would prevent lags in child development that might be affected by environment. Over the past 30 years, this program has helped children reach important and measurable gains (Currie & Thomas, 1995; Rudolph, 1991). In 1973, the landmark supplemental food program for women, infants, and children (WIC) began, the goal of which was to provide food assistance for lower-income pregnant women, nursing mothers, infants, and children under 5 years of age. WIC has grown from a $20 million demonstration project into a $3.8 billion (requested 1997 budget) mainstay for at least 7 million women and children (Richardson, 1996).

During the Reagan administration, significant changes were made in health policies. All MCH funds were consolidated, and primary care grants were funded directly to the states in the form of block grants. Services covered under these grants were those for crippled children and programs such as genetic disease, adolescent pregnancy, and hemophilia. Once these designated programs received funding, remaining grant monies could be directed based on individual states' preferences. For example, many states used these funds to develop or enlarge neonatal intensive care units (NICUs). Interestingly, during this time many voiced concern that tertiary care programs, such as NICUs, took precedence over primary care.

This marks another critical theme in the government's approach to child health and welfare programs: lack of attention to prevention-focused services. Tertiary-focused programs are expensive and meet the needs of only a small percentage of the pediatric population.

Although it has been documented that prevention programs, such as Head Start and immunization programs, are cost-effective and efficient, these programs have not historically been widely supported.

Adequate funding continues to plague federally sponsored health programs. Over the past several years, the costs of Medicaid programs have grown in excess of 10% per year. Outlays for fiscal year (FY) 1995 were approximately $156 billion (Ford, 1996). The budget resolution for FY 1997-2002 recommends reducing Medicaid spending by $72 billion through the implementation of a bipartisan Medicaid reform plan adopted by the National Governors' Association on February 6, 1996 (Ford, 1996).

In hope of capping Medicaid increases, managed care is implemented for some recipients. This form of health care delivery requires that the Medicaid program be responsible for both the organization and the delivery of care (Ferguson, 1996). Many states have begun implementing Medicaid managed care programs to improve access and continuity of care and to contain costs by reducing inappropriate and unnecessary utilization.

Critics suggest that, for its beneficiaries, Medicaid managed care is not a workable solution (Sharp, 1995). Many Medicaid dollars are used for long-term care for the elderly, which would not be included in managed care contracts. One estimate is that redirecting the entire Medicaid population into managed care would result in only a 2% budget savings (Sharp, 1995). However, in the wake of several failed health care reform proposals, managed care is currently driving health care reform.

It is unclear how maternal and child health services will be influenced by the current health reform movement. The government has played an instrumental role in the development of programs and the delivery of health care services to children and their families. Although great strides have been made, a primary care approach that supports a continuum of care approach to health care for children has yet to be achieved. The challenge is to shift the current focus on child health care during this era of cost containment. This challenge can be better addressed when the history of traditional delivery systems is understood.

■ *Hospital Care of Children: Early History*

Prior to the 19th century, there were no institutions whose care was limited to sick children, and hospitals did not encourage physicians to admit children. In fact, when Pennsylvania Hospital opened, it "abhorred children, admitting only older ones or accident cases for emergency care" (Radbill, 1976, p. 753). Children of wealthy families received care and treatment at home.

Poor sick children, if they were treated at all, frequently had no place to go when ill, except the almshouse. Almshouses of the 18th century gave shelter and support to poor adults whose children often accompanied them and also frequently served as hospitals for the sick and asylums for the "idiotic" and orphaned or abandoned children. Almshouses provided general hospital care, medical, surgical, obstetrical, and psychiatric care. Sick children could be found throughout the various departments of the almshouse/hospital, even alongside newborns in the maternity department (Hendricks & Foster, 1994; Radbill, 1955, 1976).

However, almshouses had little to offer anyone, especially children, in the way of healing, for they were filthy and infested with vermin. Hospital fever from louse-borne typhus infected many of the residents. Nursing care was most often provided by other residents of the almshouse, the elderly and illiterate paupers. Because alcoholism was so prevalent, the "nurses" were frequently drunk while provid-

ing care. No one would send a child to a hospital, except in the most extreme cases (Hendricks & Foster, 1994; Radbill, 1976).

The first medical care available exclusively for children was an outpatient dispensary built in London in 1769. George Armstrong opened his Dispensary for the Infant Poor because he felt strongly that inpatient care for children was not practical and that outpatient care was an ideal way to meet the needs of sick children. Although the dispensary closed in 1782 for lack of interest and public support, the idea of a separate hospital for sick children in America had its beginnings in this early London-based facility.

■ *Children and Hospitals: Academics and Specialization*

The development of specialty hospitals in the United States, including children's hospitals, began in the mid-1800s. Sometimes, a specialty hospital was developed out of a recognition of need, particularly among the city's poor. Often, hospitals were built by physicians who had developed a particular specialty and were anxious to control their own clinical facilities, as they had little support or encouragement to practice in older, established hospitals. A few socially conscious physicians were aware of the importance of improved facilities for abandoned and orphaned infants other than the traditional almshouse. Female philanthropists became interested in the health of women and children and therefore figured prominently in the development of both children's and women's hospitals. Advocates for children's hospitals began to preach the benefits of rest, suitable food, and soothing surroundings as essential in effecting successful medical treatment. Curing an illness brought permanent benefits such as being able to resist future infections and diseases, particularly for children (Rosenberg, 1987).

The children's hospitals of the 1850s through 1870s tended to be private institutions in converted family residences and could accommodate only about 20 patients. Financial support was provided by trustees, and medical support was provided by outside physicians working with a minimal budget. Some hospitals had full-time matrons providing custodial care, but most care was provided by the volunteer lady visitors (Hendricks & Foster, 1994; Radbill, 1955).

By the end of the 19th century, many hospitals, both general and children's, were continuing to refuse admission to infants under the age of 2 years. Among wealthier families, the mortality rate from all causes during infancy was approximately 2% to 3%. Among all classes, mortality was about 20%. Pediatrician L. Emmett Holt, in discussing these statistics in his presidential address to the American Pediatric Society in 1898, stated that, although they were late in coming, "provision for the hospital treatment of sick infants . . . is coming fast, both in the organization of separate hospitals and in the addition to many of our general hospitals of a ward for infants" (Holt, 1898, p. 148).

Children's hospitals were important because they were needed as places of research, as places for teaching physicians and students, for training nurses, and as places for the care of those whose cases were better treated in institutions than homes. Separate hospitals for children were superior to having departments of pediatrics within general hospitals because it was hard to interest house physicians in children's nutrition and diseases and difficult to convince hospital boards that requirements for infants were very different from adults' (Holt, 1898).

Between 1917 and 1940, 16 new medical specialties were approved and incorporated. With the increased specialization by physicians came the demand for similar divisions of specialization in hospitals with consequent specialty clinics (Reverby, 1987). The increase in specialization of hospital medical and nursing services also increased costs, which occurred at a time of decreasing charitable contributions and inadequate payment mechanisms, resulting in an acute financial crisis. Hospital closures became common. The primary concerns for hospitals became what are the costs, how can we lower them, and how can we increase hospital income? There was a major effort to stabilize the hospital's source of income from patients. The public still perceived the hospital as a neighborhood store where credit was available. Third-party payments, in particular the Blue Cross plan, became the solution to the hospital income dilemma. Blue Cross, a product of the Depression, was endorsed by the American Hospital Association and was promoted throughout the country. By 1937, 1 million members belonged to 39 plans. By 1947, another 26 million had joined (Reverby, 1987).

■ Academy of Pediatrics: Primary Care Model

In the early 1900s, the infant death rate continued to be high. Each summer, especially in the larger cities like New York City, the mortality rate for infants would skyrocket, the cause usually diarrheal illnesses. The majority of infants were receiving milk that was usually several days old, had never been refrigerated, and was obtained under very unsanitary circumstances. Josephine Baker, a medical inspector of the New York Health Department, after being exposed to the incredible number of infant deaths, suggested a solution to the problem, the outcome of which was a significant reduction in the number of infant deaths the following summer. She sent school nurses into the slums to instruct mothers on breastfeeding, hygiene, and how to store milk in the home appropriately. Baker also increased the number of milk stations that, in time, became a network of welfare stations providing physical exams and dispensing advice. This network represents the first major involvement by American physicians in well-child care (Baker, 1994; Cone, 1979b).

The Sheppard-Towner Act (1921-1929), although short-lived, stimulated the public's desire for preventive child health care. Despite the fact that the AMA was adamantly opposed to the Sheppard-Towner Act and its associated clinics, the Act was popular with the public, prompting pediatricians not in accord with the AMA to transform the field of pediatric medicine from a predominantly academic one into a primary care specialty. In 1923, L. Emmett Holt admitted that he and other pediatricians had fallen behind public health nurses and social workers in the field of preventive care. He called for a change in medical education to develop pediatricians who could care for well children (Baker, 1994; Cone, 1979b).

By the 1930s, the foundation for today's well-child care system was in place. Middle-class families took their infants to private physicians for routine well-child care. With increasing frequency, these physicians were formally trained pediatricians, certified through a hospital-based residency system. The alternatives for infants of poor families were sparse, limited to medical school clinics or state health departments. The continued existence of a two-tiered, two-class system ensured disparity in delivering health care to children (Baker, 1994; Cone, 1979b; Scipien & Chard, 1990).

■ Children and Hospitals: Family-Centered Care

Even though the mission statements of hospitals in the mid-19th century described as primary goals the medical and surgical treatment of children's diseases, more often nurturing was noted as the more important function. Although some nurturing was important for the health and recovery of the sick child, community leaders voiced concern that the hospital staff, including physicians, should avoid spoiling these children so they could return happily to their tenement apartments: "The hospital should seek to restore children 'to their homes unspoiled by the necessary comforts its fostering care has given them' " (Rosenberg, 1987, p. 303). Attitudes toward children and families tended to be moralistic and paternalistic. Often, the parents were reviled for their ignorance and "vicious stupidity" as the cause of their children arriving at the hospital doors in dreadful conditions, in rags, and covered with lice (Hendricks & Foster, 1994; Rosenberg, 1987).

In L. Emmett Holt's presidential address to the American Pediatric Society in 1898, he discussed quite eloquently what was needed for the health and well-being of a hospitalized infant, including the importance of extra nursing care for holding and nurturing, but nowhere in his address did he mention the family or its role in caring for the infant before, during, or after the hospitalization (Holt, 1898).

At the end of the 19th century, scientists had proved that many diseases were caused by bacteria. To prevent infections, hospital wards were closed to visitors, including families. Also, because it was noted that visits by parents caused their child distress, especially when it was time to leave, hospital personnel considered such visits too emotionally stressful for hospitalized children. Thus, to prevent both infection and emotional distress, parents were prohibited from visiting their hospitalized children (Scipien & Chard, 1990; Young, 1992).

In the early to middle 1900s, researchers were becoming more aware of the emotional effects of long-term hospitalization and isolation of children from their families. As early as the 1920s, James Spence, a British pediatric surgeon, recommended allowing mothers to stay with their hospitalized child, considering this approach a humane and more appropriate way to care for children, particularly those under the age of 4 years. In the 1940s, families were sometimes tolerated in the hospital if they could afford to have their child in a private ward. The other wards had no such privileges, indicating, perhaps, that parents of patients in private wards were not an infection hazard. The attitude of the nurses and physicians toward parents who roomed in was one of tolerating but not encouraging such behavior: "Parents were considered a 'necessary nuisance', so probably a small group, similar in social class to the staff, was easier to tolerate" (Young, 1992, p. 1423).

Many nurses felt they were better able to provide care than parents, and the prevailing sentiment was that children adjusted better to hospitalization without visits from the family. Because children became quiet and resigned when the family was not around, this was taken as positive proof that the nurses' conclusion was valid. In the 1940s, children who became distressed and agitated were thought to be poorly adjusted because of a lack of home discipline. It was not until much later that withdrawn behavior was recognized as regression due to confinement and separation from family (Thompson, 1995; Young, 1992).

Spitz, in 1945, described a condition seen in infants in foundling homes that he called "hospitalism" (Thompson, 1995). Children who developed hospitalism usually received competent physical care but were rarely talked to or handled and so began to develop severe emotional problems that became irreversible after 6 months of separation. These infants failed to thrive and were more susceptible to disease than a control group of infants who received their care from their mothers, either at home or in an institution (Scipien & Chard, 1990; Thompson, 1995; Young, 1992).

In a study conducted earlier but not published until 1953, Bowlby, a British psychologist, observed the effects of maternal deprivation in children separated from their parents during World War II. These children developed severe behavioral changes, similar to those described by Spitz. In 1960, Bowlby made the connection between hospitalization and behavioral changes in children, demonstrating the need for consistent mothering. He defined three stages of separation anxiety: protest, despair and detachment (Scipien & Chard, 1990; Thompson, 1995; Young, 1992).

As a result of growing evidence of the emotional impact of illness and hospitalization on children, hospital policies have slowly changed during the late 20th century. With efforts from organizations such as the Association for the Care of Children's Health (ACCH), more humane treatment of hospitalized children has evolved including more relaxed policies about parental visitation and decreased hospital stays. The inclusion of families on the wards of children's hospitals marked a major advance in the care of children (Thompson, 1995; Young, 1992).

In their report, *Care of Children in Hospitals,* the American Academy of Pediatrics (AAP; 1960) discussed the importance of protecting the child from the traumatic dimension of hospitalization. This protection began with the child's physician helping the parents prepare the child for hospitalization. Avoiding abrupt and unannounced separations from the mother and under certain circumstances allowing the mother to stay with the child reduced stress and anxiety in both the parent and the child. In hospitals with relaxed visiting hours, it was found that visiting privileges were not being abused. It was important to be considerate and truthful and allow for regression of the hospitalized child who was sick and fearful. Although families were thought an important factor in making the hospitalization go smoothly, their roles were strictly defined and delineated (AAP, 1960, 1971).

By 1986, the AAP was encouraging all children's hospitals to implement a liberal policy for family visiting, which would include visits by younger siblings in designated areas. Rooming-in and family-assisted care for patients were encouraged. It was important to have a "receptive attitude toward families," as it enhanced the morale of children and families and also improved the interaction between the family and the in-house physician. This interaction was considered important for the education of pediatric residents.

The AAP (1986) also stated that parents of children between 6 months and 3 years of age should be encouraged to stay to prevent separation anxiety and to go with their child to all procedures, including the operating suite. Parents should be encouraged to take a reasonable amount of control over their child's treatment as they are best suited to interpret the child's responses. If the hospital involved the parents, they would be better prepared to provide care at home after discharge, an important secondary outcome.

The AAP (1986) went on to discuss how the design of pediatric environments may need to be changed to accommodate the emerging philosophies of care-by-parent and family-centered care. The four-bed ward design should be changed to private and semiprivate rooms because "(1) many parents demand the right to be near their sick child, (2) many sick children benefit emotionally and physically from having their parents participate in their hospital care, and (3) the cost of hospital care of the sick child might be reduced with parent participation" (p. 85).

Although the AAP has begun to encourage involvement of families in the care of their children, hospitals have historically excluded families from decision making and severely curtailed their involvement in their child's care

until the time of discharge. Care is often child centered but rarely family centered. The family continues to be left on the periphery during the actual planning of a child's care while hospitalized.

In 1994, the Institute for Family-Centered Care stated that the involvement of families in every phase of pediatric health care would change the care of children and improve pediatric practice for the benefit of the family, the hospital, and the community (Hanson, Johnson, Jeppson, Thomas, & Hall, 1994). The institute defined family-centered care as "a system-wide approach to pediatric care based on the assumption that the family is a child's primary source of strength and support . . . parents and other close family members are experts on their own children and hold essential information that can enhance children's health care" (Hanson et al., 1994, p. 13). By including families in every phase of a child's care—from hospital planning and policy to individual plans of care—the child benefits directly, and the hospital and community gain as well.

■ Complementary Models

Home Care

Many factors have elevated home care to a dominant position in health care delivery models, among them the rising cost of inpatient hospital care, insurance reimbursement levels, techniques that make sophisticated home care feasible, patients' preference for home services, and the belief that patient outcomes will be improved in the home (Lessing & Tatman, 1994). Delivery of health care services in patients' homes is not a new concept. Initially, hospitals, designated as charitable institutions, delivered care only to the poor and the sick, whereas the affluent were cared for in their homes.

Home care in this country has been greatly influenced by European home visiting models. In England, pioneer William Rathbone helped establish a district nursing service, the Metropolitan Nursing Association of London, in 1850. Based on personal experience with his wife's illness, Rathbone believed that people with long-term illnesses could be better cared for in the home. Florence Nightingale supported this concept and wrote a pamphlet titled *Suggestions for Improving Nursing Service,* which recommended steps for nursing care in the home (Stanhope & Lancaster, 1988).

In 1886, the first visiting nurse society began in Philadelphia to provide home health care to the sick. Ill children were routinely cared for at home by their family under the supervision of the visiting nurse. These nurses strictly adhered to physicians' orders. They gave selected treatments, kept temperature and pulse records, and taught care techniques to family members (Stanhope & Lancaster, 1988). Eventually, visiting nursing or district nursing spread across the country. By 1910, large urban visiting nurse associations had initiated prevention programs for schoolchildren, infants, mothers, and patients with tuberculosis.

An editorial published in *Public Health Nurse Quarterly* in 1915 urged public health nurses to expand their patient base by visiting the people of moderate means. Initially, only the affluent were cared for in their homes. The concern was that these families would object to having a nurse enter their home in the same uniform worn during earlier same-day visits in the filthy and squalid homes of the wretched. Assigning patients by neighborhoods and using cotton uniforms that could be washed were some initial solutions to the problem (Crandall, 1915).

The advent and proliferation of hospitals at the end of the 19th century brought about a shift in health care delivery from home to the hospital. This trend continued until the 1970s, when delivering care in the home was expanded to include (a) care for persons with complex health needs and (b) high-technology assistance. Today, home care services benefit children with a variety of complicated health needs, such as problems associated with prematurity and chronic conditions (Schuman, 1990).

It is important that home care nurses become involved in research concerning the evaluation of health care delivered in the home (Brent, 1996). For example, Brooten and colleagues (1986, 1988) used advanced practice nurses (APNs) in the home to follow-up with early discharge of very-low-birth-weight infants. It was found that infants did exceptionally well after discharge despite their low weights. These infants were discharged a mean of 11 days earlier, weighing an average of 200 grams less, and 2 weeks younger than the control group. The success of this program resulted in a mean savings of $18,560 per infant in hospital charges.

In a longitudinal study, pregnancy and infancy home visitations demonstrated improved outcomes for infants who were at risk for abuse/neglect. During and after a 2-year period, a nurse visited maltreated children who lived in homes with fewer observed safety hazards and whose mothers were less controlling. The children experienced 87% fewer visits to physicians for injuries or ingestions and 38% fewer visits to the emergency room (Olds, Henderson, & Kitzman, 1994; Olds, Henderson, Kitzman, & Cole, 1995).

In a more recent study of tracheotomy patients, specific discharge criteria were developed that led to an easier transition to home for these children and their families. The criteria addressed all facets of tracheostomy home care. Eighty percent of parents and caregivers felt well prepared by using this format (Hotaling, Zablocki, & Madgy, 1995).

Strategies used to improve health care for impoverished children with asthma have included the use of community health workers (CHWs) to bridge the gap between low-income families and the traditional health care system (Butz et al., 1994). A subset of 140 children with asthma were recruited and enrolled in a program to receive home visits by CHWs for the purposes of obtaining medical information and teaching basic asthma education to families. Data obtained by the CHWs revealed low inhaled steroid use, high beta 2 adrenergic agonist use, frequent emergency room visits, decreased primary care visits, and increased allergen and irritant exposure. This research documents the use of appropriately trained CHWs to effectively obtain useful medical information from families. When asthma management problems were identified, the trained workers provided basic asthma education in the home (Butz et al., 1994).

Nursing care delivered in the home reduces barriers to available services, such as lack of transportation, lack of child care, poor physical health, or low motivation. Home visitation also provides a unique opportunity to obtain relevant information about a family's environment, resources, and needs that will enhance the provider's ability to individualize services (Trierweiler, Cotler, & McNally, 1996).

Schools and School-Based Clinics

An increasing national emphasis on improving both education and health outcomes for children has been noted (*Goals 2000*, 1993; *Healthy People 2000*, U.S. Department of Health and Human Services [USDHHS], 1990). School-based clinics and "full service schools" can deliver effective and efficient care to a large number of children and their families. However, the delivery of health care to children in the school setting has been underutilized.

Health services in the schools began toward the end of the 19th century when public educa-

tion became compulsory through statewide legislation. During this time, immigration to the major urban areas resulted in overcrowded conditions, high rates of infant mortality, and a dramatic increase in communicable diseases. In the early 1900s, the major focus of the physician and the nurse in the schools was on identifying and removing those children considered dangerous to others due to contagion. Impetigo and pediculosis were the most frequent causes of prolonged absenteeism (Grotberg, 1976).

Once children were removed from the school it was difficult to get them to return. Based on a program developed by Lillian Wald, nurses were sent into the schools to assist students in following the physician's advice and to make follow-up home visits to encourage students to return to school. The success of this program led to the employment of school nurses throughout the country (Igoe, 1994). In 1902, the School Nursing Section of the American Association of Public Health (AAPH) was formed. The chief objective of this section was to develop public understanding of the work of the school nurse and to promote voluntary activities in connection with the school health program. Supervision standards for school nurses were also developed by this group (Palmer, 1922). The AAPH along with the American School Health Association and the National Association of School Nurses are the dominant policymaking organizations in the area of school health.

The growth of school-based programs has paralleled that of hospitals, as the early focus of both was related to infectious diseases. Gradually, both schools and hospitals have become involved in the provision of a more comprehensive type of care. Over the years, the school nurse's role evolved from screening for communicable diseases to identifying children with physical defects to providing primary prevention services, such as vision and hearing screening, and health counseling. Today, the school nurse practitioner offers services for both primary clinical prevention and complicated case management (Igoe, 1994).

School health has been defined as a broad range of school-based and community-based activities engaged in by many different persons to coordinate educational, social, and health issues to assist families and children in preventing disease, promoting and protecting health, and minimizing the complication of the problems of school-age children (AAP, 1993). The Centers for Disease Control and Prevention's Division of Adolescent Health (DASH) lists the following eight components of school health: (a) health services, (b) health education, (c) healthy school environment, (d) physical education, (e) guidance and psychological services, (f) food services, (g) school/community health promotion efforts, and (h) site health promotion for faculty and staff (Igoe, 1994). Comprehensive school health has the potential to maximize health and education outcomes for children and adolescents by attempting to focus the efforts of families and community institutions and systems that impact health (AAP, 1986).

Although nursing practice in schools was established in 1902, school-based clinics did not evolve until the late 1960s. The first two school-based clinics were located in high schools in West Dallas, Texas, and St. Paul, Minnesota. These clinics were established due to concerns about health, psychological, and educational risks associated with teenage pregnancy and parenting. The St. Paul program has received model status due to the reduction in pregnancy rates in the schools associated with it (Dryfoos & Klerman, 1988).

In a recent report to the Committee on Government Operations (U.S. General Accounting Office, [GAO], 1994), school-based health centers or clinics were identified as an effective method for delivering care to underserved children. Findings from this report suggest that school-based centers "do improve children's

access to health care and do help to overcome financial and non-financial barriers that currently limit access, including the lack of health insurance, transportation difficulties, and insufficient attention to the particular needs of adolescents" (GAO, 1994 p. 1).

School-based clinics (SBCs) increase the likelihood that children receive primary health care. Students can obtain daily, confidential, primary care at low or no cost to them at clinics conveniently located in their schools. The services are delivered in an environment that encourages students to take responsibility for their own health care. Adolescents who use SBCs demonstrate growth in their self-esteem and coping skills, improved health and nutrition status, and increased communication with their families (Harold, 1988).

Many SBCs have multidisciplinary teams that offer the following services: athletic and school physicals, immunizations, gynecological exams, pregnancy testing, and diagnosis and treatment of minor and acute illness. Other services offered are chronic illness management and education, mental health counseling, substance abuse counseling and referral (Uphold & Graham, 1993). Education is an important aspect of the services provided by SBCs. Clinic staffs are concerned not only with addressing students' physical or psychological concerns but also with increasing their knowledge and understanding of themselves and their needs.

Funding for SBCs remains a critical issue. In 1987, legislation to support SBCs was introduced in 24 states. However, only a few of these bills survived the legislative process (Dryfoos & Klerman, 1988). SBCs rely on fragmented sources of state, local, private, and federal funding to cover start-up and operating costs. Private funds from foundations have played a large role in establishing new clinics, but this is frequently short-term funding, leaving the clinics with an uncertain flow of funds. Reimbursement from Medicaid and private insurance companies has been minimal (GAO, 1994).

In some states, school health services have expanded from child-focused activities to family and community services. Dryfoos (1994) describes a concept called "full service schools." These schools house in one building the services that children, youths, and families need. Services available in these schools include physical and mental health care, employment services, child care, parent education, case management, recreation, cultural events, and community policing. The result is a seamless institution, a community-oriented school with joint governance structure that allows maximum responsiveness to the community as well as accessibility and continuity for those most in need of services. This integration of services also helps reduce the fragmentation of existing service systems.

Evaluation of services provided in the school setting is a critical issue. Many schools have adopted health-related programs that are implemented in fragmented ways instead of using a coordinated integrated program approach. Weissberg and Elias (1993) recommended synthesizing the strengths of many prevention programs into a larger coordinated effort called Comprehensive Social-Competence and Health Education (C-SCAHE) programming. C-SCAHE is built on the premise that comprehensive, multiyear prevention programs that target multiple outcomes are needed to address the social and health needs of children and adolescents.

The delivery of health care to children in the school setting offers an effective way to increase access to care while impacting large numbers of children. Efforts should be directed toward developing comprehensive integrated health programs with evaluation mechanisms in place. With the current changes in health care delivery and financing, schools have the potential to deliver child and family health care in every neighborhood.

■ Creating Integrated Systems of Child Health Care

Managed Care

Managed care encompasses any measure that favorably affects the price of services, the site at which the services are received, or their utilization. It represents a continuum of plans that range from those that do no more than require prior authorization of inpatient stays to the staff model health maintenance organization (HMO) that employs its doctors and assumes risk for delivering a comprehensive benefit package (Fox, 1990). Managed health care organizations (MCOs) provide for both the delivery and the financing of health care for their members (enrollees). These organizations are rapidly becoming a major source of health care for the beneficiaries of both employer-funded care and publicly funded Medicaid and Medicare (USDHHS, 1995).

MCOs take a variety of forms in how they deliver care and how they are financed. Besides the HMO, there are the preferred provider organization (PPO), the hospital-physician organization/combined provider organization (HPO/CPO), and point of service plans (PPS).

All of these plans involve providers who agree to deliver health services for a set fee to the purchaser of the plan. Currently, the definition of a primary provider encompasses physicians, nurse practitioners, midwives, physician assistants, a group practice, and a group of hospitals.

Primary care providers are often referred to as "gatekeepers," as they limit access to other providers of health care. Limiting referrals to specialists and decreasing admissions to hospitals are the major means to control access to care. Incentives for the primary care provider to comply vary, depending on the type of managed care (Jonas, 1995).

Nurse-Managed Care/
Case Management

Nursing's involvement with managed care has focused on not simply reducing cost but also on increasing quality and access. Federa and Camp (1994) defined managed care as an organized system of care that seeks to influence the selection and utilization of health services of an enrolled population and ensures that care is provided in a high-quality, cost-effective manner.

There is some overlap in the literature with the terms *nurse managed care* and *case management.* Nursing case management is a model of care delivery that has been identified as a process for achieving optimal patient outcomes in expected time frames while containing costs. This can be accomplished through a multidisciplinary team approach guided by a care plan or critical pathway (Elizondo, 1995).

The development of case management programs for specific pediatric populations, such as children with chronic illness, children undergoing craniofacial reconstruction, and children with heart disease, has been reported (Schryer, 1993; Smith, 1994; Uzark, LeRoy, Callow, Cameron, & Rosenthal, 1994). In these programs case management has been reviewed as an effective way to balance expected outcomes, the process of care delivery, and cost.

Case management has also been incorporated into the process of implementing and evaluating procedures, that is, preadmission services and upper endoscopy (Geeze, 1994; Lauffer, 1992). Researchers have documented the need for hospital-based ambulatory surgery programs to fully integrate some of the traditional inpatient hospital services with the needs of ambulatory surgery through the development of preadmission services as well as adopting case management theory. Using all members of the health care team, the case management process systematically moves the parents and their child through the hospital experience in an anticipated manner that is caring, efficient, and cost-effective.

Nurse-managed clinics are described by Lenz and Edwards (1992) and Katzman, Holman, and Ashley (1993). These clinics offer preventive care, health promotion, health maintenance, and health restoration services. Nurses provide over 97% of the clinic services. Unfortunately, the only variable used to evaluate these clinics to date has been client satisfaction.

Using nursing case management to improve health outcomes maximizes nurses' roles in the process. The nurse as the case manager coordinates multidisciplinary care and also acts as a liaison for patients and families through a continuum of care across settings, while maintaining a cost-conscious focus. Not only promotion of patient self-responsibility but wellness and caring are integrated into the coordinator/financial role of the case manager (Newell, 1995).

In a reformed health care delivery system, nurses play a strategic role in planning, implementing, coordinating, and evaluating a new health care delivery model—managed care. It is important to evaluate the aspect of quality in managed care as such care is defined from the perspective of the purchaser of health care (most often the employer) and not from the perspective of the provider or the patient. Research examining the quality of care delivered under a managed care system can contribute greatly to an objective evaluation of its merits or drawbacks. Ideally, managed care should not simply seek to reduce costs but, rather, should strive to maximize value, which includes a concern with quality and access (Fox, 1990).

Emerging Systems of Health Care

Historically, health care in the United States has been designed with acute illness as the central focus: "The role of the health care system was to rescue us from the illness and to take custody of us until we were well again" (Goldsmith, 1992, p. 1). This acute care model is based on the premise that illness is unpredictable. It is designed to serve only the individual. This method of delivering care is huge and costly, and by spreading the cost across a large population it has perpetuated itself for nearly 100 years (Goldsmith, 1992).

The framework for health care delivery today is changing. Chronic illness and degenerative diseases are replacing acute illnesses as our most significant health problems. The health care needs of most citizens no longer fit the health care system. Wellness education, illness prevention, and primary care along with other complex social issues are just some of the considerations for health care providers today (Beyers, 1995; Goldsmith, 1992).

In light of the multitude of changes in the health care delivery system, the requirements of the community must be addressed along with the needs of the individual. The health care delivery system, in order to survive, must develop a multidimensional focus. The driving forces behind the push for multidimensional or integrated systems include economics, competition, and unmet health care needs. The push for managed care and capitation can be attributed in some degree to the shrinking health care dollar. The purpose of managed care is to provide a continuum of care, and the role of the primary care practitioner is to provide direction for that care (Bergman, 1993; Beyers, 1995; Goldsmith, 1992).

Because there are fewer and fewer health care dollars to be spread among a similar number of providers, competition is fierce. Mergers, affiliations, or purchases, occurring on an almost weekly basis, provide some innovative ways for providers to capture market shares. By merging or affiliating, systems can provide more comprehensive care. Therefore, they can market themselves to a larger audience and provide all care for an individual (Bergman, 1993; Beyers, 1995; Goldsmith, 1992).

Unmet or poorly met health care needs of society's oldest and youngest members with acute or chronic problems are increasingly expensive issues in health care. If health care systems can move from diagnosis and treatment to prediction and early-stage management of illness, health care providers can intervene early before these problems become acute or chronic and therefore expensive and difficult to manage or cure (Bergman, 1993; Goldsmith, 1992).

The answer to many of these problems may lie in an organized system capable of managing the full range of health services needed by clients—namely, an integrated system of health care. Integrated systems bring together health care providers with the training and expertise to deliver a continuum of care, which includes basic prevention or primary care, acute care, and ongoing care for the chronically ill or disabled. This restructured system allows for more comprehensive care delivery. The goal of the system is to meet patient needs throughout the life span with a balanced allocation of scarce resources. This system addresses the needs of both the individual and the community and allows for a reallocation of resources to health issues or common problems experienced by groups of individuals. The result is quality, cost-effective, accessible care for all. The emphasis of this system is on wellness, continuity, and health promotion (Beyers, 1995; Burch, 1995; Zismer, 1994).

The National Association of Children's Hospitals and Related Institutions (NACHRI) states that an "excellent system is vertically and horizontally integrated or affiliated to facilitate comprehensive care and coordinated delivery by care givers" (Anthony, 1995, p. 1). A pediatric integrated system would take different forms based on the population and geographic region. A pediatric system might contract directly with (a) a state Medicaid agency, (b) employers, (c) managed care organizations, (d) fee-for-service plans, or (e) other health care networks. This system could either contract with payers to provide only one level of care, operate independently, or be part of a larger network serving all ages. Affiliates might belong to more than one system so as to provide their unique services to all children and families. They would take responsibility for large numbers of children over a large geographic area to achieve cost-efficiency and quality of care (Anthony, 1995; Burch, 1995).

Important attributes of any integrated system are expertise, organization, and accountability. The ideal pediatric system assesses the health of each child and provides the appropriate level of care chosen from a full scope of quality health services. The system coordinates care with providers in other systems, shares information among all providers of services, and monitors health status by gathering data on an ongoing basis. The system is accountable to families and payers for delivering effective, efficient, patient-focused care in a timely, consistent manner, with the goal of improving health status over time (Anthony, 1995; Burch, 1995). Within an integrated system, the levels of care are linked horizontally and vertically to address patient needs. The provider within the system addresses the family's needs by facilitating the child's movement back and forth through appropriate levels.

The primary care level exists throughout the system to maintain the health of each individual child. It includes health maintenance and promotion, disease prevention, information and education, and treatment for 80% of childhood illnesses. The acute care level provides for time-sensitive diagnosis and treatment of urgent, emergent, or serious diseases or conditions through the use of four processes: (a) intake, (b) stabilization, (c) treatment, and (d) discharge or episode resolution. The chronic care level is the longer-term-planned health care management of a child with one or more chronic diseases or conditions. The management includes ongoing medically necessary care and involves short- and long-term goal set-

ting and development of a holistic care plan. All sites providing any of these levels of care must have competent pediatric-trained staff. The child and family are partners with the pediatric staff throughout the care delivery process (Anthony, 1995).

Ideally, an integrated system would provide quality care within one system, making health care easily accessible and affordable for everyone. Because this is a fairly new concept in the history of health care, little research has been done to support this method of providing care as the prototype for the future. Participating in research concerning the quality of care delivered in an integrated system can contribute greatly to an objective evaluation of its merits or drawbacks. Integrated systems of care should not just provide the most streamlined care for the most people but also be concerned about providing quality, affordable, and accessible care to meet the needs of each individual.

■ *Summary*

Although the delivery of health care has evolved over the past several centuries, continued improvement is critical for the health and welfare of America's children. The evolution of health care delivery models for children has been influenced by society's lack of differentiation of the needs of children from adults. Historically, children were considered to be the property of their parents and their value was primarily economic. In recent times, we have begun to regard children as individuals with rights and privileges. It is clear that the needs of society's youngest members differ significantly from those of adults, yet we have not established a comprehensive health care plan to satisfy those needs. Children are entitled to health care that supports a healthy, productive life.

The role of nursing has also evolved over time from one of passive caregiver to that of child advocate. Because the current health care delivery system is driven by managed care, the environment supports the development of complementary models of health care delivery for children and their families, which when implemented offer promise for improved access to health care for children from all economic levels. Ongoing research and evaluation of these models of health care encourage a more predictable future for the health of children. Nursing, by its very nature, can and will be integrally involved in the continued evolution of health care for children (James, 1990).

14

■

COMMUNITY INFRASTRUCTURES

Principles and Strategies for Improving Child Health Services

■ *Susan B. Meister*

C hild health professionals have always tried to meet two goals: to provide the best possible care for individual children and their families and to promote improvements in the programs and policies that affect child health care in their communities. Today, we are trying to do so in a context that is full of contradictions.

Much has been accomplished in improving child health, and yet over 20% of our children live in poverty. Much has been learned about the organization and financing of care, and yet little is known about the effects of managed care on children. Much has been learned about the interaction between social, economic, and physical problems, and yet few have been able to translate that knowledge into effective programs.

This chapter examines "improving community infrastructure" as a strategy for resolving those contradictions. Work to improve the administrative and bureaucratic elements in the

community's infrastructure for services is, generally, unsung and time consuming—but it is work that is entirely consistent with child health practice. More to the point, in light of the current context it is work that is vital and thus must be endorsed and supported by the discipline. Until we change the environment for services, we have little hope of bringing child health services into alignment with the needs of today's children and families.

Recently, two eminent pediatricians wrote about community child health and the need to improve the infrastructure for services (Palfrey, 1994; Richmond, 1994). They pointed out that there is an urgent need for a better conceptualization of our approach to children's care, that we need a plan for action, and that these efforts involve a transformation in professional practice. Each of these points is discussed below, and the chapter concludes with a discussion of the leadership we need to move forward.

Perspective. In this chapter, four principles define the relationships between children, families, child health services, and community infrastructure (see Hamburg, 1992; Schorr, 1991):

1. All children need a broad spectrum of support if they are to achieve their potential for growth and development.
2. The family is the most elemental crucible for child growth and development.
3. Child health services should be responsive to the wide range of individual differences found in children, in families, and in the interactions between child health and family health.
4. Even the best array of services will fall short if the bureaucratic and administrative infrastructure is inadequate.

Core elements for services. Child health services have been analyzed by a number of experts and panels (Both & Garduque, 1989; Green, 1994; Hamburg, 1992; Igoe, 1992; Keniston, 1977; Palfrey, 1994). There is general agreement that the core elements of child health services include pediatric health and illness care, with early intervention; nutrition programs; housing programs; home health visiting, especially for newborns; high-quality child care; school health programs; educational systems to prepare informed, productive citizens; recreation programs; prevention programs (e.g., pregnancy, HIV, STDs, and substance abuse); integration of health, education, and human services; publicly accountable health agencies to ensure access; and support systems for parents and families.

Characteristics of effective infrastructures. First, the infrastructures are designed so that the community systems work together to integrate services, respect the principles listed above, and meet the implicit standards of quality, appropriateness, flexibility, and efficacy. Second, the infrastructures will create a convergence of services, service providers, agencies, and related policies around a well-defined goal. Third, for child health, the infrastructures link many existing providers and programs, including hospitals, nurses and physicians, welfare, food stamp programs, WIC (Women, Infants, and Children), Title V (Maternal and Child Health Services block grant), Medicaid, EPSDT (Early and Periodic Screening, Diagnosis, and Treatments), Public Laws 92-142 and 99-467, Head Start, home visiting and outreach programs, schools, and public health programs.

■ Community Infrastructure as a Strategy

Although the heart of child health services lies in interventions with one child and family, the delivery of services is organized and financed in terms of aggregates of children, programs, and providers. Federal, state, and community infrastructures affect the relationships between the individual child and family and delivery of care. Therefore, infrastructures are critical determinants of the effectiveness of each program and the system as a whole.

The frameworks and models discussed below were selected because they constitute a broad range of programs, use a variety of linkages, and focus on community levels of infrastructure. Focusing on federal and state infrastructures would result in different strategies and different evidence of progress to improve the health of children.

Frameworks and Models Using Community Infrastructure

The frameworks of *Bright Futures* (Green, 1994), the National Forum on the Future of

Children and Families, and reports from several task forces/councils of the Carnegie Corporation of New York (1994, 1995) are analyzed here because their findings illustrate the vital potential of community infrastructures. These projects also share the characteristic of being multiyear endeavors aimed at bringing diverse experts together in the interest of defining the content and organization of child health care.

For four years the *Bright Futures* (Green, 1994) project convened expert panels and sought reviews from nearly 1,000 child health professionals in an effort to define health supervision, with guidelines and standards for the role of health professionals in addressing child health in the context of families and communities.

The resulting guidelines for health supervision are designed to help promote health, prevent mortality and morbidity, and enhance subsequent development and maturation. The model, based on health diagnosis, depends on a partnership between the health professional, the child, and the family and is part of a web that includes community-based health services, education, and welfare systems. *Bright Futures* (Green, 1994) provides guidelines for infancy, early childhood, middle childhood, and adolescence while emphasizing that health services should always be matched to the child and family and organized so that they function as part of the larger group of community-based services.

The National Forum on the Future of Children and Families of the National Academy of Sciences was created as an institutional mechanism for creating sustained dialogue among scholars, experts, and leaders from science, government, and business about social policy for children and families. After grouping the findings of 22 national panels, commissions, and government agencies into four categories—education; child health, employment, and income; child poverty; and welfare—the Forum concluded that the findings demonstrate

that the community is a principal determinant of effective delivery systems, financing of those systems, ensuring quality and accountability, and staging policy development (Both & Garduque, 1989).

A third framework comes from several task forces and councils of the Carnegie Corporation of New York (1994, 1995, in press). The Task Force on Meeting the Needs of Young Children (Carnegie Corporation, 1994), Council on Adolescent Development (Carnegie Corporation, 1995), and Task Force on Learning in the Primary Grades (Carnegie, in press) all emphasize the overarching importance of "meeting the developmental needs of children and adolescents through potentially supportive institutions such as families, schools, health agencies, community organizations, and the media" (Hamburg, 1995, p. 127). Again, broad-based analyses bring the focus back to the significance of strategies to improve the community infrastructure.

Head Start (Kotelchuck & Richmond, 1987) is an exceptional example of the benefits of improving the community infrastructure. Its aims are comprehensive; improving child health and physical abilities, helping emotional and social development, improving mental processes and skills, establishing patterns of success and confidence, developing a sense of mutual responsibility between child, family, and society, and increasing the child and family's sense of dignity (Kotelchuck & Richmond, 1987). For 30 years, the program has served as a comprehensive child development program, uniting health services, dental care, nutritional services, early childhood education, and social and mental health services. These efforts exemplify optimal community infrastructure strategies in that they are grounded in parent participation, community governance, and volunteerism (Richmond, 1989).

Several years ago, the Select Panel for the Promotion of Child Health (1981) extended the concept of Head Start by endorsing the value of first arraying a wide range of child health services and then organizing services in a manner that recognizes that most will be used only by a subset of children. This vision guided a number of efforts, including community-based projects designed to bring programs and providers into the same building or complex. Although this "one-stop shopping" can improve utilization, building the physical site for it often carries enormous capital costs.

Palfrey (1994) proposed a model that avoids draining capital funds by improving the community infrastructure instead of building a physical site. In this model, the infrastructure for child health is improved by creating the administrative support for systematic assessments and referrals for children in order to create a community-based integration of intake and referral processes. Such a program can apply the model that hospitals use for rotating various clinics through the same clinic sites. It could make use of a hospital's outpatient surgery center during evening hours or of school facilities during nonschool hours. In any case, it would be open to all families, and administrative changes would make an integrated assessment a routine part of the birth of a child as well as part of school entry and transitions.

In practical terms, this means that a wide range of programs must be linked for intake and referrals and many relevant policies must be reconciled. All pertinent programs must commit to integrate their intake data and to work through the community infrastructure, which would involve many challenges (Palfrey, 1994).

A report on four major studies of the effects of 10 years of Medicaid expansions also illustrates the vital role of the community infrastructure. Findings of the Alpha Center's (1995a) integrative report demonstrate that states that increased eligibility and improved facets of the local infrastructure, such as outreach and application procedures, often had greater success in improving health outcomes.

In summary, there is a substantial knowledge base to guide efforts to improve community infrastructures.

Goals for Improving Community Infrastructures

Our efforts to improve the infrastructure can be guided by the process by which national health goals have been set. The first set of quantitative national goals was established in *Healthy People: Surgeon General's Report on Health Promotion and Disease Prevention* (U.S. Department of Health and Human Services [USDHHS], 1979). The goals were set out as 10-year goals, and in 1990 the Public Health Service repeated the process to establish goals for the year 2000 (USDHHS, 1990). In both instances, the process included comprehensive reviews by a wide range of people, including health professionals, scientists, educators, public officials, representatives from business, labor, and voluntary organizations, and representatives from governmental and private health agencies and institutions, task forces, the Institute of Medicine, and state health departments. Specifically, the goals for *Healthy People 2000* (USDHHS, 1990) were the product of 22 expert working groups, the Institute of Medicine, a consortium of 300 national organizations, and the state health departments. A similar process could be used by states and local communities.

The following generic goals for the infrastructure were developed by integrating the conclusions from recent, broad-based analyses of child health systems (Both & Garduque, 1989; Center for the Future of Children Staff, 1993; Cunningham & Hahn, 1994; Green, 1994; Keniston and the Carnegie Council, 1977; McManus, Fox, Newacheck, & Wicks, 1992; Moon, 1993; Natapoff, 1990a, 1990b; Newson & Harvey, 1994; Rosenbaum, 1993; Schorr, 1988, 1991, 1997). It is important to note that public health services are part of the analysis. For example, public health nursing was a stronger presence in earlier decades, although many of the current and emerging threats to child health cannot be ameliorated without it. The recent erosion of those services is troubling because public health services must be part of the system and must include programs for disenfranchised children and their families.

Programs must address the nonfinancial barriers to care, such as transportation, hours of operation, and language services. They must be organized so that the services needed by most children are well distributed, with a broad mix of professionals and delivery sites. Highly specialized services, needed by small numbers of children, should be regionalized in children's hospitals and academic health centers. Systems must be designed to ensure access to services and coordination of programs. Effective infrastructures will promote partnerships between and among health programs, the family, and the community alongside the integration of a range of services.

The infrastructure can also foster the use of appropriate monitoring systems. Health outcome measures for adults are not necessarily directly applicable to children, as the common illnesses of children are not the same as adults', the patterns of their responses to illnesses may vary, and, due to their developmental processes, measures may need to be taken over time in them. Therefore, child health systems need different methods and measures for monitoring the performance of service programs. Outcome measurement should differentiate between problems with programs and problems with the system surrounding the programs.

Palfrey (1994) recommended the development of consortiums as a way to foster better infrastructures for child health services. Complex, working partnerships among the wide variety of groups providing community services are essential. They can be fostered by documenting the interests of each group, creating

incentives, and providing technical assistance (Palfrey, 1994). One group of partners, children's hospitals and academic health care centers, is in the midst of fundamental change. These facilities are essential, as they provide nearly half of the uncompensated (charity) care in the country, serve as the site of many advances in knowledge, and constitute the fulcrum for regionalized neonatal and pediatric specialty care. Their viability is in question as they undergo restructuring and the center of health services shifts within communities. Child health systems must preserve these resources in newly configured relationships with their communities (Aiken & Salmon, 1994; Iglehart, 1995; Stoeckle, 1995).

Schorr (1991, 1997) defined another role for the infrastructure. She found that successful programs share a set of attributes that conflicts with the prevailing traditions for the organization and financing of care and also conflicts with the usual approaches to education and management of child health professionals. The expansion of successful programs should not compromise the reasons for their success, which include comprehensive services with a focus on prevention and flexibility at the point of service. Therefore, for development of the programs there must be alignment of the bureaucratic environment with the characteristics of successful programs as well as concordant changes in professional education and training.

Aligning Financing Policies

Although direct experience is limited, recent analyses of the history of financing child health services include several lessons to guide the development of financing policies that would support the infrastructure for child health services (Alpha Center, 1995a, 1995b, 1995c; Brown, 1992, 1994; Budetti & Feinson, 1993; Center for the Future of Children Staff, 1993; Chafel, 1993; Chafel & Condit, 1993;

Children's Defense Fund, 1994; Coughlin, Ku, & Holohan, 1994; Cunningham & Hahn, 1994; Field & Shapiro, 1993; Hill, Bartlett, & Brostrom, 1993; Meister, 1992; Moon, Ginsburg, & Young, 1993; Natapoff, 1990a, 1990b; Newson & Harvey, 1994; Newhouse, Sloss, Manning, & Keeler, 1993; Rosenbaum, 1993; Schorr, 1991; Wehr & Jameson, 1994).

First, policies are moving toward models that include prepayment for predictable care. Those benefit packages can include traditional medical services, prevention services, chronic illness services, and community-based services, such as public health and transportation to care. The policies should also allow for a range of sites for service delivery. The range would include traditional sites for individual services as well as sites for public health services.

Financing policies should also provide adequate payment for services. Because families must have adequate resources to pay for premiums, subsidies, blends of public and private resources, or other supports will be needed for some. Children's services have been financed primarily through public insurance, private insurance, and categorical programs. As about 60% of children are enrolled in private insurance plans, it is important to decide how policy should incorporate those voluntary systems and articulate them with children's needs (Ireys, Grason, & Guyer, 1996; Lewit & Schuurmann Baker, 1995).

Success in changing financing policies to suit child health services and improvements in the infrastructure will require actions guided by goals, principles, and strategies that can tailor innovations with proven value. The four innovations listed below are examples of such starting points. Each innovation is an emerging idea with enough testing to merit further consideration. Projects could test the utility of the innovations for financing community infrastructures, and these analyses would benefit from nursing science and practice. Evaluation

methods that use a strong theory base and multiple methods to describe community innovations are emerging (Schorr, 1997). We should use them.

One project would experiment with innovations in mixed payment systems for pediatric ambulatory services. Payment would be determined by the weighted average of a capitated rate adjusted for prior use and a measure of current use, so as to prevent biases against enrolling children with risks of high costs (Newhouse et al., 1993). Data collected by nurses in the course of practice can help identify, define, and capture measures of prior and current use (Meister, 1992).

Another project would develop innovations in pediatric standards to bring the special circumstances of children to bear on decisions to deny coverage because of administrative and contractual barriers. These special circumstances include growth and development, disorders requiring specialized skills for care and regionalized systems, need for ancillary services, and disproportionate representation in clinical trial populations (Budetti & Feinson, 1993; Ireys et al., 1996; Wehr & Jameson, 1994). Nursing can help identify the full range of barriers that confront families.

Another project would extend innovations in the framework for school-based child health services to make school enrollment rather than parental employment/economic status the basis for children's eligibility for health insurance (Hill et al., 1993; Igoe, 1992). School nurses have an exceptional vantage point on these issues.

Finally, projects could develop innovations in the concept of whole communities or geographical areas as the focus of funding (Hamburg, 1992; Schorr, 1991, 1997). Public health, home health, advanced practice and acute care nurses can help identify the needs and resources of communities and geographical areas.

In sum, the knowledge base helps clarify thinking about the infrastructure and child health systems in relation to complex issues of payment, benefits, and eligibility and to suggest strategies for changing financing policies. Next, work must focus on developing strategies that can transform thinking into action. Success in implementing the strategies will also depend, in large measure, on the nature of the political will.

■ Impediments to Improving the Infrastructure

Efforts to improve the community infrastructure face substantial impediments. In short, the needs of children and their families have changed dramatically in the past 25 years but without a corresponding change in the child health system. Although the infrastructure has great potential power, efforts to change it conflict with traditional ways of organizing services and place many providers and programs on unfamiliar ground. Equally important, although the funding for the infrastructure must come from the public, the public generally has limited understanding of child health systems, and there is little public leadership in this area.

Sea Changes in Children and Families

The nature of the family, the etiology of child morbidity, and the resources allocated to child health have undergone significant transformation, or sea changes, in the past 25 years. Although there have been some changes in the content, organization, and financing of services, they have not kept up with either the needs and resources of children and their families or the etiologies of the changes.

The sea change in children is related to changes in the family, as well as the causes of morbidity. Although advances in technology have helped eradicate many infectious diseases

that threatened children, those advances also result in a growing number of children with significant disabilities and chronic illness. Furthermore, increasing numbers of children are affected by morbidities related to social etiologies such as poverty, poor education, violence, and homelessness (Palfrey, 1994; Perrin et al., 1996).

The sea change in families is related to economics. Society has long held that the family is responsible for the well-being of its children, and therefore, for the provision of the broad range of resources needed by its children. Although there has always been a percentage of families struggling with or failing to meet those responsibilities, now the majority of American children spend some part of their childhood in single-parent households, and the majority of mothers work outside the home (Hamburg, 1992; Richmond, 1995). Society has failed to recognize and respond to this dramatic alteration in the needs, resources, and abilities of children's families.

Overall, child health needs spring from a broad set of etiologies. Essential resources, including community institutions and families, are under great pressure; even the most successful health service programs cannot change the system within which they operate; public leadership is lacking; and solutions must reach beyond the health system to address economic and social factors (Both & Garduque, 1989; Green, 1994; Hamburg, 1992; Kotelchuck, 1997; Palfrey, 1994; Roper, 1994; Schorr, 1991, 1997; Stein & Tassi, 1997). Therefore, for an increasing number of children, needs have become more complicated, and demands on their families have become more conflicted. The resulting gap in support for child health and development has been inadequately addressed by the child health system and community infrastructures.

For example, 10 million children were without health insurance in 1994 (Agency for Health Care Policy and Research, 1997), nearly 21% of all children were poor in 1995, and 1 in 3 children spends at least 1 year in poverty before reaching adulthood (Center for the Future of Children, 1997); nearly 25% of American families report that it has become more difficult to get medical care (Center for Studying Health Systems Change, 1997); infant mortality rates have steadily declined, but racial differences have persisted (Guyer, Strobino, Ventura, MacDorman, & Martin, 1996; Hoekelman & Pless, 1988); recent changes in welfare policy may alter the most basic aspects of life for almost 10 million children (Larner, Terman, & Behrman, 1997); about 4 in 10 girls become pregnant at least once before age 20, and in 1990, 45% of all first births were to mothers who were either teenagers, unwed, or lacking a high school diploma (National Campaign to Prevent Teen Pregnancy, 1997).

Two reports summarizing over 50 major reports about children and the opening statements of a new maternal-child health journal clarify the meaning of the sea changes in children, families, and policy. They concluded that we have accomplished a great deal and know much about regaining our momentum but that we should view with alarm what has been happening to children and recognize that we are in the midst of major funding cutbacks and massive reorganizations of health services at every level (Both & Garduque, 1989; Carnegie Corporation, 1994; Kotelchuck, 1997).

Bureaucracy and Tradition

As noted in the reviews of child health services and analyses of community infrastructures cited in this chapter, bureaucracy and tradition can be formidable obstacles. Schorr (1988, 1991, 1997) reviewed programs across the nation and determined that we do, in fact, know how to address children's most pressing needs. The next step is to "scale up" those successful programs and develop the infrastructure so that all the children who need them may receive appropriate services. Schorr also found that the characteristics of successful programs are often in conflict with bureaucratic procedures and tradition. For example, programs for the most disadvantaged children must have flexibility in drawing on a broad spectrum of services, which means that they must regularly cross traditional, professional, and bureaucratic boundaries.

Five cities—Pittsburgh (Pennsylvania), Bridgeport (Connecticut), Savannah (Georgia), Little Rock (Arkansas), and Dayton (Ohio)—have spent 5 years trying to overcome these kinds of obstacles. The project, New Futures, funded by the Annie E. Casey Foundation, is designed to support cities as they create fundamental changes in the community infrastructure as well as educational, health, and other services for at-risk youths. The Foundation published its own conclusions about the project, aptly titled *The Path of Most Resistance* (Annie E. Casey Foundation, 1995). The report emphasized three lessons: (a) it takes a long time for broadly based collaborative decision-making bodies to gel, (b) no plan can continue to guide implementation without significant rethinking and mid-course adjustments, and (c) in some communities, change strategies must go beyond the service system and include social-capital and economic-development initiatives. Yet the Foundation also emphasized that when reform efforts are characterized by comprehensive visions they can inspire tremendous energy and sustained engagement.

The Infrastructure Is Unfamiliar and Unfunded

The infrastructure provides a vehicle for supporting and potentiating successful programs by linking schools, churches, community organizations, the media, and health care systems (Hamburg, 1992; Palfrey, 1994). But what does it cost?

In Palfrey's (1994) model, infrastructure costs would include salaries for the professionals conducting the integrated assessments and referrals, establishing communication links among programs, physical space for conducting assessments and overhead for administration and management of the infrastructure.

The infrastructure must also offer benefits that will recruit successful programs into the infrastructure. For example, if the administration and management are specifically designed to make practice and integration more effective, the costs of those elements of the infrastructure secure vital benefits for the programs too.

A project to improve community infrastructure is an important innovation in service delivery and thus deserves evaluation. Evaluation of system costs and benefits should be made at the beginning of the planning process (Meister, Feetham, Girouard, & Durand, 1991). This requires defining the target population, specifying the impact model, and developing an analytic model (Rossi & Freeman, 1989; Scott, Aiken, Mechanic, & Moravcsik, 1995). Ongoing evaluation becomes a yardstick for measuring benefits to children and their families as well as the effectiveness of the infrastructure. Benefits and outcomes for children and their families will be important to the participating providers and agencies, but evidence that integrated assessments and referrals are improving practice will also be required. Therefore, evaluations should include measures of effectiveness, efficiency, and appropriateness so that they will increase knowledge about the structure, processes, and effects of the innovation (Agency for Health Care Policy and Research, 1997; Rossi & Freeman, 1989).

Public Support Is Uncertain

Attempting to improve the child health infrastructure is occurring in an era when individual states spend more on Medicaid than on higher education, the health insurance system leaves a growing minority of Americans without coverage, the health insurance model does not cover some of the most urgent problems, and health care spending has surpassed $1 trillion (Blendon et al., 1993; Keniston & the Carnegie Council, 1977).

These costs and mismatches affect families as well as health. For example, the Center for Health Economics Research (1994) analyzed the nation's health care bill and who pays it. Certainly the costs of health spending fall on individuals in terms of higher taxes, lost jobs, and lost wages, but the Center analyzed the costs for families, estimating that excess health care spending in the past decade has cost the typical American family $7,700. Such experiences blunt the political will to do better in child health services, working against our efforts.

The impediment is uncertain public support rather than a lack of scholarship about revenue sources. For example, Moon's (1993) plan calls for sources that are progressive, able to grow with programs, and related to the benefits. Creative approaches, such as Schorr's (1991, 1997) proposals for careful reformulation of financing based on categorical eligibility, pooling public and private revenue sources, and targeting geographical areas are also directly applicable to funding the infrastructure.

However, public opinion affects the political will, and public sentiment is mixed on child health. Several reports (Bales, 1993; National Campaign to Prevent Teen Pregnancy, 1997; Robert Wood Johnson, 1997; Schorr, 1991, 1997) capture the public's view:

- Americans want to see "children first," but there is great reluctance to support programs or policies that appear to diminish either the privacy or the responsibilities of the family.
- The majority of Americans do not believe that the government can solve health care problems, although they also have limited understanding of those problems or the pro-

posed solutions. Only a small percentage of individuals endorse tax increases to solve health care problems.

- The public lacks an understanding of the patchwork of children's health programs and services, and negative perceptions about links between Medicaid and welfare generally diminish public support.
- The voting public is wary of major change.
- Conflicting views of child health problems can be so intense that communities are unable to act.

Bales (1993) offered two recommendations for galvanizing political will. School-based clinics have an evident degree of local control, which could be used as the leading edge in promoting public involvement with child health. Also, polls indicate that the public is far more likely to support efforts on behalf of all children than those aimed at poor or at-risk children. Schorr (1991, 1997) recommended a focus on improving public understanding that child health is interdependent with society and the economy so that the public can see that the solutions are important but neither quick nor cheap.

Despite these impediments, there have been successes. The establishment of Hull House, the Children's Bureau in 1912 (Haggerty, Roghmann, & Pless, 1975; Richmond, 1995), comprehensive neighborhood health centers and Head Start in the 1960s (Schmidt & Wallace, 1994), and the evolution of school health services and nursing roles within them (Igoe, 1992) were all innovations that improved the community infrastructure as part of successful child health services. Their histories will serve us well.

■ *Leadership to Move Forward*

It is time to contemplate action plans, such as demonstration and pilot projects, evalu-

ation and health services research, and community-based campaigns.

Projects that demonstrate innovations in child health infrastructure and test related policies can build on examples such as Healthy Start, a national 5-year demonstration project (1991-1995) to support communities in their efforts to reduce infant mortality by 50%. The communities used intensive and innovative approaches to develop models of coordinated, comprehensive, culturally competent health and support services (McCoy-Thompson, Vanneman, & Bloom, 1994). Their approaches are instructive because they built infrastructures for existing services, employed specific social strategies, and focused on achieving a major, measurable, and clearly defined goal within an appropriate time frame.

Evaluation and health services research will help build the knowledge base in several ways. They improve our ability to expand successful innovations by quantifying impacts and efficiency for various target populations—analyses that are generally missing and yet greatly needed (Hamburg, 1992; Palfrey, 1994; Rossi & Freeman, 1989; Schorr, 1988, 1997). For example, evaluations would help guide decisions about resource allocations that are made by federal, state, and municipal agencies and institutions (Natapoff, 1990a, 1990b).

These studies also advance methods for examining the intricate relationships between policies and families (Meister, 1989). For example, Healthy Kids in Florida is evaluating an experiment with providing health insurance through the schools. The school system is used as the means for grouping children for marketing and purchasing health insurance. The project started early in 1992 and by the end of the year had expanded eligibility to include younger siblings of school-age children (Hill, Bartlett, & Brostrom, 1993). The findings will help resolve infrastructure issues because they will clarify what works well when child health financing is organized around a community agency.

Community-based campaigns for child health services and infrastructure focus on education and involvement as the pathways to increasing public support. They help the community see the relationships between costs, services, and outcomes. They can be focused on the needs of particular areas in the community, and they can explain strategies that use economic policies to address child health issues. In short, they can be a great help to many aspects of forging new alliances to create local infrastructure (Bane & Ellwood, 1994; Kessel et al., 1994; Klerman, 1994; Palfrey, 1994; Schorr, 1992).

As nursing takes part in these efforts, priorities must be chosen with care. Guidelines developed to identify priorities for the National Institute of Nursing Research (NINR) at the National Institutes of Health (NIH) are helpful here. For example, NINR leadership determined that it is important to look for opportunities to make unique contributions to resolving issues associated with costly burdens for patients, the public, and the health delivery system (NINR, 1993). The NINR symbolizes the enhanced role of nursing, reminding us to account for changes and advances in nursing practice. We must also recognize the significance of nursing in health service delivery. If programs incorporate the resources of nursing with advances in technology and health sciences, the findings from health services research, and the accrued knowledge bases and skills of other groups of providers, the resulting strategies for improving child health will be more effective (Feetham & Meister, 1994).

We can also apply the principles that have guided 15 years of interdisciplinary work in child health policy: test scholarship with practice, reach far beyond the health sector to create a collective dedicated to improving health; develop mechanisms to coordinate, focus, and, in some instances, direct the collective; and place a high value on diligence, determination, and cooperation (Meister, 1997).

■ *Conclusion*

Studies confirm the value of improving community-based infrastructures to maximize the impact of existing services. This strategy works because it links the spectrum of supports needed by children with the reality of families and their communities. This strategy is also difficult to implement.

Although such improvements add value, they will affect the organization and financing of existing services and carry their own new costs. Improving the community infrastructure for child health services can be an effective vehicle for improving child health, but it also challenges child health professionals. Furthermore, although the strategies themselves must be well developed, political will is equally important to making progress (Richmond & Kotelchuck, 1983). A strategy will not take root unless the public endorses it.

Today, health policy must grapple with a sea change in its objectives. After 25 years of policies based on a deficit model to increase the capacity of the system, it is now apparent that policies must shift to a homeostatic model to concentrate on equilibration of the system (Richmond & Fein, 1995). Child health professionals must see to it that child health is preserved throughout the impending struggle to develop policies that will correct imbalances in the distribution of services.

The central premise here is that the knowledge base regarding child health and services serves us well as the beginning point for designing strategies to improve the infrastructure for child health services.

Changing the community infrastructure will call on health professionals to hammer out concurrent changes in practice as well as changes in interdisciplinary bureaucracy and traditions. Nursing has a particularly strong history in the evolution of services and redefinition of roles and boundaries of professions.

Changing the infrastructure will carry new costs, which health professionals, among others, must address. These new strategies risk being underused or even failing unless political will is marshalled to convince families, child health professionals, and the general public to support the aims as well as the costs of those strategies.

It is time to act, and those actions must fit into well-defined goals toward which communities at all levels should work. It is important to begin with the concept of comprehensive services and build strategies that focus on improving the infrastructure to match child needs and child services, but this is not the only challenge. Child health professionals must also grapple with marshalling the political will so that the organization and financing of the infrastructure will have the support of families, child health providers, and the American people.

15
■

ISSUES IN HEALTH
SERVICES RESEARCH

Children and Families and
the Health Care System

■ *Suzanne L. Feetham and Barbara B. Frink*

C are for children and families is no less challenging at the end of the 20th century than it has been throughout this century. The current challenges, however, now include systems of delivery of care and health care policies that may discriminate, intentionally or not, against the best interests of the health of children and their families. Although we know far more about the mechanisms and treatments of specific childhood diseases and have achieved impressive results with biomedical technologies, we are just beginning to study and understand the mechanisms of health care delivery systems that contribute to or interfere with the promotion of children's health.

As noted by the authors in this section of the volume, there are significant influences on the distribution of resources for the health and health care of children and their families and for programs of research of children. These influences include the historical lack of proactive policies and initiatives to improve the health of

children and their families and the adult orientation of our society. Comprehensive policy directed to the health of children and families is not a tradition in the United States. Policy for children and families tends to be directed to specific conditions or circumstances such as pediatric AIDS or Head Start (Huston, 1994; Langley, 1991). As an adult-oriented rather than child-oriented society, risks perceived to affect adults are more often acknowledged and are more apt to receive attention and resources than risks perceived to affect children (Lum & Tinker, 1994).

The current national interest in quality and outcomes of health care delivery systems crosses all strata of the population. This chapter (a) examines the current research base for care of children and families in acute/tertiary delivery systems within the health services research frameworks of risk, quality, and outcomes, (b) identifies work in progress, and (c) recommends some future directions for pediatric systems research. It also identifies the knowledge base to differentiate the care needs of children from those of adults in the measurement of risk, quality, and outcomes in research on children and families. Some of the current concepts in health services research are reviewed, and the "outcomes movement" and the relevance of existing research to understanding pediatric outcomes are discussed.

■ Health Services Research

The primary purpose of health services research is to produce knowledge about the performance of the health care system (Aday, Begley, Lairson, & Slater, 1993): it is the structure, processes, and outcomes of personal health services (Institute of Medicine, 1979). Personal health services occur within the context of the patient provider relationship and are within the domain of the medical care system (Aday et al., 1993). This is distinguished from the public health system, which focuses on the health of communities and populations. By definition, health services research is interdisciplinary, as it includes theories and methodologies deriving from both the biomedical and nonmedical sciences. This interdisciplinary focus becomes extremely relevant to the interpretation of outcomes.

Health Services Research Definitions

Concepts used to understand performance of the care system are efficacy, effectiveness, efficiency, and equity. Related terms are risk, quality, and outcomes. The following definitions are derived from many sources (Aday et al., 1993; Blumberg, 1986; Frink, 1998; Iezzoni & Greenberg, 1994; Institute of Medicine, 1979;

Joint Commission on Accreditation of Healthcare Organizations [JCAHO], 1997; Lohr, 1990):

- *Efficacy:* The actual benefits derived from care processes under the most ideal or controlled circumstances or the degree to which a particular care objective has been achieved under ideal conditions. The most familiar methodology for determining efficacy in health care is the randomized controlled trial.
- *Effectiveness:* The actual benefits of care processes in the normal practice environment, measured by improvements in health at the aggregate level. The improvement is greater than the total improvements to the health of the individual (micro level); at a more global level (macro) it is a measure of the "distribution of disease and health such that overall economic productivity and well-being are maximized" (Aday et al., 1993, p. 1).
- *Efficiency:* The degree to which the desired care objective is achieved related to the consumption of resources. The obvious expectation is to determine the constellation of services producing the best outcomes at the least cost. Cost-benefit/cost-effectiveness analyses are methods used to measure efficiency.
- *Equity:* Determination of the fairness of the distribution of benefits and burdens of care processes at the individual and aggregate level. The ethical concept of distributive justice and the ethical and economic concepts of allocation and availability of resources underpin determinations of equity.
- *Outcome:* Endpoint of a process or cluster of processes of care. This assumes that the determination of the endpoint is well defined. The determination of the appropriate timing of measurement to best determine the endpoint of the care process effect is particularly relevant in the research of children due to their developmental processes.
- *Outcomes assessment:* Examination of the linkages between the structures and processes of care and both of these to outcomes.
- *Outcomes management:* The study and improvement of health care outcomes. Ell-

wood (1988, p. 155) recommended a plan for outcomes management: "1) Development of standards and guidelines, 2) Routine, widespread measurement of disease-specific clinical outcomes and patient functioning and well-being, 3) Collection of clinical and outcome data on a massive scale, and 4) Analysis and dissemination of findings from a continually expanding database." Another definition is published by the Joint Commission on Accreditation of Health Care Organizations (JCAHO, 1997, p. 178): "a philosophy of making health care-related choices based on better insight into and understanding of the effect of these choices on a patient's life."

- *Outcomes measure:* "The quantification of an organization's, practitioner, or community's actual results in providing services" (JCAHO, 1997, p. 179).
- *Quality:* An attribute of the clinical care process, specifically the right process or care delivered and the degree to which it is correctly delivered. Quality is also the measure of the gap between efficacy and effectiveness: what is achieved versus what is achievable (Aday et al., 1993; Brook & Lohr, 1985). Quality applies to structure, process, and outcome. One of the most frequently cited definitions of quality comes from the Institute of Medicine:

> the degree to which health services for individuals and populations increase the likelihood of desired health outcomes and are consistent with current professional knowledge. . . . How care is provided should reflect the clinical, technical, interpersonal, manual, cognitive, and organizational and managed elements of health care. (cited in Lohr, 1990, pp. 4-5)

This definition of quality, while inclusive of both process and outcomes, leaves unanswered the question of what system of monitoring will be adequate to ensure that quality of care and services is being provided. The complexity of design and monitoring of quality indicators across patient populations, care delivery venues, interventions, and technolo-

gies in a timely, cost-effective manner is daunting. Because this is such a complex endeavor, organizations, providers, payers, and consumers have begun to compare outcomes of health care. A key component of these early efforts is that the comparisons are risk adjusted. The most common of the outcomes universally measured in acute care are mortality, length of stay, and charges (Iezzoni & Greenberg, 1994).

- *Risk:* The chance for unexpected or adverse treatment outcomes. Risk can be defined in terms of patient outcomes, such as mortality, morbidity, quality of life, recurrence of symptoms, and repeated hospitalization and/or in terms of the health systems (e.g., cost). To determine risk, both administrative data and patient record data are used.
- *Risk adjustment:* "A way to remove or reduce the effects of confounding factors in studies where cases are not randomly assigned to different treatment. The key confounding factors are those aspects of health status that are causally related to the outcome under study" (Blumberg, 1986, p. 355). For example, pediatric intensive care unit (PICU) patients are often categorized by severity of illness based on physiological stability. This provides a common metric to support clinical decisions, examine variations in outcomes, and examine resource use. Although at first glance the concept of risk adjustment may seem unrelated to equity, it is important to note that methods of risk adjustment are used not only to determine individual risk but to rationalize care. That is, decisions to allocate scarce resources may be rationalized by measures of risk.

Health Services Research on Children and Families

Method of Review

To identify the state of the science in health services research on children, literature searches for reports of research related to risk assess-

TABLE 15.1 Publications Risk Assessment, Outcomes, and Quality in Pediatric Care, 1975-1995

	1975-1979	*1980-1984*	*1985-1989*	*1990-1995*
Risk assessment				
All risk assessment	552	1,457	3,624	8,444*
All pediatric risk assessment	0	0	6	30
Pediatric nursing risk assessment	0	1	7	23
Outcomes				
All outcomes	593	1,347	3,304	12,333*
All pediatric outcomes	3	15	35	213
Pediatric nursing outcomes	0	3	0	26
Quality				
All quality	10,501	12,248	21,009	44,852*
Pediatric quality	71	76	155	473
Pediatric nursing quality	15	5	30	90

*Estimate.

ment, outcomes, quality, and research on children and their families were conducted, including a search for relevant review articles (Forrest, Simpson, & Clancy, 1996; Vivier, Bernier, & Starfield, 1994). The systematic searches resulted in the identification of a limited number of studies in comparison to research with adults (see Table 15.1).

The terms used for the literature searches were (a) *pediatric,* (b) either the select term of *outcomes, quality,* or *risk assessment,* and (c) *age delineation* of all children (birth to 18 years of age). These concepts were selected as they are integral to health services research and readily identified by clinicians through their application in health delivery systems in care maps, critical paths, quality indicators, and benchmarking (Frink & Strassner, 1996). Following the searches for all pediatric literature, *nursing* was added as a search word to the select statement. For this chapter, health services research reported by nurses and other disciplines is included for several reasons:

- A broader interdisciplinary review of research was necessary to demonstrate the state of the science, as by its nature health services research is interdisciplinary and few nurse scientists are on these research teams.

- Nursing practice is interdependent with the research and policy emanating from health services research.

- Consistency with the interdisciplinary nature of the research is required for developing recommendations and directions for the future.

Numerous publications related to quality of care were in existence by 1975; however, research related to the concepts of outcomes and risk assessment are more recent and have far fewer pediatric-based than adult-based publications. The number of studies are reflective, to some degree, of the state of the science of program evaluation and health services research across all age groups and care settings. With children experiencing a lower incidence of illness than adults, the resulting lower ratio of child- to adult-based research, while not surprising, is of concern due to the critical questions to be addressed. The paucity of nursing publications and lack of nurse scientists on health services research teams is a serious limitation, as nurse scientists would add an important perspective to this research.

This trend of limited pediatric-based health services research continues to the present. In a recent publication of the research funded by the

Agency for Health Care Policy and Research (AHCPR, 1996), of the 55 studies of research about managed care organizations, only 3 were pediatric based. However, the number of studies of research on children may increase, as in 1996 Congress requested that the National Institutes of Health (NIH) examine the inclusion of children in health research. In June 1996, experts in research of children across disciplines and in areas of science (basic, clinical, and health services) and representatives from federal agencies and national organizations with an interest in child health were convened to analyze this concern and make recommendations regarding the level of support for needed areas of research on children. One outcome is a federal notice (program announcement) to the research community of the NIH and other federal agencies interested in increasing the research on children (*NIH Guide*, 26:3, January 31, 1997).

Rationale for Emphasis on Health Services Research

The rationale for health services inquiry is that variations in clinical practice are associated with differences in patients outcomes and resource use. Inappropriate practice patterns can be changed if relevant scientific evidence is effectively disseminated to health care providers and patients (Moritz, Frink, & Laughlin, 1994). At the macro level, health services research is focused on the context of care, the organization of care services, and the financing of health care services. At the micro level, it is focused on patient and family responses to care processes, and clinical and financial outcomes for patients and families (Moritz et al., 1994).

Health policy changes are affecting the care of children and families. The traditional research, focused at the level of individual children and families, must be examined from a systems perspective and the effects of the changes documented to inform policymakers, providers, and consumers. A component of this documentation is to ensure that providers and policymakers respond to the differences in the care needs and responses between children and adults.

A serious challenge for the care of children is that more is known about outcomes in relation to adults than children. One reason for this discrepancy is that the number of ill adults exceeds that of children, which supports the increased attention to adults. With the increased number of ill adults, there is a much higher ratio of adult- versus child-focused delivery systems, with a resulting smaller market incentive for developing child-based data systems. A recursive process results in a lack of data to inform policy and payers of the differences in the care needs of children and families, so changes are not made in the distribution of resources, including the development of data systems to inform policy and payers (McGlynn, Halfon, & Leibowitz, 1995; Meister, chap. 14 in this volume).

Ireys, Grason, and Guyer (1996) broadened the concerns of monitoring the effects of changes in care delivery systems for children with special health care needs. As increasing numbers of children with such needs enroll in managed care programs, it is important to determine that their health outcomes are not threatened. Is the access to comprehensive care services decreased for children with special needs? If so, how are the changes in access related to changes in their progress and health trajectory? To monitor these outcomes, Ireys and colleagues, using the Institute of Medicine's (1979) definition of quality, identified six key components for research: content of service delivery systems, the nature of desired health outcomes, risks associated with service delivery, constraints of care, interpersonal dimensions, and attention to developmental issues. They recommended that these six components be assessed at the levels of the individual, the health plan, and the community.

Exemplar

The more common health services research related to children is population based and includes studies on capitation, risk adjustments (Fowler & Anderson, 1996), and pediatric hospitalization rates (Perrin, 1994). The landmark study conducted for the National Association of Children's Hospitals and Related Institutions (NACHRI; 1978) quantified the uniqueness of children's hospitals. The purpose of that study was to identify the operating and capital cost characteristics of the care in children's hospitals and determine the causative factors underlying the cost variances. Variables examined in this study were care intensity, occupancy patterns, staffing for nursing, ancillary and support services, and costs for medical education, research, and community services. Significant cost and financial data included sources of payment, levels of uncompensated care, and space allocations. Even though this study is considered a landmark for its contribution to our understanding of services for children, it was not conducted within the framework of health services research as discussed in this chapter.

Several characteristics of nurse staffing also differentiated children's hospitals, in that young patients required 60% more direct care nursing hours per day than adult patients. For intensive care, this difference was 8%. Since the publication in 1978 of the NACHRI research, which also provided one of the first comparative studies, examination of the allocation of nursing resources in children's hospitals has continued to receive attention (Frink, 1990; Frink, Feetham, & Hougart, 1988; Hlusko & Nichols, 1996; Linden & English, 1994; Suddaby & Frink, 1991, 1993).

Key results of the NACHRI study were that children's hospitals committed a greater percentage of beds and days of care to specialized intensive care and that the severity and complexity of the conditions of the children were greater than in general hospitals. Children's hospitals, often located in academic health centers, provide services to a larger geographic area, affecting length of stay, costs, and the number of specialized services. Although much has changed in health care delivery and financing since 1978, this study provides a baseline and objective language to communicate the special needs and services required for the care of children.

■ *Clinical Information Management*

Identifying special needs populations and adjusting payment mechanisms based on financial risk require clinical and financial data support for policymakers and consumers of health care. Historically, the health care industry has developed parallel systems to manage clinical and financial data. The current environment demands that the relationships between clinical and cost data be examined. Complex health care systems can control costs to the point that care is bankrupt. Conversely, health care delivery can be funded to deliver highly effective care but at such cost that the organization is bankrupt. This is simplistically stated but does make the point that a fine balance exists between effectiveness and efficiency, and in most cases we do not have the data-based evidence to know that the care process has been optimized while balancing cost factors.

Clinical information management is a key strategic component in both the business of the health care organization and monitoring its quality program. Information systems are central to meeting the demands for accountability, measures of quality, and cost management. The demand for greater clinical and fiscal accountability is intrinsically linked to information management and system infrastructure. Building such an infrastructure is a complex interdisciplinary challenge (Frink & Johnson, 1996); it is difficult to be successful in managing quality or outcomes without clinical information support (Kelly, 1996). Traditional health care delivery systems and providers have not addressed the need for clinical and financial databases that follow the patient over a continuum instead of isolating a specific episode of care delivered in a specific place: "Efficiency issues include the complex set of clinical practice and process variables over and above the typical cost issues involving productivity, staffing ratios, and costing strategies" (Witter, 1996, p. 13). Capturing pediatric clinical data is a critical component for inclusion in these developing information systems. Nurses practicing in pediatric-based facilities have some responsibility in contributing to the development and implementation of clinical information systems.

Basic requirements of database systems are that the data are reliable and valid, can be aggregated across patient groups and the system, can inform clinical and financial decisions in pediatric settings, and can provide information to differentiate the care needs and resources of children and their families. Variables selected for study should occur with sufficient frequency to be measurable and have significant cost or other impact to warrant evaluation. In pediatric research settings, this often requires collaboration across many sites to have a sufficient sample for study. A criterion rarely applied to data from pediatric research is that they be designed to inform policy, minimally at the institutional level but preferably at the state and/or national level (Feetham, 1997; Meister, 1992; Meister, chap. 14 in this volume; Meister, Feetham, Durand, & Girouard, 1991; Milio, 1984).

Transforming variables in a database to meaningful information describing outcomes is both a methodological and clinical challenge. Well-developed and tested instruments require years of testing, usually in multiple sites. Output from such measures is tested for statistical significance but may have limited clinical utility from a clinician's perspective. There is some belief that the current state of the science in outcomes measurement is not sufficient to make substantive changes in the efficiency and quality of health care services (Brailer, 1996). Holzemer and Reilly (1995) discuss some of the methodological and informatics issues inherent in process and outcomes research. The challenge is to devise tools that have statistical significance and power to effect change and be meaningful for clinical decision support.

One of the critical challenges for physicians, nurses, and other clinicians is striking a balance between their traditional practice focus, methodological purity, and the necessity to provide risk, quality, and outcomes measures in a rapidly transforming health care system. Part of this dilemma is realized at the level of the clinician. Clinicians focus on individual patients and families or groups within their practice and make decisions on a case-by-case basis. Unless there is a systematic method of collecting data across individual patients, potential risk or outcomes measurements may not be captured.

Figure 15.1 illustrates that individual practice data from patient care are aggregated and analyzed for variables of interest and risk. With a sufficient sample, the distribution approaches a normal distribution, and outliers can be identified. From a clinical standpoint, outliers can be the most challenging and difficult to treat and may represent considerable risk either of disease or to the system, depending on the variables measured. Clinical intervention is then focused on the outlier cases to reduce the risk or improve/ameliorate the patient's condition. Data from both the focused treatment of outliers and the understanding of incidence and

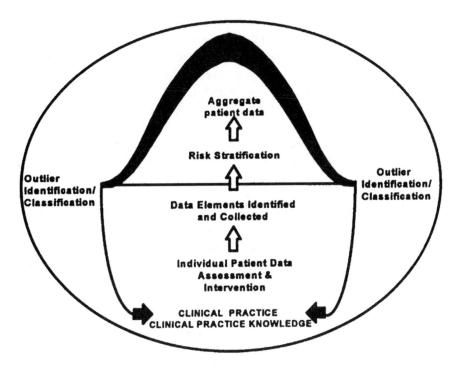

Figure 15.1. Clinical Data for Research and Evaluation
SOURCE: Barbara Frink, PhD, RN, FAAN, Director of Nursing Systems and Research, John Hopkins Hospital, Baltimore. Used with permission.

occurrence is used to update the clinical practice model or performance and may change the variables monitored. There are, of course, no perfect measures, and even in highly predictive measures, there is room for error. When focusing on outlier cases for clinical intervention or establishing incidence rates, it is important to keep in mind the following: "Whenever the focus is on outlier events, the group of outliers will be composed of 'normals' who experienced bad outcomes by chance and true 'abnormals' who actually had a high risk of bad outcomes. This problem arises particularly when patient populations are small and poor outcomes are rare" (Luft & Romano, 1993, p. 336).

One of the inherent conflicts between the population-based model and the individual-patient model is that positive outcomes or risk at the population level may not be the case at the patient level. That is, an intervention may be shown to be 98% effective in treating specific clinical conditions—a low risk from a population standpoint. However, for patients experiencing the ineffectiveness of the intervention, it is a negative outcome from the patient and clinical perspective.

An example from a quality study in an academic health center illustrates the point of the population risk versus the individual experience and opportunity for focused review of outliers. In a single-site clinical study of 3,255 individuals to establish the baseline volume of procedures in which conscious sedation was used and to determine the occurrences of critical clinical events related to conscious sedation, children represented 14% ($n = 471$) of the procedure sample. Critical events occurred in only 1.7% of the pediatric conscious sedation procedures. However, when the group of pediatric patients experiencing more than one conscious sedation procedure was analyzed, one child had experienced more than 50 procedures. A focused clinical review was then conducted in regard to the care processes in this single case (Nyberg, Frink, Nolan, & Schauble, 1996).

As providers and health care delivery systems assume more of the financial risk for patient care and move from episodic delivery to "managing lives" of care, there will be increasing pressure to obtain information that is clinically meaningful and statistically valid. The imperative for risk assessment data as evidence of quality and cost outcomes is not short term. Third-party payers, employers, regulatory bodies, and accrediting organization, such as the JCAHO, have played an important role in moving health care organizations toward the use of outcomes to measure quality and costs. Other motivating external forces are shrinking health care resources and an increasingly competitive health care environment (Johnson, 1995). Through health services research, considerable progress has been made in developing methods for assessing risk, identifying process and outcomes of care, recommending practice guidelines, and implementing methods to determine best practice. In recent sessions of Congress, private and public policymakers sent clear messages calling for accountability in health care, such as routine monitoring of quality of care and evaluating changes in access to care (McGlynn et al., 1995).

Nursing Outcomes

The use of patient outcomes to describe and measure nursing practice is not a new phenomenon. Beginning with the early efforts of Nightingale (1858), the complex issues of measuring nursing outcomes have been and continue to be addressed. In 1991, a collaborative effort of the National Center for Nursing Research and the Agency for Health Care Policy and Research produced an interdisciplinary conference devoted to patient and outcomes

and the effectiveness of nursing practice. More recently, the American Academy of Nursing conducted a second interdisciplinary conference on the state of the science in outcome measurement (Mitchell, Heinrich, Moritz, & Hinshaw, in press). Lang and Marek (1992) reviewed outcomes measured in terms of specific patient phenomenon such as physiological status, psychosocial factors, and functional status. They reported that more recent measures have included functioning in the home, family status, and patient satisfaction. Lang and Marek then proposed that the agenda for outcomes research include building on the state of the science in outcomes research in nursing and other disciplines to create an interdisciplinary effort where the effect of multiple interventions and providers can be examined. While some may not question that nursing care makes a difference in health outcomes, the data are not available on the direct effects of nursing care with children and their families and their effects on processes and functions within and across health care systems. Stewart and Archbold (1992) recommended using sensitivity to change as a criterion for selecting outcome measures of nursing processes of care or interventions. The outcome measures need to be linked conceptually and in time to the care process or intervention in order to differentiate the effects from individual differences in the child and/or family.

■ *Measurement Issues: Distinguishing Differences in Children and Adults*

The measure of risk, quality, and outcomes is confounded in the care of children and families for several reasons. Some of these reasons are based on the child, such as development, health status, and individual behavior. Still others are due to macro-changes in the health care delivery system, such as decreased length of stay, rapidly changing technology, and distribution of systems resources. The interdependence of the environment of the child, family, and family responses and resources is another reason. The differences in treatments and procedures conducted with children affect some of the process measures. For example, even children with chronic illnesses do not receive the number and variety of invasive diagnostic and monitoring procedures as adults do. What is critical in health services research on children and their families is determining the relationship of processes of care, variables of the family, child, and the system of care that affect optimal health outcomes. The definition of outcomes includes the immediate responses of the child to an episode of illness or injury (e.g., mortality or resolution of an illness), longer-term developmental and functional status, family functioning, and quality of life.

Pediatric indicators of effectiveness of care have been included in the HEDIS (Health Plan Employer Data and Information Set) 3.0 reporting measures. HEDIS is the performance measurement system of the National Committee for Quality Assurance (NCQA), which provides quality information for enrollees and purchasers of health care plans (Girouard, 1996). The Health Care Financing Administration is "strongly urging states to use the HEDIS guidelines for Medicaid managed care populations" (NACHRI, 1997, p. 10). This may affect the variables currently collected in a health care delivery information system. However, the NACHRI (1997) reported that HEDIS has not included performance measures for children with special needs or child health care across a continuum.

Children's development requires a different knowledge base for caregivers, and different data for health services research. For health professionals involved in the care of children and families, adapting their care to the different physiological and developmental needs is inherent in their clinical decisions. That the unique anatomical, physiological, and psychological development of children places them at different risks mandating different approaches and resources is well known (Graeter & Mortensen, 1996). For example, to respond to the increased vulnerability of children to rapid fluid and heat loss requires specialized equipment for intubation and the administration of fluids. When the conditions of specialized care are met, the risk of outcomes from injury, cardiac and respiratory compromise, and other sequelae can be mitigated. In the current market of managed care, the system cost for the specialized equipment and the training of health professionals may not be funded by health care delivery systems focusing on the care of adults. Therefore, data that demonstrate the difference in short-term survival and long-term morbidity and resultant cost to society are essential (Casanova & Starfield, 1995).

The potential short-term cost savings to individual health care organizations and the potential long-term costs to society raise the issue of perspective when conducting quality and outcomes studies. The perspective of the study should be explicit in effectiveness and quality studies. To whom does the risk accrue, what is the nature of the risk, to whom do the costs and benefits accrue, and for what duration are perspective questions. Framing the perspective of the analysis should assist both the public and policymakers in regard to potential risks to the health of children and their families.

Determining the timing and scope (cognitive, physical, and emotional) of measuring developmental outcomes is an additional challenge. Because of the child's development, significant outcomes may not be measurable for several years after the intervention has occurred. Not only does the passage of time become a factor, but linking the outcome back to a process of care or an intervention may not be realistic and therefore not valid. Besides using the time span between an intervention and outcome measure, the best source for measuring a relevant outcome may not be in the purview of health professionals. For example, if cognitive development is determined to be an outcome, the best assessment may be from a nonhealth professional such as a teacher.

The difference in the type, intensity, and prevalence of conditions between children and adults is a major factor affecting the data to monitor risk, quality, and outcomes. A small percentage of children with rare and often serious conditions requires the largest expenditure of health care resources (Perrin et al., 1996). This small number results in limited ability to measure effectiveness. Because the majority of children are healthy, outcome measures traditionally used for adults do not, in general, apply to children. In contrast to adults, the conditions with the highest incidence (e.g., asthma and otitis media) tend to have low severity (Homer et al., 1996). As a result, the traditional measures of morbidity and mortality frequently used in quality monitoring in adults do not apply to children (McGlynn et al., 1995).

The pattern of high usage of care resources also differs between children and adults. In adults it is known that the highest demand for care is in the final 2 weeks of life. In contrast, children with special health care needs are at increased risk of having chronic conditions requiring health services beyond what children generally require. Children with chronic illness account for 35% of pediatric hospital days, although they constitute only 2% of children with special health care needs. The cost of caring for a child with special needs is approximately seven times higher than that for a child with no disability. This pattern of care usage is significant in the current managed care environment, as nonspeciality hospitals are focusing on the care of healthy children with acute illnesses or injury. In contrast, at-risk children with chronic illnesses and disabilities are receiving their care in specialty hospitals, with accompanying higher costs.

Framing the demand for care within a cost-effective perspective to payers and policymakers is a challenge (Feeg, 1996). Health services research methods have been applied to examine capitation or risk adjustment methods as one approach to eliminate the incentive (in capitated payer systems) to discriminate against children with chronic conditions. However, in tests of five claims-based risk adjustment methods, the disincentive to enroll children with costly health conditions and special health care needs would not be eliminated by any of the capitation methods tested. Although these methods improved the payment structure, underpayment for high-risk children remained (Fowler & Anderson, 1996).

Another significant difference in children that affects risk, quality, and outcome measurement is their dependence on adults to access, receive, and monitor health care. This dependence also confounds the determination of adherence or follow-up with the recommendation of health care providers. Satisfaction with care is another recognized measure of quality with adults. However, a measure of parental satisfaction may or may not be a valid proxy for the child.

Vivier and colleagues (1994) reviewed several issues and measures related to health outcomes in children. A number of approaches have been used to measure pediatric outcomes, with the majority focusing on a subset of health concerns. They proposed a conceptualization of health that has several domains, among them longevity, disease, comfort, perceived well-being, activity, achievement, and resilience. Vivier and colleagues noted that, more recently, researchers are broadening the assessment of health outcomes in children resulting in more sensitive and comprehensive means of examining the effects of health services. However, they recommended caution in the adoption of these new measures until more data on reliability and validity are available.

Although the differences between adults and children can confound measurement in health services research, knowledgeable clinicians can contribute to the refinement and development of quality measures. For example, selecting relevant clinical data to be aggregated across conditions and/or services, documenting patient responses to changes in continuum of care, and capturing the cost of clinical data, not just charges, are areas for development. Clinicians can also systematically document changes they are seeing as a result of decreased lengths of stay and other revisions in health care delivery.

Policy and advocacy groups are also acting at the national level to ensure quality by working toward standardizing measures for health system performance. Three well-known groups are the National Committee for Quality Assurance (NCQA), the Joint Commission on Accreditation of Healthcare Organizations (JCAHO), and the Foundation for Accountability (FACCT). The NCQA and the JCAHO are standard-setting bodies, whereas the agenda for the FACCT is proposing uniform outcomes-oriented measures of quality but not setting standards nor proposing an accreditation process. The primary difference between the FACCT and the other two organizations is that it is composed solely of consumers and purchasers of health care, that, is primary employers and individual consumer groups (Graham, 1996).

■ Risk Analysis

The process of risk analysis also serves to differentiate the care of children and adults. The concept of risk has always been present in the practice and experience of health care, with risk usually handled within the clinical relationship of patient and provider. With the recent emphasis on escalation of health care costs regardless of controls and the availability of sophisticated measurement systems and analytic computer power, the focus is shifting from the analysis of individual clinical risks to the analysis of aggregate risk for strata of the population. Aggregate risk data are used in clinical decision making regarding selection of treatments, therapeutic agents, interventions, and providers.

Scenarios, or examples of children at risk within systems, are familiar to clinicians, advocacy groups, and families. Situations such as the following are not unusual:

- A new system of primary health care for children and their families is proposed under a capitated agreement with a payor and specific providers.
- Treatment for a chronic childhood disease is carved out of a provider contract for payment.
- Pediatric surgeries not deemed necessary for pediatric specialty treatment are handled in health care delivery systems not dedicated to the treatment of children and pediatric conditions.

All of the above are part of our current experience in health care delivery to children and families in the United States. The changes experienced in practice are dependent on region of the country, managed care penetration in the region, demographics, and clinical case mix. However, in each substantive change, there is inherent risk: to the patient, to the provider, to the payor, and sometimes to communities and specific groups of people. Is the risk increased? Decreased? Does it stay the same? Does the risk change for specific health care systems or groups of patients?

The measurement of risk includes both the risk factors intrinsic to the child, such as disease, genetic history, and social context, and the risk to the patient from the intervention or treatment, such as a surgical method, chemotherapy regimen, or anesthetic agent. Most recently, public concern has been raised about the risk of being treated within certain health care delivery systems due to downsizing of personnel and clinicians or methods and incentives for treatment decisions.

The current attention to outcomes research and outcomes management in health care is directly related to the concept of risk. Whether the goal of documenting outcomes is clinical and research oriented or competitive and financially driven, the need to identify the risk inherent in the outcome is critical. Determining risk is a way of "leveling the playing field" so that valid comparisons and inferences can be made. This process is often referred to as risk adjustment.

One purpose of risk adjustment is "to calculate the so-called algebra of effectiveness, the concept that patient outcomes are a complex function not only of the patient's clinical attributes and such other factors as random events, but also of the effectiveness and quality of the services provided" (Iezzoni, 1994, p. 30). Specific conceptual questions immediately come to mind: What type of risk? For what outcome? Risk to whom, and to what degree? What time period is appropriate to measure the risk? What factors contribute to the risk?

There is no universal definition of what comprises risk and therefore what should be adjusted. Iezzoni (1994, p. 31) suggested a broad set of patient characteristics that may be considered in a risk adjustment, depending on the specific aims under study. These include (a) age and gender/sex; (b) acute clinical stability, principal diagnosis (case mix), extent and severity of comorbidities, physical functional status; (c) psychological, cognitive, and psychosocial functioning; (d) cultural, ethnic, and socioeconomic attributes and behaviors; (e) health status and quality of life; and (f) patient attitudes and preferences for outcomes.

Part of the challenge of risk adjustment is to identify the relationship of the patient characteristic(s) to the outcome of study. How effective is an individual variable in predicting a specific outcome? Brailer (1996), in reporting

the work of the Corporate Hospital Rating Project (CHRP) at the University of Pennsylvania, stated that multivariate risk models are more likely to predict outcomes, given the complexity of patient characteristics. Through basic science work and literature review, the CHRP identified four categories of patient characteristics that influence outcomes, in addition to provider practice patterns. "These categories are: (a) patient clinical factors, (b) therapeutic interventions, (c) patient demographics such as market and insurance status, (d) patient selection of physicians, and (e) specialty services" (Brailer, 1996, p. 25). The CHRP work uses 40 risk adjustment variables in developing multivariate models for diagnoses and outcomes of study. Of note is how many of these characteristics are out of the control of the health care provider.

Illness Severity Exemplar of Risk Analysis

Severity is a multidimensional construct, variously defined, categorized, and measured. The term *severity* is often used as an indicator of patient risk: The more intense the severity, the greater the likelihood of a poor outcome. The focus on severity dates from the early 1980s policy issues surrounding the introduction of diagnosis-related groups (DRGs) into acute care settings. It has been a proxy for both risk adjustment and intensity of resource use, or intensity of illness. The severity of illness scoring systems have been widely used in intensive care units (ICUs) to provide a valid analysis of ICU performance at several levels (Rafkin & Hoyt, 1994). Discussions in the literature demonstrate that the term is not consistently defined. Definitions of severity range from the degree of patient physiological derangement (Jacobs, Chang, & Lee, 1987), the degree of illness within a medical diagnostic category (Horn, Sharkey, & Bertram, 1983), and the "likelihood of death or residual impairment without consideration of treatment"

(Gonella, Hornbrook, & Louis, 1984). With the development of studies on severity of illness instruments and severity risk models in the last 10 to 12 years, the definition has become more specific to the construct being measured, usually in a specific case mix or for a specific purpose (Cowen & Kelley, 1994; Kollef & Schuster, 1994; Lemeshow & Le Gall, 1994; Teres & Lemeshow, 1994; Zhu et al., 1996).

One classification of pediatric severity measures was proposed by Stein and colleagues (1987) as physiological severity, functional severity, and burden of illness. Physiological severity is usually disease specific and measured by clinical, laboratory, and medical treatment data. Functional severity is defined as the "impact of the disorder on an individual's ability to perform age-appropriate activities, irrespective of illness type and under a broad range of circumstances" (Stein et al., 1987, p. 1507): "The impact of the disease or condition on the patient, the family, or the society" is the definition of burden of illness offered by Stein and colleagues (1987, p. 1507).

Pediatric severity of illness was also examined as a correlate of nursing resource consumption and therapeutic intensity (Frink, 1990, 1991; Pollack, Wilkinson, & Glass, 1987; Yeh, Pollack, Holbrook, Fields, & Ruttimann, 1982). In the 1990s, as ICU severity measures were refined through multisite studies, they were tested to predict ICU mortality rates, ICU outcomes, and other ICU performance measures (Kollef & Schuster, 1994; Pine, Norusis, Jones, & Rosenthal, 1997; Rafkin & Hoyt, 1994).

■ Pediatric Risk of Mortality (PRISM) Severity Instrument

The most rigorously tested pediatric acute care severity instrument is PRISM (Pediatric Risk of Mortality; Pollack & Getson, 1988; Pollack, Ruttimann, Glass, & Yeh, 1985; Pol-

lack, Yeh, Ruttimann, Holbrook, & Fields, 1984), developed for use in pediatric intensive care units (PICUs). Other acute care pediatric measures of severity in earlier stages of development are the Score for Neonatal Acute Physiology (SNAP), the Perinatal Extension (SNAP-PE), and the Neonatal Therapeutic Intervention Scoring System (NTISS; Escobar, Fischer, Li, Kremers, & Armstrong, 1995; Gray, Richardson, McCormick, Workman-Daniels, & Goldmann, 1992: Perlman et al., 1995; Richardson, Gray, McCormick, Workman, & Goldmann, 1993; Richardson, Phibbs, et al., 1993; Stevens, Richardson, Gray, Goldmann, & McCormick, 1994).

PRISM is discussed here as an example of a program of research for a case-mix specific risk adjustment. This measure of severity is based on the patient's clinical status and quantity of physiological abnormalities within a 24-hour period (Pollack, Ruttimann, et al., 1987). The PRISM score consists of 14 physiological variables over 23 variable ranges that are routinely measured in a PICU or hospital laboratory. No physiological variable measured invasively is included, as such measurement may be subject to physician practice patterns. Examples of invasive physiological measures are intracranial pressure and cardiac output measurement. The PRISM score, adjusted for patient age (in months) and the operative status of the child, is used to predict mortality risk, based on a logistic regression model (Pollack, Ruttimann, & Getson, 1988).

Work in the 1980s on PRISM focused on instrument development, testing for reliability, validity, psychometrics, and predictive models in multiple PICUs (Pollack, Getson, et al., 1987; Pollack et al., 1988). Work in the 1990s has focused on refining the measure and the accuracy of PRISM in multi-institutional studies (Pollack, Patel, & Ruttimann, 1996; Pollack, Patel, Ruttimann, & Cuerdon, 1996). The program of research on the development and implementation of PRISM is frequently cited in reviews of severity of illness measurement.

However, it is one of the few instruments designed for use in pediatric acute care environments. The application and testing of this instrument continues with an international focus. More recent studies of PRISM include examining the ability to predict outcomes for children receiving extracorporeal membrane oxygenation (ECMO), children receiving emergency care in Mexico, PICU care in the Netherlands, South Africa, and Russia, and children with cancer treated in PICUs in the Netherlands (Gremke & Bonsel, 1995; Maulen-Radovan, Gutierrez-Castrellon, Zaldo-Rodriguez, & Martinez-Natera, 1996; Ruttimann, Pollack, & Fiser, 1996; van Veen et al., 1996; Wells, Riera-Fanego, Luyt, Dance, & Lipman, 1996).

When one considers the extent of testing one instrument, measuring one aspect of severity of illness in one case mix during a specific episode of care, the scope of measurement required for multiple types of risk adjustment (clinical, economic, and policy) becomes apparent—and daunting. Systematic use of well-tested risk adjustment instruments can, however, provide additional clinical decision support for interpretation of outcomes data.

■ *Benchmarking*

A less rigorous method of comparing outcomes across settings is benchmarking. This process is being used increasingly in health care to supply some measure of comparison for both competitive and quality purposes. A benchmark represents "best in class," best practice, a standard of excellence, or a "gold standard" (McKeon, 1996).

Benchmarking is included in this chapter because (a) the areas of practice examined are interdependent with system factors; (b) the concerns of individual clinical decisions are examined across the aggregate of caregivers and patients; (c) the determinations of best-practice decisions include the concepts of risk, quality, and outcomes; and (d) the most reliable/effective process of benchmarking uses empirical research data to confirm clinical judgment. Benchmarking, like health services research, is an interdisciplinary process involving experts in clinical practice, economics, systems, and research. The process of benchmarking, used in industry for several years, is now applied in health care delivery systems as one process for monitoring outcomes of quality and costs of care for children and families. Data from the processes of care maps, critical paths, and performance improvement indicators are used in benchmarking efforts internally and externally (Frink, in press; Johnson, 1995). The key to benchmarking is understanding the composition of the benchmark. Benchmarking uses measures of comparative performance to develop an understanding of what is possible and how others have achieved higher levels of performance (Czarnecki, 1996). Different types of benchmarking identified by Camp and Tweet (1994) are (a) internal, (b) competitive, (c) functional, and (d) generic. When adapting the process of benchmarking to health care, members of the participating institutions can target the business, support, and/or clinical functions for evaluation. For clinical functions, there are ready-made networks of professionals with similar problems and interests for comparisons. The network concept has been demonstrated in the children's hospitals participating in the NACHRI Patient Care FOCUS Groups 1996 benchmarking initiative (NACHRI, 1996a, 1996c).

Benchmarking in Pediatric Populations

A benchmarking effort using interdisciplinary focus groups under the auspices of the NACHRI is presented as an exemplar of the relationships between benchmarking and health

TABLE 15.2 Clinical Practices Examined in Benchmarks Across Pediatric Hospitals

Laboratory	26	Blood Products Administration	2
Diagnostic Tests	15	Pain Management	7
Bedside Testing/Point of Service Testing	6	Infection Control/Isolation	11
		Admission Criteria	2
Interdisciplinary Assessments	22	Patient Placement	3
Non-Invasive Monitoring	9	Discharge Criteria	5
Treatments/Therapies	9	Family-Centered Care	17
Nutrition Practices	4	Optimal Skill Mix	6
Medications/Fluids	17	Latex Allergy	1
Lines	6		
SUBTOTAL	**114**	**SUBTOTAL**	**54**

TOTAL BENCHMARKS = 168

SOURCE: Reproduced by permission from National Association of Children's Hospitals and Related Institutions (1996c). Areas covered in draft benchmarks. *Points of FOCUS, 2,* 1 [quarterly newsletter].

services research. One of the strengths of the NACHRI initiative is that pediatric facilities across the United States are collaborating and developing aggregate data to examine care functions. By including the assessment of quality and cost data, the functions examined in the benchmarking process can inform clinical and system-level decisions.

Historically, this effort has evolved from a long-standing committee of patient care executives. For several years, this committee guided the efforts to establish comparative data related to nursing resource consumption across the participating children's hospitals. As is critical to the work of remaining competitive in the current health care market, this interdisciplinary effort combines consultation from NACHRI staff resources with external consultative resources from the member hospitals and others with expertise in pediatric care delivery. Over 168 clinical practices have been examined, among them services for pediatric and neonatal intensive care, hematology/oncology, emergency and trauma, and medical-surgical care (see Table 15.2).

It is evident from the success of the NACHRI project that each participating institution is willing to share data openly. Another

indicator of the project's success is that as of 1996 (NACHRI, 1996b) 49 children's hospitals were participating in the program, with over 250 patient care personnel from clinicians through executives constituting 71 interdisciplinary teams.

The characteristics of this project are essential to any benchmarking program, including selection of the dimensions of care meeting the criteria of high-volume, measurable outcomes for quality and cost and the use of indicators with a clear business advantage. Another characteristic is that consensus on program goals is reached by the interdisciplinary teams. A critical characteristic of the NACHRI project is that best practice is determined through not only expert clinical judgment but is validated with empirical evidence from published clinical and health services research. For the initial care components examined in the NACHRI process, the compilation and analysis of this state-of-the-science evidence was conducted by a team led by a nurse researcher (NACHRI, 1996a). The application of these characteristics supports the integration of benchmarking into the processes and continuous quality improvement (CQI) efforts of each health system when the criterion is met of combining clinical judgment of best practice with systematic clinical data and empirical data.

A significant outcome of this collaborative program is that comparative data from a significant population of children and families across the United States are now available to be framed to inform policymakers of the significance of the difference in the care needs of children, the effectiveness of care, and improved outcomes for children and families cared for in pediatric centers.

Other evidence of benchmarking in the care of children and families has been reported by Porter (1995), Czarnecki (1996), Ellis (1995), and Igoe (1994). Porter (1995) reported on a second benchmarking program among children's hospitals (BENCHmark). The goal was for the BENCHmark effort to supplement the hospitals' CQI programs and to speed adoption of best practices from peer institutions. As an example, improvements have occurred in emergency room services in the hospitals.

Igoe (1994), an international leader in school nursing, reported that total quality management is moving into health systems in schools and recommended benchmarking as the place to start in this process. Unfortunately, the effects of school nursing services are not as well documented as the benefits of school-based student health centers. Using benchmarking to identify best practices will contribute to narrowing this information gap and demonstrate the need for combining the school health model of the population-based services of the school nurse with the individualized preventive model of school-based student health centers. Nursing can provide significant leadership in the development of these integrated systems and in the monitoring of health care delivery and quality health outcomes in schools. Benchmarking has also extended to other countries. The introduction of benchmarking in pediatric care in the northwest region of England is described as a new addition

to nursing hospital staffing (Ellis, 1995) quality initiatives.

Czarnecki (1996) reported on a collaborative effort initiated by a consortium of businesses concerned with reducing the cost of employee health care. Benchmarking was used as the process for examining best practice and possible areas for cost reductions. As part of the process, the length of stay in the neonatal intensive care unit (NICU) was studied. Although the impetus for examining care practices came from the external business community, the process was extended to include the care providers. Results of this process included improved quality outcomes for the infants and their families and a reduction in costs of care. Another significant result was that the process and data from benchmarking led to the identification of research questions for further study.

The linkages of benchmarking to nursing research of children and families occurs at two key points in the benchmarking process. First, the results of nursing research, reported in all chapters of this text, may be used as evidence for related clinical areas used in the benchmarking process. Second, additional questions for nursing and health services research can emerge from the benchmarking process. Nurses caring for children and families have the opportunity to be engaged in these significant activities.

■ *Summary and Recommendations*

Although considerable progress is evident in health services research, a strong theme of this chapter is the paucity of research related to the care of children and families in acute and tertiary care settings. Several factors have been analyzed, among them the proportionately smaller percentage of ill children in the population than adults.

Changes in health care systems will continue, coupled with the demand for integrated data systems to inform clinical, system, and policy decisions (Haggerty, 1995). Care of children will require greater knowledge of new morbidities, re-emergent old disorders, and systems to care for the increasing numbers of children with chronic illness. Data are required to measure the outcomes with children and families as alternate care systems emerge, such as pediatric subacute care (Grebin & Kaplan, 1996; NACHRI, 1996d). Clinicians and systems also need to be positioned to respond to the effects of the burgeoning knowledge and technologies emanating from the Human Genome Project.

Nurses, physicians, and other child health professionals have critical roles in contributing to outcome measurement. For example, they may ensure that policies and practices within managed care organizations promote a high quality of care for children with special care needs. Terhaar and O'Keefe (1995) framed this expected contribution in the context of a new advanced practice role focused on outcomes management in children's health. They described outcomes management as goal-directed coordination of transdisciplinary teams that focus on achieving measurable outcomes for certain populations of patients.

As the state of the science develops in the conceptualization, measurement, and analysis of risk, quality, and outcomes, it is critical that the pediatric case mix be included in health services research. Determination of the effect of child development and family orientation on both short- and long-term outcomes will both assist in refining pediatric appropriate measures and inform policymakers of issues critical to children's health.

REFERENCES

Abbot, G. (1923). *Ten years' work for children: The United States Children's Bureau, 1912-1922*. New York: Arno.

Abbott, N. C., Hansen, P., & Lewis, K. (1970). Dress rehearsal for the hospital. *American Journal of Nursing, 70,* 2360-2362.

Abrams, L. (1982). Resistance behaviors and teaching media for children in day surgery. *Journal of the Association of Operating Room Nurses, 35,* 244-258.

Abt, I. (1923). *Abt's pediatrics* (Vol. 1). Philadelphia: W. B. Saunders.

Achenbach, T. M. (1991a). *Manual for the Child Behavior Checklist/4-18 and 1991 profile*. Burlington, VT: University of Vermont Department of Psychiatry.

Achenbach, T. M. (1991b). *Manual for the Teacher's Report Form and 1991 profile*. Burlington, VT: University of Vermont Department of Psychiatry.

Achenbach, T. M., & Edelbrock, C. (1983). *Manual for Child Behavior Checklist and revised child profile*. Burlington: University of Vermont, Department of Psychiatry.

Ackerley, G. (1836). *Management of children in sickness and in health*. New York: Bancroft & Holley.

Adams, G., Bennion, L., & Huh, K. (1989). *Objective measures of ego identity status: A reference manual*. Unpublished manuscript, Utah State University, Laboratory for Research on Adolescence.

Aday, L. A., Begley, C. E., Lairson, D. R., & Slater, C. H. (1993). *Evaluating the medical care system: Effectiveness, efficiency, and equity*. Ann Arbor, MI: Health Administration Press.

Agency for Health Care Policy and Research. (1992). *Acute pain management: Operative or medical procedures and trauma* (AHCPR Publication No. 92-0032). Washington, DC: U.S. Department of Health and Human Services.

Agency for Health Care Policy and Research. (1996, December 2-4). *Research Activities, 196.*

Agency for Health Care Policy and Research. (1997). *Child health services: Building a research agenda* (AHCPR Publication No. 97-R055). Washington, DC: U.S. Department of Health and Human Services.

Aiken, L. H., & Salmon, M. E. (1994). Health care workforce priorities: What nursing should do now. *Inquiry, 31,* 318-329.

Ainsworth, M., Blehar, M., Waters, E., & Wall, S. (1978). *Patterns of attachment*. Hillsdale, NJ: Lawrence Erlbaum.

Airhihenbuwa, C. O. (1990-1991). A conceptual model for culturally appropriate health education programs in developing countries. *International Quarterly of Community Health Education, 11*(1), 53-62.

Airhihenbuwa, C. O. (1992). Health promotion and disease prevention strategies for African Americans: A conceptual model. In R. L. Braithwaite & S. E. Taylor (Eds.), *Health issues in the Black community* (pp. 267-280). San Francisco: Jossey-Bass.

Ajzen, I. (1985). From intentions to actions: A theory of planned behavior. In J. Kuhl & J. Beckman (Eds.), *Action control: From cognition to behavior* (pp. 11-39). New York: Springer-Verlag.

Ajzen, I. (1989). *Attitudes, personality and behavior*. Pacific Grove, CA: Brooks/Cole.

Ajzen, I., & Fishbein, M. (1980). *Understanding attitudes and predicting social behavior*. Englewood Cliffs, NJ: Prentice Hall.

Alex, M. R., & Ritchie, J. A. (1992). School-age children's interpretation of their experience with acute surgical pain. *Journal of Pediatric Nursing, 7,* 171-180.

Alpert, J., Kosa, J., & Haggerty, J. (1967). Medical help and maternal nursing care in the life of low income families. *Pediatrics, 39,* 749-754.

Alpha Center. (1995a). Children's health plans: Expanding coverage to the uninsured. *State Initiatives in Health Care Reform, 11,* 4-7.

Alpha Center. (1995b, March). The Medicaid expansions: Are they working? *Health Care Financing and Organization News and Progress,* pp. 1-2.

Alpha Center. (1995c). The number of Americans with health insurance coverage continues to drop. *State Initiatives in Health Care Reform, 11,* 1-3.

Altimier, L., Norwood, S., Dick, M. J., Holditch-Davis, D., & Lawless, S. (1994). Postoperative pain management in preverbal children: The prescription and administration of analgesics with and without caudal analgesia. *Journal of Pediatric Nursing, 9,* 226-232.

Altman, D., & Dore, C. J. (1985). Randomization and baseline comparisons in clinical trials. *Lancet, 335,* 149-155.

American Academy of Pediatrics. (1960). *Care of children in hospitals.* Evanston, IL: Author.

American Academy of Pediatrics. (1971). *Hospital care of children and youth.* Elk Grove Village, IL: Author.

American Academy of Pediatrics. (1986). *Care of children in hospitals* (2nd ed.). Evanston, IL: Author.

American Academy of Pediatrics. (1993). *Committee on school health* (5th ed.). Evanston, IL: Author.

American Association of Critical Care Nurses. (1997). *Thunder Project II: A study to examine pain perception and responses of critically ill pediatric and adult patients undergoing procedures.* Aliso Viejo, CA: Author.

American Heart Association. (1989). *The AHA schoolsite program: Heart decisions middle school package technical report.* Dallas, TX: Author.

American Nurses' Association Commission on Nursing Research. (1976). Priorities. *Nursing Research, 25,* 357.

Anderson, G. C. (1975). A preliminary report: Severe respiratory distress in transitional newborn lambs with recovery following nonnutritive sucking. *Journal of Nurse-Midwifery, 20*(2), 20-28.

Anderson, G. C., McBride, M. R., Dahm, J., Ellis, M. K., & Vidyasagar, D. (1982). Development of sucking in term infants from birth to four hours postbirth. *Research in Nursing and Health, 5,* 21-27.

Anderson, J. (1981). The social construction of the illness experience: Families with a chronically ill child. *Journal of Advanced Nursing, 6,* 427-434.

Anderson, J. M. (1990). Home care management in chronic illness and the self-care movement: An analysis of ideologies and economic processes influencing policy decisions. *Advances in Nursing Science, 12,* 71-83.

Anderson, J. M., & Chung, J. (1982a). The differential construction of social reality in chronically ill children: An interpretive perspective. *Human Organization, 41,* 259-262.

Anderson, J. M., & Chung, J. (1982b). Culture and illness: Parents' perceptions of their child's long term illness. *Nursing Papers, 14*(4), 40-52.

Anderson, J. M., & Elfert, H. (1989). Managing chronic illness in the family: Women as caretakers. *Journal of Advanced Nursing, 14,* 735-743.

Anderson, J. M., Elfert, H., & Lai, M. (1989). Ideology in the clinical context: Chronic illness, ethnicity and the discourse on normalization. *Sociology of Health and Illness, 11,* 253-278.

Anderson, N. L. R. (1996). Decisions about substance abuse among adolescents in juvenile detention. *Image: Journal of Nursing Scholarship, 28,* 65-70.

Andersson-Segesten, K., & Plos, K. (1989). The needs, concerns, and coping of mothers of children with cystic fibrosis. *Scandinavian Journal of Caring Science, 3*(1), 35-41.

Angst, D. B., & Deatrick, J. A. (1996). Involvement in health care decisions: Parents and children with chronic illness. *Journal of Family Nursing, 2,* 174-194.

Annie E. Casey Foundation. (1995). *The path of most resistance.* Baltimore: Author.

Anthony, M. A. (Ed.). (1995). *Pediatric excellence in delivery systems.* Alexandria, VA: National Association of Children's Hospitals and Related Institutions.

Aradine, C. (1980). Home care for young children with long-term tracheostomies. *MCN: American Journal of Maternal-Child Nursing, 5,* 121-125.

Aradine, C., Uman, H., & Shapiro, V. (1978). The infant with a long-term tracheostomy and the parents: A collaborative treatment. *Issues in Comprehensive Pediatric Nursing, 3*(1), 29-41.

Arbeit, M. L., Johnson, C. C., Mott, D. S., Harsha, D. W., Nicklas, T. A., Webber, L. S., & Berenson, G. S. (1992). The Heart Smart cardiovascular school health promotion: Behavior correlates of risk factor change. *Preventive Medicine, 21,* 18-32.

Arbeit, M. L., Johnson, C. C., Mott, D. S., Harsha, D. W., Nicklas, T. A., Webber, L. S., & Berenson, G. S. (1992). The Heart Smart Cardiovascular School Health Promotion Program: Behavior correlates of risk factor change. *Preventive Medicine, 21,* 18-32.

Asprey, J. R. (1994). Postoperative analgesic prescription and administration in a pediatric population. *Journal of Pediatric Nursing, 9,* 150-157.

Atkinson, B. A., & Day, S. A. (1981a, December 9). Paediatrics past. *Nursing Times,* pp. 1-4.

Atkinson, B. A., & Day, S. A. (1981b, December 9). Paediatric nursing: An historical view. *Nursing Times,* pp. 4-7.

Attala, J. M., Gresley, R. S., McSweeney, M., & Jobe, M. A. (1993). Health needs of school-age children in two midwestern counties. *Issues in Comprehensive Pediatric Nursing, 16,* 51-60.

Austin, J. K. (1988). Childhood adaptation and family resources. *Journal of Child and Adolescent Psychiatric and Mental Health Nursing, 1,* 18-24.

Austin, J. K. (1989). Predicting parental anticonvulsant medication compliance using the Theory of Reasoned Action. *Journal of Pediatric Nursing, 4,* 88-95.

Austin, J. K. (1990). Assessment of coping mechanisms used by parents and children with chronic illness.

MCN: American Journal of Maternal-Child Nursing, 15, 98-100.

Austin, J. K. (1991). Family adaptation to a child's chronic illness. In J. J. Fitzpatrick, R. L. Taunton, & A. K. Jacox (Eds.), *Annual review of nursing research* (Vol. 9, pp. 103-120). New York: Springer.

Austin, J. K., McBride, A. B., & Davis, H. W. (1984). Parental attitude and adjustment in childhood epilepsy. *Nursing Research, 33,* 92-96.

Austin, J. K., & McDermott, N. (1988). Parental attitude and coping behaviors of children with epilepsy. *Journal of Neuroscience Nursing, 20,* 174-179.

Austin, J. K., Risinger, M. W., & Beckett, L. A. (1992). Correlates of behavior problems in children with epilepsy. *Epilepsia, 33,* 1115-1122.

Austin, J. K., Smith, M. S., Risinger, M. W., & McNelis, A. M. (1994). Childhood epilepsy and asthma: Comparison of quality of life. *Epilepsia, 35,* 608-615.

Bailey, T. F. (1967). Puppets teach young patients. *Nursing Outlook, 15,* 36-37.

Baker, J. P. (1994). Women and the invention of well child care. *Pediatrics, 94,* 527-531.

Baker, S. J. (1918). Lessons from the draft. *Transactions of the American Association for the Study and Prevention of Infant Mortality, 9,* 181-188.

Baker, S. J. (1939). *Fighting for life.* New York: Macmillan.

Bales, S. N. (1993). Public opinion and health care reform for children. *The Future of Children, 3,* 184-197.

Bandura, A. (1972). *Psychological modeling: Connecting theories.* Chicago: Aldine/Atherton.

Bandura, A. (1977). Self-efficacy: Toward a unifying theory of behavioral change. *Psychological Review, 84,* 191-215.

Bandura, A. (1986). *Social foundations of thought and action: A social cognitive theory.* Englewood Cliffs, NJ: Prentice Hall.

Bandura, A. (1995). *Moving into forward gear in health promotion and disease prevention* [Keynote address] (Cassette Recording No. 27-9-95). Rockville, MD: Society of Behavioral Medicine.

Bane, M. J., & Ellwood, D. T. (1994). *Welfare realities: From rhetoric to reform.* Cambridge, MA: Harvard University Press.

Barnard, K. E. (1972). The effect of stimulation on the duration and amount of sleep and wakefulness in the premature infant (Doctoral dissertation, University of Washington, 1968). *Dissertation Abstracts International, 33,* 2167B.

Barnard, K. E. (1978). *Nursing child assessment training project learning resource manual.* Seattle: University of Washington School of Nursing.

Barnard, K. E., & Bee, H. L. (1983). The impact of temporally patterned stimulation on the development of preterm infants. *Child Development, 54,* 1156-1167.

Barnard, K. E., & Neal, M. V. (1977). Maternal-child nursing research: Review of the past and strategies for the future. *Nursing Research, 26,* 193-200.

Barnard, K. E., Snyder, C., & Spietz, A. (1991). Supportive measures for high-risk infants and families. In A. L. Whall & J. Fawcett (Eds.), *Family theory development in nursing: State of the science and art* (pp. 139-176). Philadelphia: F. A. Davis.

Barnes, C. M. (1975a). School-age children's recall of the intensive care unit. In American Nurses' Association (Ed.), *ANA clinical sessions, San Francisco, 1974* (pp. 73-91). New York: Appleton-Century-Crofts.

Barnes, C. M. (1975b). Levels of consciousness indicated by responses of children to phenomena in the intensive care unit. *Maternal-Child Nursing Journal, 4,* 215-285.

Barnes, C. M., Bandak, A. G., & Beardslee, C. I. (1990). Content analysis of 186 descriptive case studies of hospitalized children. *Maternal-Child Nursing Journal, 19,* 281-296.

Barnes, C. M., Kenney, F. M., Call, T., & Reinhart, J. B. (1972). Measurement in management of anxiety in children for open heart surgery. *Pediatrics, 9,* 250-259.

Barton, W. (1911). The work of infant milk stations in relation to infant mortality. *Transactions of the American Association for Study and Prevention of Infant Mortality, 1,* 299-300.

Bates, J. E., Freeland, C. A. B., & Lounsbury, M. L. (1979). Measurement of infant difficulties. *Child Development, 63,* 380-387.

Batey, M. V. (1977). Conceptualization: Knowledge and logic guiding empirical research. *Nursing Research, 26,* 10-29.

Bauman, K. E., & Udry, J. R. (1981). Subjective utility and adolescent sexual behavior. *Adolescence, 16,* 527-535.

Baumrind, D. (1991). The influence of parenting style on adolescent competence and substance use. *Journal of Early Adolescence, 11,* 56-95.

Beal, J. A., & Betz, C. L. (1992). Intervention studies in pediatric nursing research: A decade of review. *Pediatric Nursing, 18,* 586-590.

Beal, J. A., & Betz, C. L. (1993). Sampling issues in parent-child nursing research: Implications for nursing practice. *Journal of Pediatric Nursing, 8,* 261-262.

Beaven, P. W. (1957). History of the Boston Floating Hospital. *Pediatrics, 19,* 629-638.

Beaver, C. F. (1995). Environmental health hazards: How children are different from adults. *The Future of Children, 5*(2), 8-10.

Beck, A. T., Ward, C. H., Mendelson, M., Mock, J., & Erbaugh, J. (1961). An inventory for measuring depression. *Archives of General Psychiatry, 4,* 53-63.

Beck, C. T. (1988). Pediatric nursing research published from 1977 to 1986. *Issues in Comprehensive Pediatric Nursing, 11,* 261-270.

Beck, C. T. (1995). The effects of postpartum depression on maternal-infant interaction: A meta-analysis. *Nursing Research, 44,* 298-304.

Beck, C. T. (1996). Postpartum depressed mothers' experiences interacting with their children. *Nursing Research, 45,* 98-104.

Beck, M. (1973). Attitudes of pediatric heart patients towards patient care units. *Nursing Research, 22,* 234-239.

Becker, M. H. (Ed.). (1974). The Health Belief Model and personal health behavior. *Health Education Monographs, 2,* 324-473.

Becker, M. H., & Maiman, L. A. (1980). Strategies for enhancing patient compliance. *Journal of Community Health, 6,* 113-135.

Becker, P. T., Chang, A., Kameshima, S., & Bloch, M. (1991). Correlates of diurnal sleep patterns in infants of adolescent and adult single mothers. *Research in Nursing and Health, 14,* 97-108.

Beckstrand, J., Ellett, M., Welch, J., Dye, J., Games, C., Henrie, S., & Barlow, R. S. (1990). The distance to the stomach for feeding tube placement in children predicted from regression on height. *Research in Nursing and Health, 13,* 411-420.

Behar, L., & Stringfield, S. (1974). A behavior rating scale for the preschool child. *Developmental Psychology, 10,* 601-610.

Bell, J. (1995). Editorial wanted: Family nursing interventions. *Journal of Family Nursing, 1,* 355-358.

Bell, J. (1996). Advanced practice in family nursing: One view. *Journal of Family Nursing, 2,* 244-247.

Bennett, D. S. (1994). Depression among children with chronic medical problems: A meta-analysis. *Journal of Pediatric Psychology, 19,* 149-169.

Benoliel, J. Q. (1970). The developing diabetic identity: A study of family influence. In M. V. Batey (Ed.), *Communicating nursing research: Methodological issues in research* (pp. 14-32). Boulder, CO: Western Interstate Commission for Higher Education.

Benoliel, J. Q. (1975). Childhood diabetes: The commonplace in living becomes uncommon. In A. L. Strauss (Ed.), *Chronic illness and the quality of life* (pp. 89-98). St. Louis: Mosby.

Benoliel, J. Q. (1977). Role of the family in managing young diabetics. *The Diabetes Educator, 3*(2), 5-8.

Benoliel, J. Q. (1983). Grounded theory and qualitative data: The socializing influence of life-threatening disease on identity development. In P. J. Woolridge, M. H., Schmitt, J. K. Skipper, & R. C. Leonard (Eds.), *Behavioral science and nursing theory* (pp. 141-187). St. Louis: Mosby.

Berenson, G. S. (1980). *Cardiovascular risk factors in children.* New York: Oxford University Press.

Berg, C. L., Swanson, D. J., & Juhl, N. (1992). Total blood cholesterol and contributory risk factors in an adolescent population. *Journal of School Health, 62,* 64-66.

Bergman, R. L. (1993, October, 5). Quantum leaps. *Hospitals and Health Networks,* pp. 28-35.

Best, J. A. (1989). Intervention perspectives on school health promotion research. *Health Education Quarterly, 16,* 299-306.

Betz, C. L., & Beal, J. (1993). *Use of nursing models in pediatric nursing research: A decade of review.* Unpublished manuscript.

Beyer, J. E., & Aradine, C. R. (1986). Content validity of an instrument to measure young children's perceptions of the intensity of their pain. *Journal of Pediatric Nursing, 1,* 386-395.

Beyer, J. E., & Aradine, C. R. (1988). Convergent and discriminant validity of a self-report measure of pain intensity in children. *Children's Health Care, 16,* 274-283.

Beyer, J. E., & Byers, M. L. (1985). Knowledge of pediatric pain: The state of the art. *Children's Health Care, 13,* 150-159.

Beyer, J. E., DeGood, D. E., Ashley, L. C., & Russell, G. A. (1983). Patterns of postoperative analgesic use with adults and children following cardiac surgery. *Pain, 17,* 71-81.

Beyer, J. E., Villarruel, A., & Denyes, M. (1995). *The Oucher: User's manual and technical report.* Bethesda, MD: Association for the Care of Children's Health.

Beyers, M. (1995). Public policy and the nurse administrator. *Nursing Policy Forum, 1*(1), 28-33.

Bibace, R., & Walsh, M. W. (1980). Development of children's concepts of illness. *Pediatrics, 66,* 912-917.

Bixler, G. K. (1942). Research and problems in nursing. *American Journal of Nursing, 42,* 676-679.

Black, M., Nair, P., Knight, C., Wachtel, R., Roby, P., & Schuler, M. (1994). Parenting and early development among children of drug-abusing women: Effects of home intervention. *Pediatrics, 94,* 440-448.

Black, M. M., & Danesco, E. R. (1994). The impact of ecological theory on intervention research in maternal and child health. In G. Lamberty & K. Barnard (Eds.), *Research priorities: Fourth National Title V Maternal and Child Health Research Priorities Conference [Proceedings].* Washington, DC: Maternal and Child Health Bureau, Health, Resources, and Services Administration, Public Health Service, U.S. Department of Health and Human Services, and the National Center for Education in Maternal and Child Health.

Blackburn, S., & Patteson, D. (1991). Effects of cycled light activity state and cardiorespiratory function in preterm infants. *Journal of Perinatal and Neonatal Nursing, 4*(4), 47-54.

Blake, F., & Wright, H. (1963). *Essential of pediatric nursing.* Philadelphia: J. B. Lippincott.

Blendon, R. J., Donelan, K. , Hill, C., Scheck, A., Carter, W., Beatrice, D., & Altman, D. (1993). Medicaid beneficiaries and health reform. *Health Affairs, 12,* 132-151.

Bloom, K. C. (1995). The development of attachment behaviors in pregnant adolescents. *Nursing Research, 44,* 284-289.

Blumberg, M. S. (1986). Risk adjusting health care outcomes: A methodologic review. *Medical Care Review, 43,* 351-393.

Blumenthal, S. J., Matthews, K., & Weiss, S. M. (1994). *New research frontiers in behavioral medicine: Proceedings of the national conference* (NIH publication No. 94-3772). Bethesda, MD: National Institutes of Health, Health and Behavior Coordinating Committee, and the National Institute of Mental Health.

Bolduan, C. (1942). The public health of New York City: A retrospect. *Bulletin of the New York Academy of Medicine, 19*, 423.

Bomar, P., McNeeley, G., & Palmer, I. (1989). Family health nursing: History and role. In P. Bomar (Ed.), *Nurses and family and health promotion: Concepts assessment and intervention* (pp. 1-12). Baltimore: Williams & Wilkins.

Bossert, E. (1994). Factors influencing the coping of hospitalized school-age children. *Journal of Pediatric Nursing, 9*, 299-306.

Bossert, E., Holaday, B., Harkins, A., & Turner-Henson, A. (1990). Strategies of normalization used by parents of chronically ill school age children. *Journal of Child Psychiatric Nursing, 3*(2), 57-61.

Both, D. R., & Garduque, L. (Eds.). (1989). *Social policy for children and families: Creating an agenda.* Washington, DC: National Academy Press.

Botvin, G. J., & Tortu, S. (1988). Preventing adolescent substance abuse through life skills training. In R. H. Price, E. L. Cowen, R. P. Lorion, & J. Ramos-McKay (Eds.), *14 ounces of prevention: A casebook for practitioners* (pp. 98-110). Washington, DC: American Psychological Association.

Bowlby, J. (1951). *Maternal care and mental health* (Monograph Series No. 2). Geneva, Switzerland: World Health Organization.

Bowlby, J. (1953). *Child care and the growth of love.* Harmondsworth, England: Penguin.

Bowlby, J. (1960). Separation anxiety. *International Journal of Psychoanalysis, 41*, 81-113.

Bowlby, J. (1969). *Attachment and loss: Volume 1. Attachment.* New York: Basic Books.

Bowlby, J. (1982). *Attachment and loss: Volume 1. Attachment* (2nd ed.). New York: Basic Books.

Bowlby, J. (1988). *A secure base: Parent-child attachment and healthy human development.* New York: Basic Books.

Boyce, W., Jenson, E., James, S., & Peacock, J. (1983). The Family Routines Inventory. *Social Science and Medicine, 17*, 193-200.

Bradbury, D. (1962). *Five decades of action for children: Department of Health, Education, and Welfare, Children's Bureau* (pp. 1-5). Washington, DC: Government Printing Office.

Bradley, R. H., & Caldwell, B. M. (1984). 174 children: A study of the relationship between home environment and cognitive development during the first 5 years. In A. W. Gottfried (Ed.), *Home environment and early cognitive development* (pp. 2-56). New York: Academic Press.

Brailer, D. J. (1996). Clinical decision support: Managing quality in integrated delivery systems. *Quality Management in Health Care, 4*(2), 24-33.

Braithwaite, F. L., & Lythcott, N. (1989). Community empowerment as a strategy for health promotion for Black and other minority populations. *Journal of the American Medical Association, 262*, 282-283.

Brandt, P. A., & Magyary, D. L. (1993). The impact of a diabetes education program on children and mothers. *Journal of Pediatric Nursing, 8*, 31-40.

Brandt, P. A., & Weinert, C. (1981). The PRQ-A social support system. *Nursing Research, 30*, 277-280.

Bransetter, E. (1969a). The young child's response to hospitalization: Separation anxiety or lack of mothering care? *American Journal of Public Health, 59*, 92-97.

Bransetter, E. (1969b). The young child's response to hospitalization: Separation anxiety or lack of mothering care? *Communicating Nursing Research, 2*, 13-25.

Brazelton, T. B. (1984). *Neonatal Behavioral Assessment Scale* (2nd ed.). London: Spastics International.

Breitmayer, B. J., Gallo, A. M., Knafl, K. A., & Zoeller, L. H. (1992). Social competence of school-age children with chronic illnesses. *Journal of Pediatric Nursing, 7*, 181-188.

Brennan, A. (1994). Caring for children during procedures: A review of the literature. *Pediatric Nursing, 20*, 451-458.

Brent, N. (1996). Managed health care and the home health care nurse in the 1990's. *Home Health Care Nurse, 14*, 100-101.

Bretherton, I. (1995). A communication perspective on attachment relationships and internal working models. In E. Waters, B. E. Vaughn, G. Posada, & K. I. Kiyomi (Eds.), Caregiving, cultural, and cognitive perspectives on secure-base behavior and working models: New growing points of attachment theory and research. *Monographs of the Society for Research in Child Development, 60*(2-3, Serial No. 244).

Brimmer, P. F. (1978). Research and the American Nurses' Association. *Nursing Administration Quarterly, 2*(4), 43-52.

Brittain, E., & Schesselman, J. J. (1982). Optimal allocation for the comparison of proportions. *Biometrics, 38*, 1003-1009.

Brodie, B. (1982). Yesterday, today, and tomorrow's pediatric world. *Children's Health Care, 14*, 168-173.

Brodie, B. (1986). Impact of doctoral programs on nursing education. *Journal of Professional Nursing, 2*, 350-357.

Brodie, B. (1988). Voices in distant camps: The gap between nursing research and nursing practice. *Journal of Professional Nursing, 4*, 320-328.

Brodie, B. (1991). Baby's milk: A source of trust between mothers and nurses. *Public Health Nursing, 8*, 161-165.

Bronfenbrenner, U. (1979). *The ecology of human development: Experiments by nature and design.* Cambridge, MA: Harvard University Press.

Bronfenbrenner, U. (1993). Ecological systems theory. In R. H. Wozniak & K. W. Fischer (Eds.), *Development in context: Acting and thinking in specific environments* (pp. 3-44). Hillsdale, NJ: Lawrence Erlbaum.

Brook, R., & Lohr, K. (1985). Efficacy, effectiveness, variations, and quality: Boundary-crossing research. *Medical Care, 23*(Suppl.), 710-722.

Broome, M. (1995). Research-based practice in nursing education. *Capsules and Comments in Pediatric Nursing, 1*(4), 8-9.

Broome, M., & Knafl, K. (1994). Back to the future: Building on the past. *Journal of Pediatric Nursing, 9* (3), 208-210.

Broome, M., Hellier, A., Wilson, T., Dale, S., & Glenville, C. (1988). Development and testing of an instrument to measure children's fears of medical experiences. In C. Waltz & O. Strickland (Eds.), *Measurement of clinical and educational outcomes: Client-centered outcomes* (Vol. 1, pp. 201-214). New York: Springer.

Broome, M., Rehwaldt, M., & Foley, M. (1995). Utilization of cognitive-behavioral pain interventions by children and parents. In S. Funk, E. Tournquist, M. Champagne, & R. Weise (Eds.), *Key aspects of caring for the acutely ill: Technological aspects, patient education and quality of life* (pp. 146-151). New York: Springer.

Broome, M., Woodring, B., & O'Connor-Von, S. (1996). Research priorities for the nursing of children and their families: A Delphi study. *Journal of Pediatric Nursing, 11*(5), 281-287.

Broome, M. E. (1993). Integrative literature reviews in the development of concepts. In B. L. Rodgers & K. A. Knafl (Eds.), *Concept development in nursing: Foundations, techniques, and applications* (pp. 193-215). Philadelphia: W. B. Saunders.

Broome, M. E., & Endsley, R. C. (1987). Group preparation of young children for painful stimulus. *Western Journal of Nursing Research, 9,* 484-502.

Broome, M. E., & Endsley, R. C. (1989). Maternal presence, childrearing practices, and children's response to an injection. *Research in Nursing and Health, 12,* 229-235.

Broome, M. E., & Hellier, A. P. (1987). School-age children's fears of medical experiences. *Issues in Comprehensive Pediatric Nursing, 10,* 77-86.

Broome, M. E., Carlson, K., & Vessey, J. (1997). *A research utilization project using distraction to reduce pain, anxiety, and behavioral distress on children and adolescents during venipuncture or IV catheter insertion in the emergency room.* Denver, CO: Society of Pediatric Nurses.

Broome, M. E., Lillis, P. P., & Smith, M. C. (1989). Pain interventions with children: A meta-analysis or research. *Nursing Research, 38,* 154-158.

Brooten, D., & Naylor, M. (1995). Nurses' effect on changing patient outcomes. *Image: Journal of Nursing Scholarship, 27,* 95-99.

Brooten, D., Kumar, S., Brown, L., Butts, P., Finkler, S., Bakewell-Sachs, S., Gibbons, A., & Delivoria-Papadopoulos, M. (1986). A randomized clinical trial of early hospital discharge and home follow-up of very low birthweight infants. *New England Journal of Medicine, 315,* 934-939.

Brooten, D., Monroe, B. H., York, R., Cohens, N., Rancoli, M., & Hollingsworth, A. (1988). Early discharge and specialist transitional care. *Image: Journal of Nursing Scholarship, 20*(2), 64-68.

Brown, J. S., Tanner, C. A., & Padrick, K. P. (1984). Nursing's search for scientific knowledge. *Nursing Research, 33,* 26-32.

Brown, P., Rustia, J., & Schappert, P. (1991). A comparison of fathers of high-risk newborns and fathers of healthy newborns. *Journal of Pediatric Nursing, 6,* 269-273.

Brown, S. S. (Ed.). (1992). *Including children and pregnant women in health care reform.* Washington, DC: National Academy Press.

Brown, S. S. (1994). Implications for mothers and children of the health care reform movement. In H. M. Wallace, R. P. Nelson, & P. J. Sweeney (Eds.), *Maternal and child health practices* (4th ed., pp. 30-39). Oakland: Third Party Publishing Company.

Bru, G., Carmody, S., Donohue-Sword, B., & Bookbinder, M. (1993). Parental visitation in the post-anesthesia care unit: A means to lessen anxiety. *Children's Health Care, 22,* 217-226.

Brubaker, B. H. (1983). Health promotion: A linguistic analysis. *Advances in Nursing Science, 5*(1), 1-14.

Bruhn, J. G., & Parcel, G. S. (1982). Current knowledge about the health behavior of young children: A conference summary. *Health Education Quarterly, 9,* 143-165.

Bryant, G. (1985). Preventive health care for preschool children or health surveillance. *Child: Care, Health and Development, 12,* 195-206.

Budetti, P., & Feinson, C. (1993). Ensuring adequate health care benefits for children and adolescents. *The Future of Children, 3*(2), 37-59.

Burch, S. (Ed.). (1995). The making of an integrated child health care network. In *Children's hospitals today.* Alexandria, VA: National Association of Children's Hospitals and Related Institutions.

Burke, M. L., Hainsworth, M. N., Eakes, G. G., & Lindgren, C. L. (1992). Current knowledge and research on chronic sorrow: A foundation for inquiry. *Death Studies, 16,* 231-245.

Burke, S. O. (1980). The invulnerable child. *Nursing Papers, 12*(2), 48-54.

Burke, S. O. (1986a). Resilience, vulnerability, and risk in children: A conceptual model. In K. King, E. Prodrick, & B. Bauer (Eds.), *Nursing research: Science for quality care: Proceedings of the 10th National Research Conference* (pp. 349-354). Toronto, Ontario: University of Toronto Press.

Burke, S. O. (1986b). Risk and competence: A model and studies with handicapped children. *Canadian Journal of Public Health, 77,* 40-45.

Burke, S. O., Costello, E. A., & Handley-Derry, M. H. (1989). Maternal stress and repeated hospitalizations of children who are physically disabled. *Children's Health Care, 18,* 82-90.

Burke, S. O., Kauffmann, E., Costello, E. A., & Dillon, M. C. (1991). Hazardous secrets and reluctantly taking charge: Parenting a child with repeated hospitalizations. *Image: Journal of Nursing Scholarship, 23,* 39-45.

Burke, S. O., Kauffmann, E., Wiskin, N. M., & Harrison, M. B. (1995). Children with chronic illness and their parents in the community. In M. J. Stewart (Ed.), *Community nursing: Promoting Canadians' health* (pp. 284-313). Toronto: W. B. Saunders.

Burke, S. O., & Roberts, C. A. (1990). Nursing research and the care of chronically ill and disabled children. *Journal of Pediatric Nursing, 5,* 316-327.

Burke, S. O., & Wiskin, N. (1984). Invulnerable handicapped children: Clinical validation of characteristics and amenability to change. In M. Kravis & J. Laurin (Eds.), *Nursing papers (Special suppl.). Nursing research: A base for practice* (pp. 51-61). Montreal: McGill University Press.

Burkhardt, P. V. (1993). Health perceptions of mothers of children with chronic conditions. *Maternal-Child Nursing Journal, 21,* 122-129.

Burns, A. C. (1992). The expanded Health Belief Model as a basis for enlightened preventive health care practice and research. *Journal of Health Care Marketing, 12*(3), 32-45.

Burns, C. (1992). A new assessment model and tool for pediatric nurse practitioners. *Journal of Pediatric Health Care, 6,* 73-81.

Burns, C. (1993). Using a comprehensive taxonomy of diagnoses to describe the practice of pediatric nurse practitioners: Findings of a field study. *Journal of Pediatric Health Care, 7,* 115-121.

Bush, P. J., & Iannotti, R. J. (1985). The development of children's health orientations and behaviors: Lessons for substance abuse prevention. In C. L. Jones & R. J. Battjes (Eds.), *National Institute on Drug Abuse Monograph 56* (DHHS No. ADM 85-2335, pp. 45-54). Washington, DC: Government Printing Office.

Bush, P. J., & Iannotti, R. J. (1988). Origins and stability of children's health beliefs relative to medicine use. *Social Science and Medicine, 27,* 345-352.

Bush, P. J., & Iannotti. R. J. (1990). A Children's Health Belief Model. *Medical Care, 28,* 69-80.

Butcher, A. H., Frank. G. C., Harsha, D. W., Serpas, D. C., Little, S. D., Nicklas, T. A., Hunter, S. M., & Berenson, G. S. (1988). Heart Smart: A school health program meeting the 1990 objectives for the nation. *Health Education Quarterly, 5,* 17-34.

Butz, A. M., Malveaux, F., Eggleston, P., Thompson, L., Schneider, S., Weeks, K., Huss, K., Murigande, C., & Rand, C. (1994). Use of community health workers with inner-city children who have asthma. *Clinical Pediatrics, 34,* 581-590.

Caire, J. B., & Erickson, S. (1986). Reducing distress in pediatric patients undergoing cardiac catheterization. *Children's Health Care, 14,* 146-152.

Callery, P., & Smith, L. (1991). A study of role negotiation between nurses and the parents of hospitalized children. *Journal of Advanced Nursing, 16,* 772-781.

Camp, R. C., & Tweet, A. G. (1994). Benchmarking applied to health care. *Joint Commission Journal on Quality Improvement, 20*(5), 229-238.

Campbell, L. (1990). The not-so-ancient history of neonatal research. *Neonatal Network, 9*(3), 82-84.

Caplan, G. (1959). *Concepts of mental health and consultation: Their application in public health and social work.* Washington, DC: U.S. Department of Health, Education and Welfare.

Capuzzi, C. (1989). Maternal attachment to handicapped infants and the relationship to social support. *Research in Nursing and Health, 12,* 161-167.

Carabott, J. A., Javaheri, Z., Keilty, K., & Manger, G. (1992). Oral fluid intake in children following tonsillectomy and adenoidectomy. *Pediatric Nursing, 18,* 124-127.

Carey, M. E. (1976). A child's struggle for independence following kidney transplantation. *Maternal-Child Nursing Journal, 5,* 45-54.

Carey, W. B., & McDevitt, S. C. (1978). Revision of the Infant Temperament Questionnaire. *Pediatrics, 61,* 137-142.

Carnegie, M. E. (1991). Research in nursing: Then and now. *Research Notes: Indiana University School of Nursing, 2*(2), 6.

Carnegie Corporation of New York. (1994). *Starting points: Meeting the needs of our youngest children.* New York: Author.

Carnegie Corporation of New York. (1995). *Great transitions: Preparing adolescents for a new century.* New York: Author.

Carnegie Corporation of New York. (in press). *Task force on learning in the primary grades.* New York: Author.

Carrieri, V. K., Kieckhefer, G., Janson-Bjerklie, S., & Souza, J. (1991). The sensation of pulmonary dyspnea in school-age children. *Nursing Research, 40,* 81-85.

Carter, M. C., & Miles, M. S. (1983). *Parental stressor scale: Pediatric intensive care unit.* Unpublished manual, University of Kansas School of Nursing, Kansas City.

Carter, W. B. (1990). Health behavior as a rational process: Theory of Reasoned Action and multiattribute utility theory. In K. Glanz, F. M. Lewis, & B. K. Rimer (Eds.), *Health behavior and health education:*

Theory, research, and practice (pp. 63-91). San Francisco: Jossey-Bass.

Carty, R. M. (1977). Identification of behavioral responses of preschool-age children before, during, and after hospitalization in a pediatric intensive care unit (Doctoral dissertation, Catholic University of America). *Dissertation Abstracts International, 38,* 1380-1381B.

Casanova, C., & Starfield, B. (1995). Hospitalizations of children and access to primary care: A cross-national comparison. *International Journal of Health Services, 25,* 283-294.

Cassetta, R. A. (1994). Children: A community in crisis. *The American Nurse, 26*(10), 1, 20-21.

Caty, S., Ellerton, M. L., & Ritchie, J. A. (1984). Coping in hospitalized children: An analysis of published case studies. *Nursing Research, 33,* 277-282.

Caty, S., Ritchie, J. A., & Ellerton, M. L. (1989). Mothers' perceptions of coping behaviors in hospitalized preschool children. *Journal of Pediatric Nursing, 4,* 403-410.

Center for Health Economics Research. (1994). *The Nation's health care bill: Who bears the burden?* Waltham, MA: Center for Health Economics Research.

Center for the Future of Children. (1993). Health care reform: Recommendations and analysis. *The Future of Children, 4*(2), 4-22.

Center for the Future of Children. (1997). Children and poverty. *The Future of Children, 7,* 1-148.

Center for Studying Health Systems Change. (1997). *Data Bulletin, 1,* 1-2.

Chafel, J. A. (1993). Child poverty: Overview and outlook. In J. A. Chafel (Ed.), *Child poverty and public policy* (pp. 1-8). Washington, DC: Urban Institute Press.

Chafel, J. A., & Condit, K. (1993). Advocacy for children in poverty. In J. A. Chafel (Ed.), *Child poverty and public policy* (pp. 273-326). Washington, DC: Urban Institute Press.

Chamberlin, R. W. (1994). Primary prevention: The missing piece in child development legislation. In R. J. Simeonsson (Ed.), *Risk, resilience, and prevention: Promoting the well-being of children* (pp. 33-51). Baltimore: Paul H. Brookes.

Charron-Prochownik, D., Kovacs, M., Obrosky, D. S., & Ho. V. (1995). Illness characteristics and psychosocial and demographic correlates of illness severity at onset of insulin-dependent diabetes mellitus among school-age children. *Journal of Pediatric Nursing, 10,* 354-359.

Children's Defense Fund. (1994). *The state of America's children: Yearbook 1994.* Washington, DC: Author.

Childs, R. E. (1985). Maternal psychological conflicts associated with the birth of a retarded child. *Maternal-Child Nursing Journal, 5,* 39-44,

Christian, B. J. (1994). Quality of life and family relationships in families coping with their child's chronic illness. In S. G. Funk, E. M. Tornquist, M. T. Champagne, & R. A. Wiese (Eds.), *Key aspects of caring for the chronically ill: Hospital and home* (pp. 304-312). New York: Springer.

Clatworthy, S. (1978). The effect of therapeutic play on the anxiety behaviors of hospitalized children (Doctoral dissertation, Boston University, 1978). *Dissertation Abstracts International, 38,* 6142B.

Clatworthy, S. (1981). Therapeutic play: Effects on hospitalized children. *Children's Health Care, 9,* 108-113.

Clayton, S. L. (1927). Standardizing nursing techniques, its advantages and disadvantages. *American Journal of Nursing, 27,* 939-943.

Clements, D. B., Copeland, L. G., & Loftus, L. G. (1990). Critical times for families with a chronically ill child. *Pediatric Nursing, 16,* 157-161.

Clubb, R. L. (1991). Chronic sorrow: Adaptation patterns of parents with chronically ill children. *Pediatric Nursing, 17,* 461-466.

Coffman, S., Levitt, M. J., & Guacci-Franco, N. (1993). Mothers' stress and close relationships: Correlates with infant status. *Pediatric Nursing, 19,* 135-140.

Coffman, S., Levitt, M. J., & Guacci-Franco, N. (1995). Infant-mother attachment: Relationships to maternal responsiveness and infant temperament. *Journal of Pediatric Nursing, 10,* 9-18.

Cohen, D. C., Richardson, J., & LaBree, L. (1994). Parenting behaviors and the onset of smoking and alcohol use: A longitudinal study. *Pediatrics, 94,* 368-375.

Cohen, F., Nehring, W., Malm, K. C., & Harris, D. M. (1995). Family experiences when a child is HIV-positive: Report of natural and foster parents. *Pediatric Nursing, 21,* 248-254.

Cohen, M. H. (1993a). Diagnostic closure and the spread of uncertainty. *Issues in Comprehensive Pediatric Nursing, 16,* 135-146.

Cohen, M. H. (1993b). The unknown and the unknowable: Managing sustained uncertainty. *Western Journal of Nursing Research, 15,* 77-96.

Cohen, M. H. (1995a). The stages of the prediagnostic period in chronic, life-threatening childhood illness: A process analysis. *Research in Nursing and Health, 18,* 39-48.

Cohen, M. H. (1995b). The triggers of heightened parental uncertainty in chronic, life-threatening childhood illness. *Qualitative Health Research, 5,* 63-77.

Cohen, M. H., & Martinson, I. M. (1988). Chronic uncertainty: Its effects on parental appraisal of a child's health. *Journal of Pediatric Nursing, 3,* 89-96.

Cohen, S. (1964). *Progressives and urban school reform: The Public Education Association of New York City, 1895-1954.* New York: Teachers College Press.

Coie, J. D., Watt, N. F., West, S. G., Hawkins, D., Asarnow, J. R., Markman, H. J., Ramey, S. L., Shure, M. B., & Long, B. (1993). The science of prevention: A conceptual framework and some directions for a national research program. *American Psychologist, 48,* 1013-1022.

Cole, M., John-Steiner, V., Scribner, S., & Souberman, E. (Eds.). (1978). *Mind in society: The development of higher psychological processes.* Cambridge, MA: Harvard University Press.

Committee on Bioethics. (1995). Informed consent, parental permission, and assent in pediatrics. *Pediatrics, 95,* 314-317.

Cone, T. E., Jr. (1979a). *History of American pediatrics.* Boston: Little, Brown.

Cone, T. E., Jr. (1979b). Pediatrics comes of age: The twentieth century. In T. E. Cone Jr., *History of American pediatrics* (pp. 159-199). Boston: Little, Brown.

Connell, D. B., Turner, R., & Mason, E. (1985). Summary of findings of school health education evaluation: Health promotion effectiveness, implementation, and costs. *Journal of School Health, 55,* 316-321.

Conway, A. E. (1989). Young infants' feeding patterns when sick and well. *Maternal-Child Nursing Journal, 18,* 255-350.

Coontz, S. (1992). *The way we never were: America, families and the nostalgia trap.* New York: Basic Books.

Coopersmith, S. (1967). *The antecedents of self-esteem.* San Francisco: Freeman.

Copeland, L. (1993). Caring for children with chronic conditions: Model of critical times. *Holistic Nursing Practice, 8*(1), 45-55.

Copeland, L., & Clements, D. B. (1993). Parental perceptions and support strategies for caring for a child with a chronic condition. *Issues in Comprehensive Pediatric Nursing, 16,* 109-121.

Corbo-Richert, B. H. (1994). Coping behaviors of young children during a chest tube procedure in the pediatric intensive care unit. *Maternal-Child Nursing Journal, 22,* 134-146.

Corbo-Richert, B. H., Caty, S., & Barnes, C. M. (1993). Coping behaviors of children hospitalized for cardiac surgery: A secondary analysis. *Maternal-Child Nursing Journal, 21,* 27-36.

Cormier, P. P. (1979). Identification of typologies derived from child behaviors in the hospital as predictors of psychological upset. *Journal of Psychiatric Nursing and Mental Health Services, 17*(6), 28-35.

Coughlin, T. A., Ku, L., & Holohan, J. (1994). *Medicaid since 1988: Costs, coverage and the shifting alliance between the Federal government and the states.* Washington, DC: Urban Institute.

Covington, C., Cronenwett, L., & Loveland-Cherry, C. (1991). Newborn behavioral performance in colic and non-colic infants. *Nursing Research, 40,* 292-296.

Covotsos, L. (1976). *Child welfare and social progress: A history of the United States Children's Bureau, 1912-1935.* Unpublished doctoral dissertation, University of Chicago.

Cowell, J. M., Montgomery, A. C., & Talashek, M. (1992). Cardiovascular risk stability: From grade school to high school. *Journal of Pediatric Health Care, 6,* 349-354.

Cowen, E. L. (1991). In pursuit of wellness. *American Psychologist, 46,* 404-408.

Cowen, J. S., & Kelley, M. A. (1994). Errors in bias in using predictive scoring systems. *Critical Care Clinics, 10*(1), 53-72.

Cox, C. L. (1982). An interaction model of client health behavior: Theoretical prescription for nursing. *Advances in Nursing Science, 5,* 41-56.

Cox, C. L., Cowell, J., Marion, L., & Miller, E. (1990). The Health Self-Determinism Index for Children. *Research in Nursing and Health, 13,* 267-271.

Craft, M. J., Lakin, J. A., Oppliger, R. A., Clancy, G. M., & Vanderlinden, D. W. (1990). Siblings as change agents for promoting the functional status of children with cerebral palsy. *Developmental Medicine and Child Neurology, 32,* 1049-1057.

Craft, M. J., & Willadsen, J. A. (1992). Interventions related to the family. *Nursing Clinics of North America, 27,* 517-540.

Crain, W. (1980). *Theories in development.* Englewood Cliffs, NJ: Prentice Hall.

Crandall, E. (1915). Care of the sick in their homes. *Public Health Nurse Quarterly, 7*(1), 10-15.

Cranley, M. S. (1981). Development of a tool for the measurement of maternal attachment during pregnancy. *Nursing Research, 30,* 281-284.

Cravens, H. (1985). Child-saving in the age of professionalism, 1915-1930. In J. Hawes & N. R. Hiner (Eds.), *American childhood: A research guide and historical handbook* (pp. 287-312). Westport, CT: Greenwood.

Crockett, L. J., & Petersen, A. C. (1993). Adolescent development: Health risks and opportunities for health promotion. In S. G. Millstein, A. C. Petersen, & E. O. Nightingale (Eds.), *Promoting the health of adolescents: New directions for the twenty-first century* (pp. 13-37). New York: Oxford University Press.

Crooks, C. E., Lammarino, N. K., & Weinberg, A. D. (1987). The family's role in health promotion. *Health Values, 11*(2), 7-12.

Cross, T. L., Bazron, B. J., & Dennis, K. (1989). *Towards a culturally competent system of care: 1.* Washington, DC: National Institute of Mental Health: Child and Adolescent Service System Program.

Crummette, B. (1979). The maternal care of asthmatic children. *Maternal-Child Nursing Journal, 14,* 103-109.

Cunningham, P. J., & Hahn, B. A. (1994). The changing American family: Implications for children's health insurance coverage and the use of ambulatory care services. *The Future of Children, 4*(3), 24-42.

Currie, J., & Thomas, D. (1995). Does Head Start make a difference? *American Economic Review, 85,* 341-364.

Cutler, B. A., Smith, K. E., & Kilmon, C. (1995). Characteristics of fifth-grade children in relation to the type of after-school care. *Journal of Pediatric Health Care, 9,* 167-171.

Cystic Fibrosis Foundation. (1992). *CFR mortality: Patient registry 1991 annual data report.* Bethesda, MD: Author.

Czarnecki, M. T. (1996). Benchmarking: A data-oriented look at improving health care performance. *Journal of Nursing Care Quality, 10*(3), 1-6.

Dabbs, J. M., Johnson, J. E., & Leventhal, H. (1968). Palmar sweating: A quick and simple measure. *Journal of Experimental Psychology, 78,* 347-350.

D'Antonio, I. (1976). Mother's responses to the functioning and behavior of cardiac children in child-rearing situations [Monograph]. *Maternal-Child Nursing Journal, 5,* 207-261.

Damrosch, S. P., & Perry, L. A. (1989). Self-reported adjustment, chronic sorrow, and coping of parents of children with Down syndrome. *Nursing Research, 38,* 25-30.

Danek, G. D., & Noris, E. M. (1992). Pediatric IV catheters: Efficacy of saline flush. *Pediatric Nursing, 18,* 111-113.

Dashiff, C. (1993). Parents' perceptions of diabetes in adolescent daughters and its impact on the family. *Journal of Pediatric Nursing, 8,* 361-369.

Davidson, D. M., Van Camp, J., Iftner, C. A., Landry, S. M., Bradley, B. J., & Wong, N. D. (1991). Family history fails to detect the majority of children with high capillary blood total cholesterol. *Journal of School Health, 61,* 75-80.

Davies, B., & Eng, B. (1993). Survey of nursing research programs in children's hospitals. *Journal of Pediatric Nursing, 8* (3), 159-166.

Davies, L. K. (1993). Comparison of dependent-care activities for well siblings of children with cystic fibrosis and well siblings in families without children with chronic illness. *Issues in Comprehensive Pediatric Nursing, 16,* 91-98.

Davis, J. H. (1985). Children and pets: A therapeutic connection. *Pediatric Nursing, 11,* 377-379.

Davis, K. (1993). The accuracy of tympanic temperature measurement in children. *Pediatric Nursing, 19,* 267-272.

Deatrick, J., Feetham, S., Hayman, L., & Perkins, M. (1993). Development of a model to guide advanced practice in family nursing. In S. Feetham, S. Meister, J. Bell, & C. Gilliss (Eds.), *The nursing of families: Theory/research/education/practice* (pp. 147-154). Newbury Park, CA: Sage.

Deatrick, J., & Knafl, K. (1988). Developing programs for hospitalized children: Clinical significance of qualitative research. *Journal of Pediatric Nursing, 3,* 123-126.

Deatrick, J. A. (1984). It's their decision now: Perspectives of chronically disabled adolescents concerning surgery. *Issues in Comprehensive Pediatric Nursing, 7,* 17-31.

Deatrick, J. A., Angst, D. B., & Madden, M. (1994). Promoting self care with adolescents. *Capsules and Comments in Pediatric Nursing, 1*(2), 11-18.

Deatrick, J. A., Faux, S. A., & Moore, C. M. (1993). The contribution of qualitative research to the study of families' experiences with childhood illness. In S. L. Feetham, S. B. Meister, J. M. Bell, & C. L. Gilliss (Eds.), *The nursing of families* (pp. 61-69). Newbury Park, CA: Sage.

Deatrick, J. A., & Knafl, K. A. (1990). Management behaviors: Day-to-day adjustments in childhood chronic conditions. *Journal of Pediatric Nursing, 5,* 15-22.

Deatrick, J. A., Knafl, K. A., & Walsh, M. (1988). The process of parenting a child with a disability. *Journal of Advanced Nursing, 13,* 15-21.

DeMaio-Esteves, M. (1990). Mediators of daily stress and perceived health status in adolescent girls. *Nursing Research, 39,* 360-364.

Denehy, J. A. (1990). Anticipatory guidance. In M. J. Craft & J. A. Denehy (Eds.), *Nursing interventions for infants and children* (pp. 53-67). Philadelphia: W. B. Saunders.

Denyes, M. J. (1980). Development of an instrument to measure self-care agency in adolescents. *Dissertation Abstracts International, 4,* 1716-B. (University Microfilms No. 8025672)

Denyes, M. J. (1983). Nursing research related to schoolage children and adolescents. In *Annual review of nursing research* (Vol. 1, pp. 27-53). New York: Springer.

Dewis, M. E. (1989). Spinal cord injured adolescents and young adults: The meaning of body changes. *Journal of Advanced Nursing, 14,* 389-396.

DiClemente, R. J., Zorn, J., & Temoshok, L. (1986). Adolescents and AIDS: A survey of knowledge, attitudes, and beliefs about AIDS in San Francisco. *American Journal of Public Health, 76,* 1443-1445.

DilOrio, C., Parsons, M., Lehr, S., Adame, D., & Carlone, J. (1992). Measurement of safe sex behavior in adolescents and young adults. *Nursing Research, 41,* 203-208.

Dittemore, I. L. (1983). Behavioral responses in the early recovery of a severely burned 4-year-old child. *Maternal-Child Nursing Journal, 12,* 21-34.

Dixon, D. (1996). Unifying concepts in parents' experiences with health care providers. *Journal of Family Nursing, 2,* 111-132.

Dixon, P. (1995). Parent and nurse interaction during acute care pediatric hospitalization. *Capsules and Comments in Pediatric Nursing, 2*(2), 91-99.

Dixon, S., & Stein, M. (1987). *Encounters with children.* Chicago: Yearbook Medical Publishers.

Doherty, W., & McCubbin, H. (1985). Families and health care: An emerging arena of theory, research and clinical intervention. *Family Relations, 34*(1), 5-12.

Donnelly, E. (1994). Parents of children with asthma: An examination of family hardiness, family stressors, and family functioning. *Journal of Pediatric Nursing, 9*, 398-408.

Dryfoos, J. (1994). *Full service schools.* San Francisco: Jossey-Bass.

Dryfoos, J., & Klerman, L. (1988). School-based clinics: Their role in helping students meet the 1990 objective. *Health Education Quarterly, 15*(1), 71-80.

Duffy, J. (1974). *A history of public health in New York City, 1866-1966.* New York: Russell Sage.

Duffy, J. (1992). *The sanitarians.* Urbana: University of Illinois Press.

Dusenbury, L., & Botvin, G. J. (1992). Substance abuse prevention: Competence enhancement and the development of positive life options. *Journal of Addictive Diseases, 11*(3), 29-45.

Duvall, E. M. (1977). *Marriage and family development* (5th ed.). Philadelphia: Lippincott.

Eakes, G. G. (1995). Chronic sorrow: The lived experience of parents of chronically, mentally ill individuals. *Archives of Psychiatric Nursing, 2,* 74-84.

Ebmeier, C., Lough, M. A., Huth, M. M., & Autio, L. (1991). Hospitalized school-age children express ideas, feelings, and behaviors toward God. *Journal of Pediatric Nursing, 6,* 337-349.

Edwards-Beckett, J., & Cedargren, D. (1995). The sociocultural context of families with a child with myelomeningocele. *Issues in Comprehensive Pediatric Nursing, 18,* 27-42.

Egan, E., Snyder, M., & Burns, K. (1992). Intervention studies in nursing: Is the effect due to the independent variable? *Nursing Outlook, 40*(4), 187-190.

Egeland, B., Carlson, E., & Sroufe, L. A. (1993). Resilience as process. *Development and Psychopathology, 5,* 517-528.

Eland, J. M. (1981). Minimizing pain associated with prekindergarten intramuscular injections. *Issues in Comprehensive Pediatric Nursing, 5,* 361-372.

Elander, G., Hellstrom, G., & Qvarnstrom, B. (1993). Care of infants after major surgery: Observation of behavior and analgesic administration. *Pediatric Nursing, 19,* 221-226.

Elder, G. H., Eccles, J. S., Ardelt, M., & Lord, S. (1995). Inner-city parents under economic pressure: Perspectives on the strategies of parenting. *Journal of Marriage and the Family, 57,* 771-784.

Elder, J. P., McGraw, S. A., Stone, E. J., Harsha, D., Wambsgans, K., & Green, T. (1994). CATCH: Process evaluation of tobacco policies, food services, and secular trends in CATCH. *Health Education Quarterly,* Suppl. 2, S107-S127.

Elfert, H., Anderson, J. M., & Lai, M. (1991). Parents' perception of children with chronic illness: A study of immigrant Chinese families. *Journal of Pediatric Nursing, 6,* 114-120.

Elizondo, A. P. (1995). Nursing case management in the neonatal intensive care unit, Part 2: Developing critical pathways. *Neonatal Network, 14*(1), 11-19.

Elkind, D. (1985). Cognitive development and adolescent disease. *Journal of Adolescent Health Care, 6,* 84-89.

Ellerton, M., Caty, S., & Ritchie, J. A. (1985). Helping young children master intrusive procedures through play. *Children's Health Care, 13,* 167-173.

Ellerton, M.-L., Ritchie, J. A., & Caty, S. (1994). Factors influencing young children's coping behaviors during stressful healthcare encounters. *Maternal-Child Nursing Journal, 22,* 74-82.

Ellett, M., Beckstrand, J., Welch, J., Dye, J., & Games, C. (1992). Predicting the distance for gavage tube placement in children. *Pediatric Nursing, 18,* 119-121.

Ellickson, P. L., & Hays, R. D. (1991). Beliefs about resistance self-efficacy and drug prevalence: Do they really affect drug use? *International Journal of the Addictions, 25,* 1353-1378.

Ellis, J. (1995). Using benchmarking to improve practice. *Nursing Standards, 9*(35), 25-28.

Ellsworth, R. B. (1981). *Child and adolescent adjustment profile (CAAP).* Palo Alto, CA: Consulting Psychologists Press.

Ellwood, P. (1988). Shattuck lecture—outcomes management: A technology of patient experience. *New England Journal of Medicine, 318,* 1549-1556.

Epstein, L. H., Valoski, A., Wing, R. R., & McCurley, J. (1994). Ten-year outcomes of behavioral family-based treatment for childhood obesity. *Health Psychology, 13,* 373-383.

Erickson, R. S., & Moser Woo, T. (1994). Accuracy of infrared ear thermometry and traditional temperature methods in young children. *Heart and Lung, 23,* 181-195.

Erikson, E. (1963). *Childhood and society* (Rev. ed.). New York: Norton.

Escobar, G. J., Fischer, A., Li, D. K., Kremers, R., & Armstrong, M. A. (1995). Score for neonatal acute physiology: Validation in three Kaiser Permanente neonatal intensive care units. *Pediatrics, 96,* 918-922.

Ewen, E. (1985). *Immigrant women in the land of dollars: Life and culture on the lower east side.* New York: Monthly Review Press.

Faber, H., & McIntosh, R. (1966). *History of the American Pediatric Society, 1887-1965.* New York: McGraw-Hill.

Fagin, C. M. (1965). Rooming in and its effects on the behavior of young children: A comparative survey on the effects of maternal attendance during hospitalization on the post hospital behavior of young children (Doctoral dissertation, New York University, 1964). *Dissertation Abstracts International, 25,* 4657-4658.

Fagin, C. M. (1966). *The effects of maternal attendance during hospitalization on the posthospital behavior of young children.* Philadelphia: F. A. Davis.

Fagin, C. M., & Nusbaum, J. G. (1978). Parental visiting privileges in pediatric units: A survey. *Journal of Nursing Administration, 8,* 24-27.

Farrand, L. L., & Cox, C. L. (1993). Determinants of positive health behavior in middle childhood. *Nursing Research, 42,* 208-213.

Faulkner, M. S. (1996). Family responses to children with diabetes and their influence on self-care. *Journal of Pediatric Nursing, 11,* 82-93.

Faux, S. A. (1986). Parental child-rearing practices as perceived by siblings of chronically impaired children. In K. King, E. Prodrick, & B. Bauer (Eds.), *Nursing research: Science for quality care: Proceedings of the 10th National Research Conference* (pp. 308-314). Toronto, Ontario: University of Toronto Press.

Faux, S. A. (1991). Sibling relationships in families of congenitally impaired children. *Journal of Pediatric Nursing, 6,* 175-184.

Faux, S. A., & Deatrick, J. (1991, February 23). *The illness experiences of children and their families: An analysis of qualitative research.* Paper presented at the Qualitative Health Research Conference, Edmonton, Alberta.

Faux, S. A., & Knafl, K. A. (1996). Family-health care provider relationships: The new paradigm. *Journal of Family Nursing, 2,* 107-110.

Feather, N. T. (Ed.). (1982). *Expectations and actions: Expectancy-value models in psychology.* Hillsdale, NJ: Lawrence Erlbaum.

Federa, R. D., & Camp, T. L. (1994). The changing managed care market. *Journal of Ambulatory Care Management, 17,* 1-7.

Feeg, V. D. (1996). Now is the time for a kid version of Medicare [Editorial]. *Pediatric Nursing, 22,* 466, 499.

Feetham, S. (1992). Family outcomes: Conceptual and methodological issues. In Proceedings of the State of the Science Conference sponsored by the National Center for Nursing Research, *Patient outcomes research: Examining the effectiveness of nursing practice* (NIH Publication No. 93-3411, pp. 103-111). Washington, DC: Government Printing Office.

Feetham, S. (1997). Families and health in the urban environment: Implications for programs, research and policy. In H. J. Wallberg, O. Reyes, & R. P. Weissberg (Eds.), *Children and youth: Interdisciplinary perspectives* (Issues in Children's and Families' Lives, Vol. 7, pp. 321-362). Thousand Oaks, CA: Sage.

Feetham, S., Keefe, M., & Barnsteiner, J. (1987, September). *The development of nursing research activities in children's hospitals.* Paper presented at the annual meeting of the National Association of Children's Hospitals and Related Institutions, Denver, CO.

Feetham, S. L. (1984). Family research: Issues and directions for nursing. In H. H. Werley & J. J. Fitzpatrick (Eds.), *Annual review of nursing research* (Vol. 2, pp. 3-25). New York: Springer.

Feetham, S. L., & Meister, S. B. (1994). Innovations in providing maternal and child health nursing services. In H. M. Wallace, R. P. Nelson, & P. J. Sweeney (Eds.), *Maternal and child health practices* (4th ed., pp. 149-159). Oakland: Third Party Publishing Company.

Feetham, S. L., Meister, S. B., Bell, J. M., & Gilliss, C. L. (Eds.). (1993). *The nursing of families: Theory, research, education, practice.* Newbury Park, CA: Sage.

Fegley, B. J. (1988). Preparing children for radiologic procedures: Contingent versus noncontingent instruction. *Research in Nursing and Health, 11,* 3-9.

Ferguson, B. G. (1979). Preparing young children for hospitalization: A comparison of two methods. *Pediatrics, 64,* 656-664.

Ferguson, S. (1996). The use of Medicaid managed care: A case study of two states. *Journal of Pediatric Nursing, 11*(3), 65-67.

Ferketich, S. L., & Mercer, R. T. (1995a). Paternal-infant attachment of experiences and inexperienced fathers during infancy. *Nursing Research, 44,* 31-37.

Ferketich, S. L., & Mercer, R. T. (1995b). Predictors of role competence for experiences and inexperienced fathers. *Nursing Research, 44,* 89-95.

Feroli, K., & Hobson, S. (1995). Defining anemia in a preadolescent African American population. *Journal of Pediatric Health Care, 9,* 199-204.

Ferrell, B. R., Rhiner, M., Shapiro, B., & Dierkes, M. (1994). The experience of pediatric cancer pain, Part I: Impact of pain on the family. *Journal of Pediatric Nursing, 9,* 368-379.

Feshbach, S. (1956). The catharsis hypothesis and some consequences of interaction with aggressive and neutral play objects. *Journal of Personality, 24,* 449-462.

Feshbach, S. (1982). Sex differences in empathy and aggression in two age groups. *Developmental Psychology, 1,* 102-107.

Field, M. J., & Shapiro, H. T. (Eds.). (1993). *Employment and health benefits: A connection at risk.* Washington, DC: Institute of Medicine and National Academy Press.

Fine, G., & Sandstrom, K. (1988). *Knowing children: Participant observation with minors.* Newbury Park, CA: Sage.

Fink, A. (1993). *Evaluation fundamentals.* Newbury Park, CA: Sage.

Finney, J. W., & Bonner, M. J. (1992). The influence of behavioral family interventions on the health of chronically ill children. *Behavioral Change, 9,* 157-170.

Fishbein, M., & Ajzen, I. (1975). *Beliefs, attitudes, intention, and behavior: An introduction to theory and research.* Reading, MA: Addison-Wesley.

Fisher, K. W., Bullock, D. H., Rotenberg, E. J., & Raya, P. (1993). The dynamics of competence: How context contributes directly to skill. In R. H. Wozniak & K. W. Fischer (Eds.), *Development in context: Acting and thinking in specific environments* (pp. 93-117). Hillsdale, NJ: Lawrence Erlbaum.

Fisher, M. D. (1994). Identified needs of parents in a pediatric intensive care unit. *Critical Care Nurse, 14,* 82-90.

Fitzgerald, M. (1982). A 50 years' overview of paediatric nursing practice. *Australian Nurses Journal, 12,* 63-64.

Flaherty, M. (1986). Preschool children's conceptions of health and health behaviors. *Maternal-Child Nursing Journal, 15,* 205-206.

Flaskerud, J., & Nyamathi, A. (1990). Effects of an AIDS education program on the knowledge, attitudes, and practices of low-income Black and Latina women. *Journal of Community Health, 15,* 343-355.

Fleming, J. W., Holmes, S., Barton, L., & Osbahr, B. (1993). Differences in color preferences of well school-age children and those in varying stages of illness. *Maternal-Child Nursing Journal, 21,* 130-142.

Flynn, B. S., Worden, J. K., Seckler-Walker, R. H., Badger, G. J., & Geller, B. M. (1995). Cigarette smoking prevention effects of mass media and school interventions targeted to gender and age groups. *Journal of Health Education, 26*(2), 45-51.

Folkman, S., & Lazarus, R. (1985). Consistency in coping. *Journal of Health and Social Behavior, 27,* 456-459.

Foltz, A. T. (1993). Parental knowledge and practices of skin cancer prevention: A pilot study. *Journal of Pediatric Health Care, 7,* 220-225.

Ford, M. (1996, July 19). *Medicaid reform.* Washington, DC: Congressional Research Services, Library of Congress.

Forrest, C. B., Simpson, L., & Clancy, C. (1996). Child health services research: Challenges and opportunities. In U.S. Department of Health and Human Services, *Child health: Building a research agenda* (AHCPR Publication No. 97-R022). Rockville, MD: U.S. Department of Health and Human Services.

Fowler, E. J., & Anderson, G. F. (1996). Capitation adjustment for pediatric populations. *Pediatrics, 98,* 10-17.

Fox, P. D. (1990). Foreword: Overview of managed care trends. *The insider's guide to managed care.* Washington, DC: National Health Lawyers Association.

Fraley, A. M. (1986). Chronic sorrow in parents of premature children. *Children's Health Care, 15,* 114-116.

Fraley, A. M. (1990). Chronic sorrow: A parental response. *Journal of Pediatric Nursing, 5,* 268-273.

Francis, E. E., Williams, D., & Yarandi, H. (1993). Anemia as an indicator of nutrition in children enrolled in a Head Start program. *Journal of Pediatric Health Care, 7,* 156-160.

Frankel, F. (1993). Sources of family annoyance (SOFA): Development, reliability, and validity. *Journal of Pediatric Nursing, 8,* 177-184.

Freire, P. (1973). *Education for critical consciousness.* New York: Seabury.

French, J. P., & Nocera, M. (1994). Drug withdrawal symptoms in children after continuous infusions of fentanyl. *Journal of Pediatric Nursing, 9,* 107-113.

Frey, M., & Denyes, M. (1989). Health and illness self-care in adolescents with IDDM: A test of Orem's theory. *Advances in Nursing Science, 12,* 67-75.

Frey, M., & Fox, M. (1990). Assessing and teaching self-care to youths with diabetes mellitus. *Pediatric Nursing, 16,* 587-599.

Friedemann, M. L., & Andrews, M. (1990). Family support and child adjustment in single parent families. *Issues in Comprehensive Pediatric Nursing, 13,* 289-301.

Friedman, L. M., Furberg, C. D., & DeMets, D. L. (1996). *Fundamentals of clinical trials.* St. Louis: C. V. Mosby.

Frink, B. B. (1990). The relationship of clinical status/severity and ICU therapy consumption to nursing resource consumption in a pediatric intensive care unit. *Dissertation Abstracts International.* (University Microfilms No. 9101155)

Frink, B. B. (1991). Evaluation of intensive care with the use of ICUES software [Abstract]. In O. Rienhoff & D. A. B. Lindberg (Eds.), *Lecture notes in medical informatics: No. 42. Nursing informatics* (pp. 248-249). New York: Springer-Verlag.

Frink, B. B. (1998). Evaluation, quality, and outcomes. In J. Dienemann (Ed.), *Nursing administration: Managing patient care* (2nd ed., pp. 493-509). Englewood Cliffs, NJ: Prentice Hall.

Frink, B. B., Feeg, V., & Dienneman, N. (1992). *The development of nursing research activities in children's hospitals.* Unpublished manuscript.

Frink, B. B., Feetham, S. L., & Hougart, M. K. (1988). A management data base for staffing analysis. *Applied Nursing Research, 1,* 98.

Frink, B. B., & Johnson, K. (1996). Infrastructure to support guidelines based pediatric care. In *Quality improvement workshop proceedings* (pp. 1-10). Alexandria, VA: National Association of Children's Hospitals and Related Institutions.

Frink, B. B., & Strassner, L. (1996). Variance analysis. In D. Flarey & S. S. Blancett (Eds.), *Handbook of nursing case management: Health care delivery in a world of managed care* (pp. 194-223). Gaithersburg, MD: Aspen.

Fullard, W., McDevitt, S. C., & Carey, W. B. (1984). Assessing temperament in 1 to 3 year old children. *Journal of Pediatric Psychology, 9,* 205-217.

Fuller, P. W., Wenner, W. H., & Blackburn, S. (1978). Comparison between time-lapse video recordings of behavior and polygraphic state determinations in premature infants. *Psychophysiology, 15,* 594-598.

Fulton, R. A. B., & Moore, C. M. (1995). Spiritual care of the school-age child with a chronic condition. *Journal of Pediatric Nursing, 10,* 224-231.

Gagliardi, B. A. (1991a). The family's experience of living with a child with Duchenne Muscular Dystrophy. *Applied Nursing Research, 4,* 159-164.

Gagliardi, B. A. (1991b). The impact of Duchenne Muscular Dystrophy on families. *Orthopaedic Nursing, 10*(5), 41-49.

Gallagher, J. J. (1990). The family as a focus for intervention. In S. J. Meisels & J. P. Shonkoff (Eds.), *Handbook of early childhood intervention* (pp. 540-559). New York: Cambridge University Press.

Gallo, A. M. (1990). Family management style in juvenile diabetes: A case illustration. *Journal of Pediatric Nursing, 5,* 23-32.

Gallo, A. M., Breitmayer, B., Knafl, K. A., & Zoeller, L. (1991). Stigma in childhood chronic illness: A well sibling perspective. *Pediatric Nursing, 17,* 21-25.

Gallo, A. M., Breitmayer, B., Knafl, K. A., & Zoeller, L. (1992). Well siblings of children with chronic illness: Parents' reports of their psychological adjustment. *Pediatric Nursing, 18,* 23-27.

Gallo, A. M., Breitmayer, B., Knafl, K. A., & Zoeller, L. (1993). Mothers' perceptions of sibling adjustment and family life childhood chronic illness. *Journal of Pediatric Nursing, 8,* 318-324.

Ganong, L. H. (1995). Current trends and issues in family nursing research. *Journal of Family Nursing, 1,* 171-206.

Garcia, A. W., Norton-Broda, M. A., Frenn, M., Coviak, C., Pender, N. J., & Ronis, D. L. (1995). Gender and developmental differences in exercise beliefs among youth and prediction of their exercise behavior. *Journal of School Health, 65,* 213-219.

Garlinghouse, J., & Sharp, L. J. (1968). The hemophiliac child's self-concept and family stress in relation to bleeding episodes. *Nursing Research, 17,* 32-37.

Gaut, D. A., & Kieckhefer, G. M. (1988). Assessment of self-care agency in chronically ill adolescents. *Journal of Adolescent Health Care, 9,* 55-60.

Gedaly-Duff, V. (1984). Preparing the young child for a painful procedure: The dental extraction. *Dissertation Abstracts International, 45,* 513B. (University Microfilm No. 84-11065)

Geeze, M. A. (1994). Pediatric outpatient upper endoscopy: Perioperative case management. *Seminars in Perioperative Nursing, 3,* 27-39.

Gennaro, S. (1988). Postpartal anxiety and depression in mothers of preterm infants. *Nursing Research, 37,* 82-85.

Gesell, A., & Ilg, F. (1943). *Infant and child in the culture of today.* New York: Harper.

Gibbons, C. L. (1985). Deaf children's perception of internal body parts. *Maternal Child Nursing Journal, 14,* 19-27.

Gibson, C. (1986). Relationships between family-related factors, parent's appraisal of coping, parental coping behaviors, and the impact on the family of a child with cystic fibrosis. In K. King, E. Prodrick, & B. Bauer (Eds.), *Nursing research: Science for quality care: Proceedings of the 10th National Research Conference* (pp. 267-278). Toronto, Ontario: University of Toronto Press.

Gibson, C. (1988). Perspective in parental coping with a chronically ill child: The case of cystic fibrosis. *Issues in Comprehensive Pediatric Nursing, 11,* 33-41.

Gibson, C. H. (1995). The process of empowerment in mothers of chronically ill children. *Journal of Advanced Nursing, 21,* 1201-1210.

Gilhooly, J., & Hellings, P. (1992). Breast feeding problems and telephone consultation. *Journal of Pediatric Health Care, 6,* 343-340.

Gilliss, C. L., & Davis, L. L. (1992). Family nursing research: Precepts from paragons and peccadilloes. *Journal of Advanced Nursing, 17,* 28-33.

Gilliss, J. R. (1996, August 2). The study of families needs more relevant questions. *Chronicle of Higher Education,* p. A40.

Gillon, J. E. (1972). Family stresses when a child has congenital heart disease. *Maternal-Child Nursing Journal, 1,* 265-272.

Gilmer, M. J., Speck, B. J., Bradley, C., Harrell, J. S., & Belyea, M. (1996). The Youth Health Survey: Reliability and validity of an instrument for assessing cardiovascular health habits in adolescents. *Journal of School Health, 66,* 106-111.

Ginzberg, E. (1994). Improving health care for the poor: Lessons from the 1980s. *Journal of the American Medical Association, 271,* 464-467.

Ginzburg, H., & Opper, S. (1979). *Piaget's theory of intellectual development.* Englewood Cliffs, NJ: Prentice Hall.

Girouard, S. (1996). HEDIS 3.0: Another piece of the quality puzzle. *Children's Hospitals Today, 6,* 20-21.

Glenister, A. M., Castiglia, P., Kanski, G., & Haughey, B. (1990). AIDS knowledge and attitudes of primary grade teachers and students. *Journal of Pediatric Health Care, 4,* 77-85.

Goals 2000, Educate America Act of 1993: Title I, Section 102, Public Law 103-227.

Gochman, D. S., & Saucier, J. (1982). Perceived vulnerability in children and adolescents. *Health Education Quarterly, 9,* 142-155.

Godfrey, A. E. (1955). A study of nursing care designed to assist hospitalized children and their parents in their separation. *Nursing Research, 4,* 52-70.

Goldman, L. R. (1995). Case studies of environmental risks to children. *The Future of Children, 5*(2), 27-33.

Goldsmith, J. C. (1992, May/June). The reshaping of health care. *Health Care Forum Journal,* pp. 19-27.

Gonella, J. S., Hornbrook, M. D., & Louis, D. Z. (1984). Staging of diseases: A case-mix measurement. *Journal of the American Medical Association, 251,* 637-644.

Gordon, M. (1982). *Nursing diagnosis: Process and application.* New York: McGraw-Hill.

Gortmaker, S., Walker, D., Weitzman, M., & Sobol, A. (1990). Chronic conditions, socioeconomic risks, and behavioral problems in children and adolescents. *Pediatrics, 85,* 267-276.

Gortmaker, S. L. (1985). Demography of chronic childhood diseases. In N. Hobbs & J. M. Perrin (Eds.), *Issues in the care of children with chronic illness* (pp. 135-154). San Francisco: Jossey-Bass.

Gortner, S. R. (1983). The history and philosophy of nursing science and research. *Advances in Nursing Science, 5*(2), 1-8.

Gortner, S. R., & Nahm, H. (1977). An overview of nursing research in the United States. *Nursing Research, 26,* 10-33.

Gott, M., & O'Brien, M. (1990). The role of the nurse in health promotion. *Health Promotion International, 5*(2), 137-143.

Gottlieb, L. N., & Baillies, J. (1995). Firstborn's behaviors during a mother's second pregnancy. *Nursing Research, 44,* 356-362.

Gottlieb, L. N., & Mendelson, M. J. (1990). Parental support and first-born girls' adaptation to the birth of a sibling. *Journal of Applied Developmental Psychology, 11,* 29-48.

Graeter, L. J., & Mortensen, M. E. (1996). Kids are different: Developmental variability in toxicology. *Toxicology, 111*(1-3), 15-20.

Graham, J. (1996). Foundation for accountability (FAACT): A major new voice in the quality debate. In S. Vibbert (Ed.), *Medical outcomes and guidelines sourcebook: 1997.* New York: Faulkner & Gray.

Graham, M. V. (1993). Parental sensitivity to infant cues: Similarities and differences between mothers and fathers. *Journal of Pediatric Nursing, 8,* 376-384.

Gray, J. E., Richardson, D. K., McCormick, M. C., Workman-Daniels, K., & Goldmann, D. A. (1992). Neonatal therapeutic intervention scoring system: A therapy-based severity of illness index. *Pediatrics, 90,* 561-567.

Grebin, B., & Kaplan, S. C. (1996). Pediatric subacute care: An introduction. In M. W. Kelly (Ed.), *Subacute care services: The opportunities and challenges* (pp. 93-107). Chicago: Irwin.

Green, L. W., & Frankish, C. J. (1994). Theories and principles of health education applied to asthma. *Chest, 106,* 219S-230S.

Green, L. W., Kreuter, M. W., Deeds, S. G., & Partridge, K. B. (1980). *Health education planning: A diagnostic approach.* Palo Alto, CA: Mayfield.

Green, M. (Ed.). (1994). *Bright futures: Guidelines for health supervision of infants, children and adolescents.* Arlington, VA: National Center for Education in Maternal and Child Health.

Gremke, R. J., & Bonsel, G. J. (1995). Comparative assessment of pediatric intensive care: A national multicenter study. Pediatric Intensive Care Assessment of Outcome (PICASSO) [see comments]. *Critical Care Medicine, 23,* 238-245.

Grey, M., Cameron, M. E., & Thurber, F. W. (1991). Coping and adaptation in children with diabetes. *Nursing Research, 40,* 144-149.

Grey, M., Cameron, M. E., Lipman, T. H., & Thurber, F. W. (1994). Initial adaptation in children with newly diagnosed diabetes and healthy children. *Pediatric Nursing, 20,* 17-22.

Grey, M., & Flint, S. (1989). 1988 NAPNAP membership survey: Characteristics of members' practice. *Journal of Pediatric Health Care, 3,* 336-341.

Grey, M., & Thurber, F. W. (1991). Adaptation to chronic illness in childhood: Diabetes mellitus. *Journal of Pediatric Nursing, 6,* 302-309.

Grey, M. J., Genet, M., & Tamborlane, W. V. (1980). Psychosocial adjustment of latency-aged diabetics: Determinants and relationship to control. *Pediatrics, 65,* 69-73.

Grobe, S. (1990). Nursing intervention lexicon and taxonomy study: Language and classification methods. *Advanced Nursing Science, 13*(2), 22-33.

Gröer, M. W., Thomas, S. P., & Shoffner, D. (1992). Adolescent stress and coping: A longitudinal study. *Research in Nursing and Health, 15,* 209-217.

Gross, D., Conrad, B., Fogg, L., Willis, L., & Garvey, C. (1993). What does the NCATS measure? *Nursing Research, 42,* 260-265.

Gross, D., Conrad, B., Fogg, L., Willis, L., & Garvey, C. (1995). A longitudinal study of maternal depression and preschool children's mental health. *Nursing Research, 44,* 96-101.

Grossman, D. G. S. (1991). Circadian rhythms in blood pressure in school-age children of normotensive and hypertensive parents. *Nursing Research, 40,* 28-34.

Grossman, D. G. S., Jorda, M. L., & Farr, L. A. (1993). Blood pressure rhythms in early school-age children of normotensive and hypertensive parents: A replication study. *Nursing Research, 43,* 232-237.

Grossman, M., & Rowat, K. M. (1995). Parental relationships, coping strategies, received support, and well-being in adolescents of separated or divorced and married parents. *Research in Nursing and Health, 18,* 249-261.

Grotberg, E. (Ed.). (1976). *200 years of children.* Washington, DC: U.S. Department of Health and Human Services.

Grotevant, H. D. (1989). The role of theory in guiding family assessment. *Journal of Family Psychology, 3,* 104-117.

Gureno, M. A., & Reisinger, C. L. (1991). Patient controlled analgesia for the young pediatric patient. *Pediatric Nursing, 17,* 251-254.

Guyer, B., Strobino, D. M., Ventura, S. J., MacDorman, M., & Martin, J. A. (1996). Annual summary of vital statistics—1995. *Pediatrics, 88,* 1007-1019.

Haase, J. (1987). Components of courage in chronically ill adolescents: A phenomenological study. *Advances in Nursing Science, 9*(2), 64-80.

Haddock, B. J., Merrow, D. L., & Swanson, M. S. (1996). The falling grace of axillary temperatures. *Pediatric Nursing, 22,* 121-125.

Hader, D. F., & Sorensen, E. R. (1988). The effects of body position of transcutaneous oxygen tension. *Pediatric Nursing, 14,* 469-472.

Haggerty, R. J. (1995). Child Health 2,000: New pediatrics in the changing environment of children's needs in the 21st century. *Pediatrics, 96,* 804-812.

Haggerty, R. J., Roghmann, K. J., & Pless, I. B. (Eds.). (1975). *Child health and the community.* New York: John Wiley.

Hahn, E. J. (1995). Predicting Head Start parent involvement in an alcohol and other drug prevention program. *Nursing Research, 44,* 45-51.

Hahn, E. J., Simpson, M. R., & Kidd, P. (1966). Cues to parent involvement in drug prevention and school activities. *Journal of School Health, 66,* 165-170.

Hainsworth, M. A., Burke, M. L., Lindgren, E. L., & Eakes, G. G. (1994). Coping with chronic sorrow. *Issues in Mental Health Nursing, 15,* 59-64.

Hall, C. (1954). *A primer of Freudian psychology.* New York: Mentor Books.

Hall, G. S. (1905). *Adolescence: Its psychology and its relationship to physiology, anthropology, sociology, sex, crime, religion, and education.* New York: Appleton.

Hall, L. A., Gurley, D. N., Sachs, B., & Kryscio, R. J. (1991). Psychosocial predictors of maternal depressive symptoms, parenting attitudes, and child behavior in single-parent families. *Nursing Research, 40,* 214-220.

Hall, L. A., Sachs, B., Rayans, M. K., & Lutenbacher, M. (1993). Childhood physical and sexual abuse: Their relationship with depressive symptoms in adulthood. *Image: Journal of Nursing Scholarship, 25,* 317-323.

Halpern, S. (1988). *American pediatrics: Social dynamics of professionalism, 1880-1980.* Berkeley: University of California Press.

Hamburg, D. A. (1992). *Today's children: Creating a future for a generation in crisis.* New York: Random House.

Hamburg, D. A. (1995). [Epilogue]. In Carnegie Corporation of New York, *Great transitions: Preparing adolescents for a new century* (pp. 125-135). New York: Carnegie Corporation of New York.

Hampshire, S. (1959). *Thought and action.* New York: Viking.

Hanson, J. L., Johnson, B. H., Jeppson, E. S., Thomas, J., & Hall, J. H. (1994). *Hospitals: Moving forward with family-centered care.* Bethesda, MD: Institute for Family-Centered Care.

Harder, L., & Bowditch, B. (1982). Siblings of children with cystic fibrosis: Perceptions of the impact of disease. *Children's Health Care, 10,* 116-120.

Harlan, W. R., Kalberer, J. T., & Vogel, M. A. (1994). Disease prevention research at NIH: An agenda for all. *Preventive Medicine, 23,* 547-548.

Harold, N. (1988). School-based clinics. In *Health and social work* (GAO/HEHS Publication No. 94-166, pp. 303-306). Washington, DC: U.S. General Accounting Office.

Harrell, J. S., McMurray, R. G., Bangdiwala, S. J., Frauman, A. C., Gansky, S. A., & Bradley, C. B. (1995). The effects of a school-based intervention to reduce cardiovascular disease risk factors in elementary school children: The Cardiovascular Health in Children (CHIC) study. *Journal of Pediatrics, 128,* 797-805.

Harrell, J. S., McMurray, R. G., Frauman, A. G., Bangdiwala, S. I., & Levine, A. (1995, February). *Cardiovascular health in children and youth in North Carolina (CHIC): Implications for state-wide intervention.* Paper presented at the Adolescent Health Forum: Health Problems, Health Behaviors, and Behavioral Risk in North Carolina Youth, Chapel Hill.

Hart, D., & Bossert, E. (1994). Self-reported fears of hospitalized school-age children. *Journal of Pediatric Nursing, 9,* 83-90.

Harter, S. (1985). *Manual for the Self-Perception Profile for Children.* Denver, CO: University of Denver Press.

Hasselmeyer, E. G. (1961). *Behavior patterns of premature infants: A study of the relationship between a specific nursing procedure and general well-being of the prematurely born infant* (PHS Publication No. 840). Washington, DC: Government Printing Office.

Hasselmeyer, E. G., de LaPuente, J., Lundeen, E. C., & Morrison, M. (1963). A weight chart for premature infants. *Nursing Research, 12,* 222-231.

Hatton, D., Canam, C., Thorne, S., & Hughes, A. M. (1995). Parents' perceptions of caring for an infant or toddler with diabetes. *Journal of Advanced Nursing, 22,* 569-577.

Hauck, M. R. (1991). Mothers' descriptions of the toilet training process: A phenomenologic study. *Journal of Pediatric Nursing, 6,* 80-86.

Haugh, K. H., & Claxton, G. J. (1993). Guaranteed coverage with multiple insurers: Closing gaps and easing transitions. *The Future of Children, 3*(2), 123-141.

Hawkins, J., Hayes, E., & Corliss, L. (1994). School nursing in America, 1902-1994: A return to public health nursing. *Public Health Nursing, 2,* 416-425.

Hayes, V. E., & Knox, J. E. (1984). The experience of stress in parents of children hospitalized with long-term disabilities. *Journal of Advanced Nursing, 9,* 333-341.

Hayman, L. L., Meininger, J. C., Coates, P. M., & Gallagher, P. R. (1995). Nongenetic influences of obesity on risk factors for cardiovascular disease during two phases of development. *Nursing Research, 44,* 277-283.

Hayman, L. L., Meininger, J. C., Gallagher, P. R., & Whalen, K. (1994). Familial resemblance of the lipid profile [Abstract]. *Circulation, 90,* 590.

Hayman, L. L., Meininger, J. C., Stashinko, E. E., Gallagher, P. R., & Coates, P. M. (1988). Type A behavior and physiological cardiovascular risk factors in school-age twin children. *Nursing Research, 37,* 290-296.

Hayman, L. L., & Ryan, E. A. (1994). The cardiovascular health profile: Implications for health promotion and disease prevention. *Pediatric Nursing, 20,* 509-515.

Heamon, D. J. (1995). Perceived stressors and coping strategies of parents who have children with developmental disabilities: A comparison of mothers with fathers. *Journal of Pediatric Nursing, 10,* 311-320.

Hedrick, G. (1979). Mothering conjoined twins. *Maternal-Child Nursing Journal, 8,* 125-133.

Heiney, S., Goon-Johnson, K., Ettinger, R. S., & Ettinger, S. (1990). The effects of group therapy on siblings of pediatric oncology patients. *Journal of Pediatric Oncology Nursing, 7*(3), 95-100.

Heller, D. A., DeFaire, U., Pedersen, N. L., Dahlen, G., & McClearn, G. E. (1993). Genetic and environmental influences on serum lipid levels in twins. *New England Journal of Medicine, 328,* 1150-1156.

Hendricks, R., & Foster, M. S. (Eds.). (1994). *For a child's sake.* Niwot: University Press of Colorado.

Hennessey, J. A. (1974). Hospitalized toddlers, responses to mothers' tape recordings during brief separations (Doctoral dissertation, University of Pittsburgh). *Dissertation Abstracts International, 35,* 1766-1767B.

Hennessey, J. A. (1976). Hospitalized toddlers; responses to mothers' tape recordings during brief separations. *Maternal-Child Nursing Journal, 5,* 69-91.

Hess, C. A. (1994). The organization of maternal and child health services. In H. M. Wallace, R. P. Nelson, & P. J. Sweeney (Eds.), *Maternal and child health practices* (4th ed., pp. 131-148). Oakland, CA: Third Party Publishing Company.

Hester, L., & White, M. (1996). Perceptions of practicing CNSs about their future role. *Clinical Nurse Specialist: Journal of Advanced Practice Nursing, 10*(4), 190-193.

Hester, N. K. (1979). The preoperational child's reaction to immunization. *Nursing Research, 28,* 250-255.

Hester, N., Foster, R., & Kristensen, K. (1990). Measurement of pain in children: Generalizability and validity of the pain ladder and the Poker Chip Tool. In D. Tyler & E. Krane (Eds.), *Advances in pain research and therapy: Vol. 15. Pediatric pain* (pp. 79-84). New York: Raven.

Hester, N. O. (1984). The child's health self-concept scale: Its development and psychometric properties. *Advances in Nursing Science, 7,* 45-55.

Hester, N. O. (1992). Children's health research. *Communicating Nursing Research, 25,* 103-122.

Heuer, L. (1993). Parental stressors in a pediatric ICU. *Pediatric Nursing, 19,* 128-131.

Higgins, S. S., & Kayser-Jones, J. (1996). Factors influencing parent decision making about pediatric cardiac transplantation. *Journal of Pediatric Nursing, 11,* 152-160.

Hill, I. T., Bartlett, L., & Brostrom, M. B. (1993). State initiatives to cover uninsured children. *The Future of Children, 3*(2), 142-163.

Hill, P. D., & Aldag, J. C. (1996). Smoking and breast-feeding status. *Research in Nursing and Health, 19,* 125-132.

Hills, M. D., & Lindsey, E. (1994). Health promotion: A viable curriculum framework for nursing education. *Nursing Outlook, 42,* 158-162.

Hills, R. G., & Lutkenhoff, M. L. (1993). Social skills group for physically challenged school-age children. *Pediatric Nursing, 19,* 573-577.

Hinds, P. S. (1984). Inducing a definition of hope through the use of grounded theory methodology. *Journal of Advanced Nursing, 9,* 64-80.

Hinds, P. S. (1988). Adolescent hopefulness in illness and health. *Advances in Nursing Science, 10*(3), 79-88.

Hinds, P. S., & Martin, J. (1988). Hopefulness and the self-sustaining process in adolescents with cancer. *Nursing Research, 37,* 336-340.

Hirose, T., & Ueda, R. (1990). Long-term follow-up study of cerebral palsy children and coping behavior of parents. *Journal of Advanced Nursing, 15,* 762-770.

Hlusko, D. L., & Nichols, B. S. (1996). Can you depend on your patient classification system? *Journal of Nursing Administration, 26*(4), 39-44.

Hobbs, N., Perrin, J., & Ireys, H. (1985). *Chronically ill children and their families.* San Francisco: Jossey-Bass.

Hobdell, E. F., Adamo, F., Caruso, J., Dihoff, R., Neveling, E., & Roncoli, M. (1989). The effect of nursing activities on the intracranial pressure of children. *Critical Care Nurse, 9,* 75-79.

Hochbaum, G. M. (1958). *Public participation in medical screening programs: A sociopsychological study* (PHS Publication No. 572). Washington, DC: U.S. Department of Health, Education, and Welfare.

Hodges, L. C., & Parker, J. (1987). Concerns of parents with diabetic children. *Pediatric Nursing, 13,* 22-24.

Hoekelman, R. A., & Pless, B. P. (1988). Infant mortality in the United States, 1915-1988. *Pediatrics, 82,* 582-595.

Holaday, B. (1974). Achievement behavior in chronically ill children. *Nursing Research, 23,* 25-30.

Holaday, B. (1978). Parenting the chronically ill child. In P. Brandt, P. Chinn, & V. Hung (Eds.), *Current practices in pediatric nursing* (pp. 101-105). St. Louis: Mosby.

Holaday, B. (1981). Maternal response to their chronically ill infants' attachment behavior of crying. *Nursing Research, 30,* 343-348.

Holaday, B. (1982). Maternal conceptual set development: Identifying patterns of maternal response to chronically ill infant crying. *Maternal-Child Nursing Journal, 11,* 47-59.

Holaday, B. (1987). Patterns of interaction between mothers and their chronically ill infants. *Maternal-Child Nursing Journal, 16,* 29-46.

Holaday, B., & Turner-Henson, A. (1987). Chronically ill school-age children's use of time. *Pediatric Nursing, 13,* 410-414.

Holaday, B., Turner-Henson, A., Harkins, A., & Swan, J. (1993). Chronically ill children in self care: Issues for pediatric nurses. *Journal of Pediatric Health Care, 7,* 256-263.

Holaday, B., Turner-Henson, A., & Swan, J. H. (1991). Stability of schoolage children's survey responses. *Image: Journal of Nursing Scholarship, 23,* 109-114.

Holaday, B., Turner-Henson, A., & Swan, J. H. (1994). Chronically ill latchkey children. *Clinical Pediatrics, 33,* 303-306.

Hollen, P. J., & Hobbie, W. L. (1993). Risk taking and decision making of adolescent long-term survivors of cancer. *Oncology Nursing Forum, 20,* 769-776.

Holt, J. L. (1968a). Children's recall of a pre-school age hospital experience after an interval of five years (Doctoral dissertation, University of Pittsburgh, 1967). *Dissertation Abstracts International, 28,* 3352B.

Holt, J. L. (1968b). Discussion of the method and clinical implications from the study "Children's Recall of a Pre-School Age Hospital Experience After an Interval of Five Years." *Communicating Nursing Research, 1,* 56-81.

Holt, L. E. (1898). The scope and limitations of hospitals for infants. *Transactions of the American Pediatric Society, 10,* 147-160.

Holt, L. E. (1922). *The care and feeding of children: A catechism for the use of mothers and children's nurses.* New York: Appleton. (Original work published 1894)

Holt, L. E. (1933). *Diseases of infancy and childhood.* New York: Appleton. (Original work published 1897)

Holzemer, W. L., & Reilly, C. A. (1995). Variables, variability, and variations research: Implications for medical informatics. *Journal of the American Medical Informatics Association, 2,* 169-182.

Homer, C. J., Szilagyi, P., Rodewald, L., Bloom S. R., Greenspan, P., Yazdgerdi, S., Leventhal, J. M., Finkelstein, D., & Perrin, J. M. (1996). Does quality of care affect rates of hospitalization for childhood asthma? *Pediatrics, 98,* 18-23.

Horn, S. D., Sharkey, P. D., & Bertram, D. A. (1983). Measuring severity of illness: Homogeneous case-mix groups. *Medical Care, 21,* 14-30.

Horsley, J., Crane, J., Crabtree, M. K., & Wood, D. J. (Eds.). (1983). *Using research to improve nursing practice: A guide.* Orlando, FL: Grune & Stratton.

Hotaling, A. J., Zablocki, H., & Madgy, D. N. (1995). Pediatric tracheotomy discharge teaching: A comprehensive checklist format. *International Journal of Pediatric Otorhinolaryngology, 33,* 113-126.

Houtrouw, S. M., & Carlson, K. L. (1993). The relationship between maternal characteristics, maternal vulnerability beliefs, and immunization compliance. *Issues in Comprehensive Pediatric Nursing, 16,* 41-50.

Hovestadt, A. J., Anderson, W. T., Piercy, F. P., Cochran, S. W., & Fine, M. (1985). A family-of-origin scale.

Journal of Marriage and Family Therapy, 11, 287-297.

Howard, J. K. H., Bindler, R. M., Dimico, G. S., Norwood, S. L., Nottingham, J. P., Synoground, G., Trilling, J. A., Van Gemert, F. C., Kirk, M. C., Newkirk, G. R., Leaf, D. A., & Cleveland, P. D. (1991). Cardiovascular risk factors in children: A Bloomsday report. *Journal of Pediatric Nursing, 6,* 222-229.

Hudson, W. (1982). *The clinical measurement package: A field manual.* Homewood, IL: Dorsey.

Hurrelmann, K. (1990). Health promotion for adolescents: Preventive and corrective strategies against problem behavior. *Journal of Adolescence, 13,* 231-250.

Huston, A. C. (1994). Children in poverty: Designing research to affect policy. *Social Policy Report: Society for Research in Child Development, 8*(2), 1-12.

Huston, A. C., McLoyd, V. C., & Garcia Coll, C. (1994). Children and poverty: Issues in contemporary research. *Child Development, 65,* 275-282.

Hutchins, V. (1994). Maternal and Child Health Bureau: Roots. *Pediatrics, 94,* 695-699.

Huttlinger, K., Wesley, R., & Kulwicki, A. (1996). Multicultural research. In *Proceedings from the 20th Annual Midwest Nursing Research Society Conference* (p. 18). Glenview, IL: Midwest Nursing Research Society.

Hymovich, D. P. (1976). Parents of sick children: Their needs and tasks. *Pediatric Nursing, 2,* 9-13.

Hymovich, D. P. (1984). Development of the Chronicity Impact and Coping Instrument–Parent Questionnaire (CICI–PQ). *Nursing Research, 33,* 218-222.

Hymovich, D. P., & Baker, C. D. (1985). The needs, concerns and coping of parents of children with cystic fibrosis. *Family Relations, 34*(1), 91-98.

Hymovich, D. P., & Hagopian, G. A. (1992). *Chronic illness in children and adults: A psychosocial approach.* Philadelphia: W. B. Saunders.

Iezzoni, L. I. (Ed.). (1994). *Risk adjustment for measuring health care outcomes.* Ann Arbor, MI: Health Administration Press.

Iezzoni, L. I., & Greenberg, L. G. (1994). Risk adjustment and current health policy debates. In L. I. Iezzoni (Ed.), *Risk adjustment for measuring health outcomes.* Ann Arbor, MI: Health Administration Press.

Iffrig, S. M. C. (1956). Nursing observations of one hundred premature infants and their feeding programs. *Nursing Research, 5,* 71-81.

Iglehart, J. K. (1995). Rapid changes for academic medical centers. *New England Journal of Medicine, 332,* 407-411.

Igoe, J. B. (1991). Empowerment of children and youth for consumer self-care. *American Journal of Health Promotion, 6,* 55-64.

Igoe, J. B. (1992). Is health a school issue? School-based health services. In L. Aiken & C. Fagin (Eds.), *Charting nursing's future: Agenda for the 1990s* (pp. 279-286). New York: J. B. Lippincott.

Igoe, J. B. (1994). School nursing. *Nursing Clinics of North America, 29,* 443-458.

Inhelder, B., & Piaget, J. (1985). *The growth of logical thinking from childhood to adolescence.* New York: Basic Books.

Institute of Medicine. (1979). *Report on health services research.* Washington, DC: National Academy of Sciences.

Ireys, H. T., Grason, H. A., & Guyer, B. (1996). Assuring quality of care for children with special needs in managed care organizations: Roles for pediatricians. *Pediatrics, 98*(2, Pt. 1), 178-185.

Jackson, P. L., & Vessey, J. A. (1996). *Primary care of the child with a chronic condition* (2nd ed.). St. Louis: Mosby.

Jacobs, S., Chang, W. S., & Lee, B. (1987). One year's experience with the APACHE II severity of disease classification system in a general intensive care unit. *Anesthesia, 42,* 738-744.

Jacobson, D., & Melvin, D. (1995). A comparison of temperament and maternal bother in infants with and without colic. *Journal of Pediatric Nursing, 10,* 181-188.

Jaloweic, A., Murphy, S. P., & Powers, M. J. (1984). Psychometric assessment of the Jaloweic Coping Scale. *Nursing Research, 33,* 157-161.

James, S. R. (1990). Perspectives in child health care. In S. R. Mott, S. R. James, & A. M. Sperhac (Eds.), *Nursing care of children and families* (2nd ed., pp. 3-22). Redwood City, CA: Benjamin/Cummings.

Jean, S. L. (1949). The past as a springboard to the future. *Journal of School Health, 19*(1), 3-10.

Jeans, P. C., Rand, W., & Blake, F. G. (1946). *Essentials of pediatrics.* Philadelphia: J. B. Lippincott.

Jemmott, J. B., III, & Jemmott, L. S. (1994). Interventions for adolescents in community settings. In R. J. DiClemente & J. L. Peterson (Eds.), *Preventing AIDS: Theories and methods of behavioral interventions* (pp. 141-174). New York: Plenum.

Jemmott, J. B., III, Jemmott, L. S., Spears, H., Hewitt, N., & Cruz-Collins, M. (1992). Self-efficacy, hedonistic expectancies, and condom-use intentions among inner city Black adolescent women: A social-cognitive approach to AIDS risk behavior. *Journal of Adolescent Health, 13,* 512-519.

Jemmott, L. S., & Jemmott, J. B., III. (1991). Applying the Theory of Reasoned Action to AIDS risk behavior: Condom use among Black women. *Nursing Research, 40,* 228-235.

Jemmott, L. S., & Jemmott, J. B., III. (1992). Increasing condom-use intentions among sexually active Black adolescent women. *Nursing Research, 41,* 273-279.

Jerrett, M. D. (1985). Children and their pain experience. *Children's Health Care, 14,* 83-89.

Jerrett, M. D. (1994). Parents' experience of coming to know the care of a chronically ill child. *Journal of Advanced Nursing, 19,* 1050-1056.

Jerrett, M. D., & Evans, K. (1986). Children's pain vocabulary. *Journal of Advanced Nursing, 11,* 403-408.

Jessop, D. J., & Stein, R. E. K. (1989). Meeting the needs of individuals and families. In R. E. K. Stein (Ed.), *Caring for children with chronic illness: Issues and strategies* (pp. 63-74). New York: Springer.

Jessop, D. J., & Stein, R. K. (1988). Essential concepts in the care of children with chronic illness. *Pediatrician, 15,* 5-12.

Jessor, S., & Jessor, R. (1977). *Problem behavior and psychological development: A longitudinal study of youth.* New York: Cambridge University Press.

Jimmerson, K. R. (1991). Maternal, environmental, and temperamental characteristics of toddlers with and toddlers without sleep problems. *Journal of Pediatric Health Care, 5,* 71-77.

Johnson, B., Jeppson, E., & Redburn, L. (1992). *Caring for children and families: Guidelines for hospitals.* Washington, DC: Association for Care of Children's Health.

Johnson, C. C., Nicklas, T. A., Arbeit, M. L., Harsha, D., Mott, D. S., Hunter, S. M., Wattigney, W., & Berenson, G. S. (1991). Cardiovascular intervention for high risk families: The Heart Smart program. *Southern Medical Journal, 84,* 1305-1312.

Johnson, D. I. (1995). Using external data and databases: Issues and sources. *Journal of Nursing Care Quality, 10*(1), 31-39.

Johnson, J. E., & Dabbs, J. M. (1967). Enumeration of active sweat glands: A simple physiological indicator of psychological changes. *Nursing Research, 16,* 273-275.

Johnson, J. E., Kirchhoff, K. T., & Endress, M. P. (1975). Altering children's distress behavior during orthopedic cast removal. *Nursing Research, 24,* 404-410.

Johnson, J. L., Ratner, P. A., Bottorff, J. L., & Hayduk, L. A. (1993). An exploration of Pender's Health Promotion Model using LISREL. *Nursing Research, 42,* 121-138.

Johnson, W. L. (1977). Research programs of the National League for Nursing. *Nursing Research, 26,* 172-176.

Joint Commission for the Accreditation of Healthcare Organizations. (1996). *Comprehensive accreditation manual for hospitals.* Oakbrook Terrace, IL: Author.

Joint Commission for the Accreditation of Healthcare Organizations. (1997). *Nursing practice and outcomes measurement.* Oakbrook Terrace, IL: Author.

Jonas, S. (1995). *An introduction to the U.S. health care system.* New York: Springer.

Jones, D. C. (1994). Effect of parental participation on hospitalized child behavior. *Issues in Comprehensive Pediatric Nursing, 17,* 81-92.

Jones, N. E. (1992). Injury prevention: A survey of clinical practice. *Journal of Pediatric Health Care, 6,* 182-186.

Kachoyeanos, M. (1995). An evaluation of the research on tympanic thermometry for pediatric use. *Capsules and Comments in Pediatric Nursing, 2*(1), 9-15.

Kagan, B. M., Hess, J. H., Lundeen, E., Shafer, K., Parker, J. B., & Steigall, C. (1955). Feeding premature infants: A comparison of various milks. *Pediatrics, 15,* 373-381.

Kaiser Commission on the Future of Medicaid. (1995, February). *Medicaid facts.* Washington, DC: Author.

Kalisch, P., & Kalisch, B. (1978). *The advance of American nursing.* Boston: Little, Brown.

Kanner, A. D., Coyne, J. C., Schaefer, C., & Lazarus, R. (1981). Comparison of two models of stress measurement: Daily hassles and uplifts versus major life events. *Journal of Behavioral Medicine, 4,* 1-39.

Karl, D. (1995). Maternal responsiveness of socially high-risk mothers to the elicitation cues of their 7-month old infants. *Journal of Pediatric Nursing, 10,* 254-263.

Katz, V. (1971). Auditory stimulation and development behavior of the premature infant. *Nursing Research, 20,* 196-201.

Katzman, E., Holman, E., & Ashley, J. (1993). A nurse managed center's client satisfaction survey. *Nursing and Health Care, 14,* 420-425.

Kazdin, A. E., Esveldt-Dawson, K., French, N. H., & Unis, A. S. (1987). Problem-solving skills training and relationship therapy in the treatment of antisocial child behavior. *Journal of Consulting and Clinical Psychology, 55,* 76-85.

Keith, R. A., & Lipsey, M. W. (1993). The role of theory in rehabilitation assessment, treatment, and outcomes. In R. L. Glueckauf, L. B. Sechrest, G. R. Bond, & E. C. McDonel (Eds.), *Improving assessment in rehabilitation and health* (pp. 33-58). Newbury Park, CA: Sage.

Kelder, S. H., & Perry, C. L. (1993). Prevention of substance abuse. In D. S. Glenwick & L. A. Jason (Eds.), *Promoting health and mental health in children, youth, and families* (pp. 75-97). New York: Springer.

Keller, C., & Nicholls, R. (1990). Coping strategies of chronically ill adolescents and their parents. *Issues in Comprehensive Pediatric Nursing, 13,* 73-80.

Kelly, J. (1996). Clinical information management: An essential foundation for quality management in health care. *Quality Management in Health Care, 4*(2), v-vi.

Kelly, L. E. (1995). Adolescent mothers: What factors relate to level of preventive health care sought for their infants? *Journal of Pediatric Nursing, 10,* 105-113.

Keltner, B. R. (1992). Family influences on child health status. *Pediatric Nursing, 18,* 128-131.

Keniston, K., & Carnegie Council on Children. (1977). *All our children.* New York: Carnegie Corporation of New York.

Kennedy, C. M., & Riddle, I. I. (1989). The influence of the timing of preparation on the anxiety of preschool children experiencing surgery. *Maternal-Child Nursing Journal, 18,* 117-131.

Kennedy-Malone, L. (1996). Evaluation strategies for CNS's: Application of an evaluation model. *Clinical Nurse Specialist: The Journal of Advanced Practice Nursing, 10*(4), 195-198.

Kerner, J. F., Dusenbury, L., & Mandelblatt, J. S. (1993). Poverty and cultural diversity: Challenges for health promotion among the medically underserved. *Annual Review of Public Health, 14,* 355-357.

Kessel, S. S., Soto-Torre, L. E., Kogan, M. D., Koontz, A. M., Fingerhut, L. A., & Ellison, B. P. (1994). America's children: Disparities among key maternal and child health measures. In H. M. Wallace, R. P. Nelson, & P. J. Sweeney (Eds.), *Maternal and child health practices* (4th ed., pp. 48-62). Oakland, CA: Third Party Publishing Company.

Khampalikit, S. (1983). The interrelationship between the asthmatic child's dependency behavior, his perception of his illness, and his mother's perception of his illness. *Maternal-Child Nursing Journal, 12,* 221-296.

Kiburz, J. A. (1994). Perceptions and concerns of the school-age siblings of children with myelomeningocele. *Issues in Comprehensive Pediatric Nursing, 17,* 223-231.

Kieckhefer, G. M. (1987). Testing self-perception of health theory to predict health promotion and illness management behavior in children with asthma. *Journal of Pediatric Nursing, 2,* 381-391.

Kieckhefer, G. M. (1988). The meaning of health to children with asthma. *Journal of Asthma, 25,* 325-333.

Kikuchi, J. F. (1986). Assimilative and accommodative responses of mothers to their newborn infants with congenital defects [Monograph]. *Maternal-Child Nursing Journal, 9,* 141-219.

King, C. (1993). *Children's health in America: A history.* New York: Twayne.

King, E. H. (1981). Child-rearing practices: Child with chronic illness and well sibling. *Issues in Comprehensive Pediatric Nursing, 5,* 185-194.

King, I. (1981). *A theory for nursing: Systems, concepts, and process.* New York: John Wiley.

Kirschbaum, M. S., & Knafl, K. A. (1996). Major themes in parent-provider relationships: A comparison of life-threatening and chronic illness experiences. *Journal of Family Nursing, 2,* 195-216.

Kleiber, C., Halm, M., Titler, M., Montgomery, L. A., Johnson, S. L., Niholson, A., Craft, M., Buckwalter, K., & Megivern, K. (1994). Emotional responses of family members during a critical care hospitalization. *American Journal of Critical Care, 3,* 70-76.

Kleiber, C., Hanrahan, K., Fagan, C. L., & Zittergruen, M. A. (1993). Heparin vs. saline for peripheral IV locks in children. *Pediatric Nursing, 19,* 405-409.

Kleiber, C., & Montgomery, L. (1995). Information needs of the siblings of critically ill children. *Children's Health Care, 24,* 47-60.

Klerman, L. (1994). Relationship between economic status and health of women and children. In H. M. Wallace, R. P. Nelson, & P. J. Sweeney (Eds.), *Mater-*

nal and child health practices (4th ed., pp. 63-72). Oakland, CA: Third Party Publishing Company.

Klerman, L. V. (1991). *Alive and well? A research and policy review of health programs for poor young children.* New York: National Center for Children in Poverty, Columbia University School of Public Health.

Knafl, K. A. (1992). Family outcomes: Family-practitioner interface. In U.S. Department of Health and Human Services (Ed.), *Patient outcomes research: Examining the effectiveness of nursing practice* (NIH Publication No. 93-3411, pp. 97-102). Proceedings of a conference sponsored by the National Center for Nursing Research, September 1991. Rockville, MD: U.S. Department of Health and Human Services.

Knafl, K. A., Ayres, L., Gallo, A. M., Zoeller, L. H., & Breitmayer, B. J. (1995). Learning from stories: Parents' accounts of the pathway to diagnosis. *Pediatric Nursing, 21,* 411-415.

Knafl, K. A., Breitmayer, B., Gallo, A., & Zoeller, L. (1992). Parents' views of health care providers: An exploration of the components of a positive working relationship. *Children's Health Care, 21,* 90-95.

Knafl, K. A., Breitmayer, B., Gallo, A., & Zoeller, L. (1994). *Final report: How families define and manage a child's chronic illness.* Submitted to National Institute of Health for funded Grant No. NR01594.

Knafl, K. A., Breitmayer, B., Gallo, A., & Zoeller, L. (1996). Family responses to childhood chronic illness: Description of management styles. *Journal of Pediatric Nursing, 11,* 315-326.

Knafl, K. A., Cavillari, K., & Dixon, D. (1988). *Pediatric hospitalization: Family and nurse perspectives.* Glenview, IL: Scott, Foresman.

Knafl, K. A., & Deatrick, J. A. (1986). How families manage chronic conditions: An analysis of the concept of normalization. *Research in Nursing and Health, 9,* 215-222.

Knafl, K. A., & Deatrick, J. A. (1990). Family management style: Concept analysis and development. *Journal of Pediatric Nursing, 5,* 4-14.

Knafl, K. A., Deatrick, J., & Moore, C. (1996, April). *Normalization: Reanalysis and further development of the concept.* Paper presented at the 20th Annual Conference of the Midwest Nursing Research Association, Detroit, MI.

Knafl, K. A., & Dixon, D. M. (1983). The role of siblings during pediatric hospitalization. *Issues in Comprehensive Pediatric Nursing, 6,* 13-22.

Knafl, K. A., Gallo, A., Breitmayer, B., Zoeller, L., & Ayres, L. (1993). One approach to conceptualizing family response to illness. In S. Feetham, J. Bell, S. Meister, & K. Gilliss (Eds.), *The nursing of families: Theory/research/education/practice* (pp. 70-78). Newbury Park, CA: Sage.

Koizumi, S. (1992). Japanese mothers' responses to the diagnosis of childhood diabetes. *Journal of Pediatric Nursing, 7,* 154-159.

Kolbe, L. J. (1990). An epidemiological surveillance system to monitor the prevalence of youth behaviors that most affect health. *Health Education, 21,* 44-48.

Kollef, M. H., & Schuster, D. P. (1994). Predicting intensive care unit outcome with scoring systems. Underlying concepts and principles. *Critical Care Medicine, 10,* 1-18.

Koniak-Griffin, D., & Brecht, M. (1995). Linkages between sexual risk taking, substance use, and AIDS knowledge among pregnant adolescents and young mothers. *Nursing Research, 44,* 340-346.

Kornguth, M. L. (1990). School illnesses: Who's absent and why? *Pediatric Nursing, 16,* 95-99.

Kotelchuck, M. L. (1997). *Maternal and Child Health Journal:* "In the beginning . . . " *Maternal and Child Health Journal, 1,* 1-4.

Kotelchuck, M. L., & Richmond, J. B. (1987). Head Start: Evolution of a successful comprehensive child development program. *Pediatrics, 79,* 441-445.

Kovacs, M. (1980-1981). Rating scales to assess depression in school-age children. *Acta Paedopsychiatrica, 46,* 305-315.

Kovacs, M. (1985). The Children's Depression Inventory (CDI). *Psychopharmacology Bulletin, 21,* 995-998.

Kozlowski, L. J., DiMarcello, K. J., Stashinko, E. E., & Phifer, L. C. (1994). Pulse oximetry in a pediatric medical-surgical population. *Journal of Pediatric Nursing, 9,* 199-204.

Kramer, M. (1992). Barriers to the primary prevention of mental, neurological, and psychosocial disorders of children: A global perspective. In G. W. Albee, L. A. Bond, & T. V. C. Monsey (Eds.), *Improving children's lives: Global perspectives on prevention* (pp. 3-36). Newbury Park, CA: Sage.

Kramer, M., Chamorro, I., Green, D., & Knudtson, F. (1975). Extra tactile stimulation of the premature infant. *Nursing Research, 24,* 324-334.

Kristensen, K. L. (1995). The lived experience of childhood loneliness: A phenomenological study. *Issues in Comprehensive Pediatric Nursing, 18,* 125-137.

Kristjansdottir, G. (1991). A study of the needs of parents of hospitalized 2- to 6-year old children. *Issues in Comprehensive Pediatric Nursing, 14,* 49-64.

Kruger, S. (1992). Parents in crisis: Helping them cope with a seriously ill child. *Journal of Pediatric Nursing, 7,* 133-140.

Krulik, T. (1980). Successful "normalizing" tactics of parents of chronically ill children. *Journal of Advanced Nursing, 5,* 573-578.

Kueffner, M. (1975). Passage through hospitalization of severely burned, isolated school-age children. In M. Batey (Ed.), *Communicating nursing research* (Vol. 7, pp. 181-197). Boulder, CO: Western Interstate Commission on Higher Education.

Kyngas, H., & Barlow, J. (1995). Diabetes: An adolescent's perspective. *Journal of Advanced Nursing, 22,* 941-947.

L'Abate, L., & Bagarozzi, D. A. (1993). *Sourcebook of marriage and family evaluation.* New York: Brunner/Mazel.

La Greca, A. M. (1994). Editorial: Assessment in pediatric psychology: What's a researcher to do? *Journal of Pediatric Psychology, 19,* 283-290.

Ladd-Taylor, M. (1986). *Raising a baby the government way.* New Brunswick, NJ: Rutgers University Press.

Laffrey, S. C., Loveland-Cherry, C. J., & Winkler, S. J. (1986). Health behavior: Evolution of two paradigms. *Public Health Nursing, 3,* 92-100.

Lakatos, I. (1970). Falsification and the methodology of scientific research programmes. In I. Lakatos & A. Musgrave (Eds.), *Criticism and the growth of knowledge* (pp. 91-195). Cambridge, England: Cambridge University Press.

Lambert, S. A. (1984). Variables that affect the school-age child's reaction to hospitalization and surgery: A review of the literature. *Maternal-Child Nursing Journal, 13,* 1-18.

LaMontagne, L. L. (1984). Children's locus of control beliefs as predictors of preoperative coping behavior. *Nursing Research, 33,* 76-79.

LaMontagne, L. L., Hepworth, J. T., Pawlak, R., & Chiafery, M. (1992). Parental coping and activities during pediatric critical care. *American Journal of Critical Care, 1,* 76-80.

LaMontagne, L. L., Johnson, B. D., & Hepworth, J. T. (1991). Children's ratings of postoperative pain compared to ratings by nurses and physicians. *Issues in Comprehensive Pediatric Nursing, 14,* 241-247.

LaMontagne, L. L., & Pawlak, R. (1990). Stress and coping of parents of children in a pediatric intensive care unit. *Heart and Lung, 19,* 416-421.

Lamberty, G., & Barnard, K. (Eds.). (1994). *Research priorities: Fourth National Title V Maternal and Child Health Research Priorities Conference [Proceedings].* Washington, DC: Maternal and Child Health Bureau, Health, Resources, and Services Administration, Public Health Service, U.S. Department of Health and Human Services, and the National Center for Education in Maternal and Child Health.

Lang, N. M., & Marek, K. D. (1992). Outcomes that reflect clinical practice. In P. Moritz (Ed.), *Patient outcomes research: Examining effectiveness of nursing practice* (pp. 27-38). Bethesda, MD: National Center for Nursing Research.

Langley, P. A. (1991). The coming of age of family policy. *Families in Society: The Journal of Contemporary Human Services, 72,* 116-120.

Larner, M. B., Terman, D. L., & Behrman, R. E. (1997). Welfare to work: Analysis and recommendations. *The Future of Children, 7,* 4-19.

Larson, J. (1915). New York's balance sheet of infant life saving. *American City, 12,* 193-194.

Latham, H. C., & Heckel, R. N. (1972). *Pediatric nursing.* St. Louis: C. V. Mosby.

Lauer, M. E., Mulhern, R. K., Wallskog, J. M., & Camitta, B. M. (1983). A comparison study of parental adaptation following a child's death at home or in the hospital. *Pediatrics, 71,* 107.

Lauffer, D. (1992). Integrated preadmission services and case management: The foundation for achievable patient outcomes in a hospital-based ambulatory surgery setting. *Seminars in Perioperative Nursing, 1,* 136-141.

LaVigne, J., & Faier-Routman, J. (1993). Correlates of psychosocial adjustment to pediatric physical disorders: A meta-analytic review. *Developmental and Behavioral Pediatrics, 14,* 117-123.

Lavin, A. T., Shapiro, G. R., & Weill, K. S. (1992). Creating an agenda for school-based health promotion: A review of 25 selected reports. *Journal of School Health, 62,* 212-228.

Lawler, M. K. (1977). An adolescent's behavioral responses to a second renal transplant. *Maternal-Child Nursing Journal, 6,* 51-63.

Lawler, M. K., Volk, R., Viviani, N., & Mengel, M. B. (1990). Individual and family factors impacting diabetic control in the adolescent: A preliminary study. *Maternal-Child Nursing Journal, 19,* 331-345.

Lawrence, M., Arbeit, M., Johnson, C. C., & Berenson, G. S. (1991). Prevention of adult heart disease beginning in childhood: Intervention programs. In E. Saunders (Ed.), *Cardiovascular diseases in Blacks* (pp. 249-261). Philadelphia: F. A. Davis.

Lazarus, R., & Folkman, S. (1984). *Stress, appraisal, and coping.* New York: Springer.

Leahey, M., & Harper-Jacques, S. (1996). Family-nurse relationships: Core assumptions and clinical implications. *Journal of Family Nursing, 2,* 133-151.

Lederer, S. E., & Grodin, M. A. (1994). Historical overview: Pediatric experimentation. In M. A. Grodin & L. H. Glanz (Eds.), *Children as research subjects: Science, ethics, and law* (pp. 3-28). New York: Oxford University Press.

Lee, C. M., Picard, M., & Blain, M. D. (1994). A methodological and substantive review of intervention outcome studies for families undergoing divorce. *Journal of Family Psychology, 8,* 3-15.

Lee, E. J., & Bass, C. (1990). Survey of accidents in a university day care center. *Journal of Pediatric Health Care, 4,* 18-23.

Leff, P., & Walizer, E. (1992). *Building the healing partnership: Parents, professionals, and children with chronic illnesses and disabilities.* Cambridge, MA: Brookline.

Leger, R. R., & Meeropol, E. (1992). Children at risk: Latex allergy and spina bifida. *Journal of Pediatric Nursing, 7,* 371-376.

Lemeshow, S., & Le Gall, J. R. (1994). Modeling the severity of illness of ICU patients: A systems update. *Journal of the American Medical Association, 272,* 1049-1055.

Lenart, J. C., St. Clair, P. A., & Bell, M. A. (1991). Child-rearing knowledge, beliefs, and practices of Cambodian refugees. *Journal of Pediatric Health Care, 5,* 299-305.

Lenz, C., & Edwards, J. (1992). Nurse-managed primary care. *Journal of Nursing Administration, 22*(9), 57-61.

Lessick, M., & Forsman, I. (1995). Advances in genetic health care; New challenges for pediatric nursing. *Capsules and Comments in Pediatric Nursing, 1*(3), 3-12.

Lessing, D., & Tatman, M. A. (1994). Paediatric home care in the 1990s. *Archives of Disease in Childhood, 66,* 994-996.

Lewandowski, L. A. (1980). Stresses and coping styles of parents of children undergoing open-heart surgery. *Critical Care Quarterly, 3,* 75-84.

Lewin, D. J. (1996). Meta-analysis: A new standard or clinical fool's gold? *Journal of NIH Research, 8,* 30-31.

Lewis, C. E., & Lewis, M. A. (1982). Determinants of children's health-related beliefs and behavior. *Family and Community Health, 4,* 44-85.

Lewis, C. E., & Lewis, M. A. (1989). Educational outcomes and illness behaviors of participants in a child-initiated care system: A 12-year follow-up study. *Pediatrics, 84,* 845-850.

Lewis, C. E., Siegal, J. M., & Lewis, M. A. (1984). Feeling bad: Exploring sources of distress among preadolescent children. *American Journal of Public Health, 74,* 117-121.

Lewis, M. A., Hatton, C., Salas, I., Leake, B., & Chiofalo, N. (1991). Impact of the children's epilepsy program on parents. *Epilepsia, 32,* 365-374.

Lewis, M. A., & Lewis, C. E. (1990). Consequences of empowering children to care for themselves. *Pediatrician, 17,* 63-67.

Lewis, M. A., Rachelefsky, G., Lewis, C. E., Leake, C. E., Leake, B., & Richards, W. (1994). The termination of a randomized clinical trial for poor Hispanic children. *Archives of Pediatrics and Adolescent Medicine, 148,* 364-367.

Lewis, M. A., Salas, I., de la Sota, A., Chiofalo, N., & Leake, B. (1990). Randomized trial of a program to enhance the competencies of children with epilepsy. *Epilepsia, 31,* 101-109.

Lewit, E. M., & Schuurmann Baker, L. (1995). Child indicators: Health insurance coverage. *The Future of Children, 5*(3), 192-204.

Lightburn, A. (1992). Participant observation in special needs adoptive families. In J. F. Gilgun, K. Daly, & G. Handel (Eds.), *Qualitative methods in family research* (pp. 217-235). Newbury Park, CA: Sage.

Linden, L., & English, K. (1994). Adjusting the cost-quality equation: Utilizing work sampling and time study data to redesign clinical practice. *Journal of Nursing Care Quality, 8*(3), 34-42.

Lindgren, C. L., Burke, M. L., Hainsworth, M. H., & Eakes, G. (1992). Chronic sorrow: A lifespan concept. *Scholarly Inquiry for Nursing Practice: An International Journal, 6,* 27-39.

Lindley, P., & Walker, S. N. (1993). Theoretical and methodological differentiation of moderation and mediation. *Nursing Research, 42,* 276-279.

Lindsay, E. (1943). *Origins and development of the school health movement in the United States.* Unpublished doctoral dissertation, Stanford University.

Lipshitz, M., Marino, B. L., & Sanders, S. T. (1993). Chloral hydrate side effects in young children: Causes and management. *Heart and Lung, 22,* 408-414.

LoBiondo-Wood, G., Bernier-Henn, M., & Williams, L. (1992). Impact of the child's liver transplant on the family. *Pediatric Nursing, 18,* 461-466.

Lockwood, N. L. (1970). The effects of situational doll play upon the preoperative stress reactions of hospitalized children. In American Nurses' Association (Ed.), *ANA clinical sessions* (pp. 120-133). New York: Appleton-Century-Crofts.

Loehlin, J. C. (1992). *Latent variable models: An introduction to factor, path, and structural analysis* (2nd ed.). Hillsdale, NJ: Lawrence Erlbaum.

Logsdon, D. A. (1991). Conceptions of health and health behaviors of preschool children. *Journal of Pediatric Nursing, 6,* 396-406.

Lohr, K. N. (Ed.). (1990). *Medicare: A strategy for quality assurance* (Vol. 1). Washington, DC: National Academy Press.

Lorenz, F. O., & Melby, J. N. (1994). Analyzing family stress and adaptation: Methods of study. In R. D. Conger & G. H. Elder (Eds.), *Families in troubled times: Adapting to change in rural America* (pp. 21-54). New York: Aldine de Gruyter.

Losty, M., Orlofsky, I., & Wallace, H. (1950). A transport service for premature babies. *American Journal of Nursing, 50,* 10-12.

Luepker, R. V., Perry. C. L., McKinlay, S. M., Nader, P. R., Parcel, G. S., Stone, E. J., Webber, L. S., Elder, J. P., Feldman, H. A., Johnson, C. C., Kelder, S. H., & Wu, M. (1996). Outcomes of a field trial to improve children's dietary patterns and physical activity: The child and adolescent trial for cardiovascular health (CATCH). *Journal of the American Medical Association, 275,* 768-776.

Luft, H. S., & Romano, P. S. (1993). Chance, continuity, and change in hospital mortality rates: Coronary artery bypass graft patients in California hospitals, 1983 to 1989. *Journal of the American Medical Association, 270,* 331-337.

Lum, M. R., & Tinker, T. L. (1994). *A primer on health risk communication principles and practices.* Washington, DC: U.S. Department of Health and Human Services, Public Health Service, Agency for Toxic Substances and Disease Registry.

Lundeen, E. C. (1937). The premature infant at home. *American Journal of Nursing, 37,* 466-470.

Luscher, M. (1969). *Luscher color test* (I. Scott, Trans.). New York: Random House. (Original work published 1948)

Lynch, M. (1994). Preparing children for day surgery. *Children's Health Care, 23,*(2), 75-85.

Lynn, M. R. (1986). Mothers' reactions to their children's hospitalizations. *Journal of Pediatric Nursing, 1,* 274-277.

Lynn, M. R. (1989). Siblings' responses in illness situations. *Journal of Pediatric Nursing, 4,* 127-130.

Maglacas, A. M. (1988). Health for all: Nursing's role. *Nursing Outlook, 36*(2), 66-71.

Magyary, D., Brandt, P., Fleming, J., Kieckhefer, G., & Padgett, D. (1993). Nursing specialty guidelines: The implications for clinical scholarship and early intervention practice. *Journal of Pediatric Nursing, 8,* 253-260.

Mahaffy, P. R. (1965). The effects of hospitalization on children admitted for tonsillectomy and adenoidectomy. *Nursing Research, 14,* 12-19.

Mahon, N. E., & Yarcheski, A. (1992). Alternate explanations of loneliness in adolescents: A replication and extension study. *Nursing Research, 41,* 151-156.

Mahon, N. E., Yarcheski, A., & Yarcheski, T. J. (1993). Health consequences of loneliness in adolescents. *Research in Nursing and Health, 16,* 23-31.

Mahon, N. E., Yarcheski, T. J., & Yarcheski, A. (1995). Validation of the revised UCLA Loneliness Scale for adolescents. *Research in Nursing and Health, 18,* 263-270.

Main, M., Kaplan, N., & Cassidy, J. (1985). Security in infancy, childhood, and adulthood: A move to the level of representation. In J. Bretherton & E. Waters (Eds.), Growing points of attachment theory and research. *Monographs of the Society for Research in Child Development, 50*(1-2, Serial No. 209).

Maligalig, R. (1994). Parents' perceptions of stressors of ambulatory surgery. *Journal of Post-Anesthesia Nursing, 9,* 278-282.

Mansson, M. E., Fredrikzon, B., & Rosberg, B. (1992). Comparison of preparation and narcotic-sedative premedication in children undergoing surgery. *Pediatric Nursing, 18,* 337-342.

Mardiros, M. (1982). Mothers of disabled children: A study of parental stress. *Nursing Papers, 14*(3), 47-56.

Mardiros, M. (1987). *Understanding parents of children with disabilities: Developing a meaning centered approach.* Unpublished doctoral dissertation, University of Texas, Austin.

Margolis, P. A., Carey, T., Lannon, C. M., Earp, J. L., & Leininger, L. (1995). The rest of the access-to-care puzzle: Addressing structural and personal barriers to health care for socially disadvantaged children. *Archives of Pediatric and Adolescent Medicine, 149,* 541-545.

Marlow, D. (1969). *Textbook of pediatric nursing.* Philadelphia: W. B. Saunders.

Martin, K., Scheet, N., & Stegman, M. (1993). Home health clients: Characteristics, outcomes of care, and nursing interventions. *American Journal of Public Health, 83,* 1730-1734.

Martinson, E., Armstrong, G. D., Geis, D., Anglim, M. A., Gronseth, E., MacInnis, H., Kersey, J., & Nesbit, M. E. (1978). Home care for children dying of cancer. *Pediatrics, 62,* 106-113.

Martinson, I., & Yi-Hua, L. (1992). The reactions of Chinese children who have cancer. *Pediatric Nursing, 18,* 345-349.

Mason, J. O. (1991). *Healthy children 2000* (DHHS Publication No. HRSA-MCH 91-2). Washington, DC: Maternal and Child Health Bureau, U.S. Department of Health and Human Services.

Matthews, K. A., & Angulo, J. (1980). Measurement of the Type A behavior pattern in children: Assessment of children's competitiveness, impatience-anger, and aggression. *Child Development, 51,* 466-475.

Maulen-Radovan, I., Gutierrez-Castrellon, P., Zaldo-Rodriguez, R., & Martinez Natera, O. (1996). PRISM score evaluation to predict outcome in pediatric patients on admission at an emergency department. *Archives of Medical Research, 27,* 553-558.

Macbriar, B. R. (1983). Self-concept of preadolescent and adolescent children with a meningomyelocele. *Issues in Comprehensive Pediatric Nursing, 6,* 1-11.

McBride, A. B. (1994). Managing chronicity: The heart of nursing care. In S. G., Funk, E. M. Tornquist, M. T. Champagne, & R. A. Wiese (Eds.), *Key aspects of caring for the chronically ill: Hospital and home* (pp. 8-20). New York: Springer.

McCaffery, M. (1971). Children's responses to rectal temperatures: An exploratory study. *Nursing Research, 20,* 32-45.

McCain, G. C. (1982). Parent created recordings for hospitalized children. *Children's Health Care, 10,* 104-105.

McCarthy, S. M., & Gallo, A. (1992). A case illustration of family management style. *Journal of Pediatric Nursing, 7,* 395-402.

McCloskey, J. C., & Bulechek, G. M. (1994). Standardizing the language for nursing treatments: An overview of the issues. *Nursing Outlook, 42*(2), 56-64.

McCloskey, J. C., & Bulechek, G. M. (1996). *Nursing intervention classification (NIC)* (2nd ed.). St. Louis: C. V. Mosby.

McClowry, S. G. (1988). A review of the literature pertaining to the psychosocial responses of school-age children to hospitalization. *Journal of Pediatric Nursing, 3,* 296-311.

McClowry, S. G. (1990). The relationship of temperament to pre- and post-hospitalization behavioral responses of school-age children. *Nursing Research, 39,* 30-35.

McCorkle, R., Benoliel, J., Donalson, G., Georgiadon, F., Moinpour, C., & Godell, B. (1989). A randomized clinical trial of home nursing care for lung cancer patients. *Cancer, 64,* 1375-1382.

McCoy-Thompson, M., Vanneman, J., & Bloom, F. (1994). *The Healthy Start initiative: A community-driven approach to infant mortality reduction—Vol. II. Early implementation: Lessons learned.* Arlington, VA: National Center for Education in Maternal and Child Health.

McCubbin, H., Thompson, A., & McCubbin, M. (1996). *Family assessment: Resiliency, coping, and adaptation.* Madison: University of Wisconsin Press.

McCubbin, H. I., Comeau, J. K., & Harkins, J. A. (1991a). Family Inventory of Resources for Management (FIRM). In H. I. McCubbin & A. I. Thompson (Eds.), *Family assessment inventories for research and practice* (pp. 163-165). Madison, WI: Family Stress Coping and Health Project.

McCubbin, H. I., McCubbin, M. A., Nevin, R. S., & Cauble, E. (1991b). Coping Health Inventory for Parents (CHIP). In H. I. McCubbin & A. I. Thompson (Eds.), *Family assessment inventories for research and practice* (pp. 198-199). Madison, WI: Family Stress Coping and Health Project.

McCubbin, H. I., & Patterson, J. M. (1991). Family inventory of life events and changes. In H. I. McCubbin & A. I. Thompson (Eds.), *Family assessment inventories for research and practice* (pp. 79-98). Madison, WI: Family Stress Coping and Health Project.

McCubbin, H. I., Patterson, J. M., Beuman, E., & Harris, L. H. (1991d). Adolescent–Family Inventory of Life Events and Changes (AFILE). In H. I. McCubbin & A. I. Thompson (Eds.), *Family assessment inventories for research and practice* (pp. 109-110). Madison, WI: Family Stress Coping and Health Project.

McCubbin, H. I., Patterson, J. M., & Wilson, L. R. (1991e). Family Inventory of Life Events and Changes (FILE). In H. I. McCubbin & A. I. Thompson (Eds.), *Family assessment inventories for research and practice* (pp. 97-98). Madison, WI: Family Stress Coping and Health Project.

McCubbin, H. I., & Thompson, A. I. (1987). *Family assessment inventories for research and practice.* Madison: University of Wisconsin Press.

McCubbin, M. A. (1984). Nursing assessment of parental coping with cystic fibrosis. *Western Journal of Nursing Research, 6,* 407-418.

McCubbin, M. A. (1988). Family stress, resources, and family types: Chronic illness in children. *Family Relations, 37,* 203-210.

McCubbin, M. A. (1989). Family stress and family strengths: A comparison of single and two-parent families with handicapped children. *Research in Nursing and Health, 12,* 101-112.

McCubbin, M. A., & Huang, S. T. T. (1989). Family strengths in the care of handicapped children: Targets for intervention. *Family Relations, 38,* 436-443.

McCubbin, M. A., & McCubbin, H. I. (1993). Family coping with illness: The Resiliency Model of Family Stress, Adjustment, and Adaptation. In C. B. Danielson, L. Hamel-Bissell, & P. Winstead-Fry (Eds.), *Families, health, and illness: Perspectives on coping and intervention* (pp. 21-63). St. Louis: C. V. Mosby.

McCubbin, M. A., McCubbin, H. I., & Thompson, A. I. (1991c). Family Hardiness Index. In H. I. McCubbin & A. I. Thompson (Eds.), *Family assessment inventories for research and practice* (p. 133). Madison, WI: Family Stress Coping and Health Project.

MacDonald, H. (1995). Chronic renal disease: The mother's experience. *Pediatric Nursing, 21,* 503-507, 574.

MacDonald, H. (1996). "Mastering uncertainty": Mothering the child with asthma. *Pediatric Nursing, 22,* 56-59.

McGillicuddy, M. C. (1976). A study of the relationship between mothers' rooming-in during their children's hospitalization and changes in selected areas of children's behavior (Doctoral dissertation, New York University). *Dissertation Abstracts International, 37,* 700B.

McGinnis, J. M. (1992). The role of the federal government in promoting health through the schools: Report from the Office of Disease Prevention and Health Promotion. *Journal of School Health, 62*(4), 131-134.

McGinnis, J. M., Richmond, J. B., Brandt, E. N., Windom, R. E., & Mason, J. O. (1992). Health progress in the United States: Results of the 1990 objectives for the nation. *Journal of the American Medical Association, 268,* 2545-2552.

McGlynn, E. A., Halfon, N., & Leibowitz, A. (1995). Assessing the quality of care for children: Prospects under health reform. *Archives of Pediatric Adolescent Medicine, 149,* 359-368.

McGrath, P. A. (1990). *Pain in children.* New York: Guilford.

McKay, L., & Diem, E. (1995). Health concerns of adolescent girls. *Journal of Pediatric Nursing, 10,* 19-27.

McKeever, P. T. (1981). Fathering the chronically ill child. *MCN: American Journal of Maternal-Child Nursing, 6,* 124-128.

McKeon, T. (1996). Benchmarks and performance indicators: Two tools for evaluating organizational results and continuous quality improvement efforts. *Journal of Nursing Care Quality, 10*(3), 12-17.

McKinlay, J. B. (1993). The promotion of health through planned sociopolitical change: Challenges for research and policy. *Social Science in Medicine, 36,* 109-117.

McLaughlin, J. S. (1982). Toward a theoretical model for community health programs. *Advances in Nursing Science, 5*(1), 7-28.

McLeroy, K. R., Gottlieb, N. H., & Burdine, J. N. (1987). The business of health promotion: Ethics issues and professional responsibilities. *Health Education Quarterly, 14*(1), 91-109.

McManus, M., Fox, H., Newacheck, P., & Wicks, L. (1992, September). *A review of national health care reform proposals from a maternal and child health framework.* Washington, DC: Association of Maternal and Child Health Programs.

McMullen, A., Fioravanti, I. D., Pollack, V., Rideout, K., & Sciera, M. (1993). Heparinized saline or normal saline. *MCN: American Journal of Maternal Child Nursing, 18,* 78-85.

Means, R. (1962). *A history of health education in the United States.* Philadelphia: Lea & Febiger.

Measel, C. P., & Anderson, G. C. (1979). Nonnutritive sucking during tube feedings: Effect on clinical course in premature infants. *Journal of Obstetric, Gynecologic, and Neonatal Nursing, 8*(5), 265-272.

Meckel, R. (1990). *Save the babies.* Baltimore: Johns Hopkins University Press.

Medoff-Cooper, B. (1986). Temperament in very low birthweight infants. *Nursing Research, 35,* 139-143.

Meier, P. (1978). A crisis group for parents of high-risk infants. *Maternal-Child Nursing Journal, 7,* 21-30.

Meier, P. (1988). Bottle and breastfeeding: Effects on transcutaneous pressure and temperature in preterm infants. *Nursing Research, 37,* 36-41.

Meier, P., & Pugh, E. (1985). Breastfeeding behavior of small preterm infants. *Maternal-Child Nursing Journal, 10,* 396-401.

Meininger, J. C., Hayman, L. L., Coates, P. M., & Gallagher, P. R. (1988). Genetics or environment? Type A behavior and other cardiovascular risk factors in twin children. *Nursing Research, 37,* 341-346.

Meininger, J. C., Hayman, L. L., Coates, P. M., & Gallagher, P. R. (in press). Genetic and environmental influences on cardiovascular disease risk factors in adolescents. *Nursing Research.*

Meininger, J. C., Stashinko, E. E., & Hayman, L. L. (1991). Type A behavior in children: Psychometric properties of the Matthews Youth Test for Health. *Nursing Research, 40,* 221-227.

Meister, S. B. (1989). Health care financing, policy, and family nursing practice: New opportunities. In C. B. Gilliss, B. L. Highley, B. M. Roberts, & I. M. Martinson (Eds.), *Toward a science of family nursing* (pp. 146-155). Reading, MA: Addison-Wesley.

Meister, S. B. (1992). Knowledge, decisions, and the timing of policy development: Creating a strategic framework for science policy. In P. Moritz (Ed.), *Patient outcomes research: Examining effectiveness of nursing practice* (pp. 159-173). Bethesda, MD: National Center for Nursing Research.

Meister, S. B. (1997). *Policy for children's health: Scholarship, practice and principles.* Cambridge, MA: Harvard University Press.

Meister, S. B., Feetham, S. L., Durand, B. A., & Girouard, S. (1991). Creating and extending successful innovations: Practice and policy implications. In E. Groetsman (Ed.), *Differentiating nursing practice into the twenty-first century* (pp. 315-328). Kansas City, MO: American Academy of Nursing.

Melamed, B. C., & Siegel, L. J. (1975). Reduction of anxiety in children facing hospitalization and surgery by use of filmed modeling. *Journal of Clinical Psychology, 43,* 511-521.

Meleis, A. I. (1990). Being and becoming healthy: The core of nursing knowledge. *Nursing Science Quarterly, 3*(3), 107-113.

Melnyk, B. M. (1994). Coping with unplanned childhood hospitalization: Effects of informational interventions on mothers and children. *Nursing Research, 43,* 50-55.

Melvin, P. M. (1983). Milk to motherhood: The New York milk committee and the beginning of well-child programs. *Mid-American, 65*(3), 111-134.

Mendez, L., Yeaworth, R., York, J., & Goodwin, T. (1980). Factors influencing adolescents' perceptions of life change events. *Nursing Research, 29,* 384-388.

Meng, A., & Zastowny, T. (1982). Preparation for hospitalization: A stress inoculation training program for parents and children. *Maternal-Child Nursing Journal, 11,* 87-94.

Menke, E. M. (1987). The impact of a child's chronic illness on school-age children. *Children's Health Care, 15,* 132-140.

Mercer, R. T. (1974). Mothers' responses to their infants with defects. *Nursing Research, 23,* 133-137.

Mercer, R. T. (1981). A theoretical framework for studying factors that impact on the maternal role. *Nursing Research, 30,* 73-77.

Mercer, R. T., & Ferketich, S. L. (1988). Stress and social support as predictors of anxiety and depression during pregnancy. *Advances in Nursing Science, 10*(2), 26-39.

Mercer, R. T., & Ferketich, S. L. (1995). Experienced and inexperienced mothers' maternal competence during infancy. *Research in Nursing and Health, 18,* 333-343.

Mickalide, A. (1986). Children's understanding of health and illness: Implications for health promotion. *Health Values, 10*(3), 5-21.

Midence, K. (1994). The effects of chronic illness on children and their families: An overview. *Genetic, Social, and General Psychology Monographs, 120,* 311-326.

Miles, M., & D'Auria, J. (1994). Parenting the medically fragile infant. *Capsules and Comments in Pediatric Nursing, 1*(1), 2-7.

Miles, M., & Harrell, J. (1991). *Exploratory center for the study of health behaviors in vulnerable youth.* Grant Narrative No. P20 NR HD MH 0300.

Miles, M. S., & Carter, M. C. (1982). Sources of parental stress in pediatric intensive care units. *Children's Health Care, 11,* 65-69.

Miles, M. S., Carter, M. C., Hennessey, J., Eberly, T. W., & Riddle, I. (1989a). Testing a theoretical model: Correlates of parental stress responses in the pediatric intensive care unit. *Maternal-Child Nursing Journal,* *18,* 207-219.

Miles, M. S., Carter, M. C., Hennessey, J., Riddle, I., & Eberly, T. W. (1989b). Effects of the intensive care unit environment on parents of cardiac surgery children. *Maternal-Child Nursing Journal, 18,* 235-239.

Miles, M. S., Carter, M. C., Riddle, I., Hennessey, J., & Eberly, T. W. (1989c). The pediatric intensive care unit environment as a source of stress for parents. *Maternal-Child Nursing Journal, 18,* 199-206.

Miles, T. (1985, May 1). A suitable case for treatment. *Nursing Times, 81,* 48-50.

Milio, N. (1970). *9226 Kerscheval.* Ann Arbor: University of Michigan Press.

Milio, N. (1984). Nursing research and the study of health policy. In H. H. Werley & J. Fitzpatrick (Eds.), *Annual review of nursing research* (Vol. 2, pp. 3-25). New York: Springer-Verlag.

Milio, N. (1986). *Promoting health through public policy.* Ottawa: Canadian Public Health Association.

Milio, N. (1988). *Primary care and the public's health.* Ottawa: Canadian Public Health Association.

Miller, B. A., Galanter, E., & Pridham, K. H. (1960). *Plans and the structure of behavior.* New York: Holt, Rinehart & Winston.

Miller, B. C. (1986). *Family research methods.* Beverly Hills, CA: Sage.

Millstein, S. G. (1989). Challenge for the behavioral scientists. *American Psychologist, 44,* 837-842.

Millstein, S. G., Petersen, A. C., & Nightingale, E. O. (1993). Adolescent health promotion: Rationale, goals, and objectives. In S. G. Millstein, A. C. Petersen, & E. O. Nightingale (Eds.), *Promoting the health of adolescents: New directions for the twenty-first century* (pp. 3-9). New York: Oxford University Press.

Mitchell, P. H., Heinrich, J., Moritz, P., & Hinshaw, A. S. (Eds.). (in press). Outcome measures and care delivery systems. *Medical Care,* Supplment.

Mobley, C. E., Harless, L. S., & Miller, K. L. (1996). Self-perceptions of preschool children with spina bifida. *Journal of Pediatric Nursing, 11,* 217-224.

Monahan, G. H., & Schkade, J. K. (1985). Comparing care by parents and traditional nursing units. *Pediatric Nursing, 11,* 463-468.

Monsen, R. B. (1992). Autonomy, coping, and self-care agency in healthy adolescents and adolescents with spina bifida. *Journal of Pediatric Nursing, 7,* 9-13.

Moon, M. (1993). Who bears the burden? The distribution of costs and benefits. *The Future of Children,* *3*(2), 164-183.

Moon, M., Ginsburg, P. B., & Young, D. A. (1993). Paying for children's medical care: Is the Medicare experience helpful? *The Future of Children, 3*(2), 77-91.

Moore, J. B. (1995). Measuring the self-care practice of children and adolescents: Instrument development. *Maternal-Child Nursing Journal, 23,* 101-108.

Moore, J. B., & Gaffney, K. F. (1989). Development of an instrument to measure mothers' performance of self-care activities for children. *Advances in Nursing Science, 12,* 76-84.

Moos, R., & Moos, B. (1986). *Family Environment Scale manual.* Palo Alto, CA: Consulting Psychologist Press.

Moos, R. H. (1980). Social-ecological perspectives on health. In G. C. Stone, F. Cohen, & N. E. Adler (Eds.), *Health psychology: A handbook* (pp. 523-547). San Francisco: Jossey-Bass.

Moritz, P., Frink, B. B., & Laughlin, J. (1994). *The nursing systems branch* [Systems report]. Bethesda, MD: National Institute of Nursing Research.

Morris, N. M., Hatch, M. H., & Chipman, S. S. (1966). Deterrents to well-child supervision. *American Journal of Public Health, 56,* 1232-1238.

Morris, N. M., & Udry, J. R. (1980). Validation of a self-administered instrument to assess stage of adolescent development. *Journal of Youth and Adolescence, 9,* 271-280.

Morrow, J. D. (1995). Temperament of the infant with myelomeningocele. *Journal of Pediatric Nursing, 10,* 99-104.

Morton, L. I. (1987). *A medical bibliography.* Aldershot, England: Grover.

Mulligan, J. E. (1976). *Three federal interventions on behalf of childbearing women: The Sheppard-Towner Act, Emergency Maternity and Infant Care, and the Maternal and Child Health and Mental Retardation Planning Amendments of 1963.* Unpublished doctoral dissertation, University of Michigan, Ann Arbor.

Mullins, J. (1987). Authentic voices from parents of exceptional children. *Family Relations, 36,* 30-33.

Munet-Vilaro, F., & Vessey, J. A. (1990). Children's explanation of leukemia: A Hispanic perspective. *Journal of Pediatric Nursing, 5,* 274-282.

Munet-Vilaro, F., & Egan, M. (1990). Reliability issues of the Family Environment Scale for cross-cultural research. *Nursing Research, 39,* 244-247.

Murata, J. E., Mace, J. P., Strehlow, A., & Shuler, P. (1992). Disease patterns in homeless children: A comparison with national data. *Journal of Pediatric Nursing, 7,* 196-204.

Murphy, K. M. (1989). *Threatened perinatal loss: Defining and managing strategies used by parents of critically ill infants.* Unpublished doctoral dissertation, University of Illinois, Chicago.

Murphy, K. M. (1990). Interactional styles of parents following the birth of a high risk infant. *Journal of Pediatric Nursing, 5,* 33-41.

Nader, P. R., Sallis, J. F., Patterson, T. L., Abramson, I. S., Rupp, J. W., Senn, K. L., Atkins, C. J., Roppe, B. E., Morris, J. A., Wallace, J. P., & Vega, W. A. (1989). A family approach to cardiovascular risk reduction: Results from the San Diego family health project. *Health Education Quarterly, 16,* 229-244.

Namboodiri, K. K., Kaplan, E. B., Heuch, I., Elston, R. C., Green, P., Rao, D. C., Laskarzewski, P., Glueck, C. J., & Rifkind, B. M. (1985). The collaborative Lipid Research Clinics Family Study: Biological and cultural determinants of familial resemblance for plasma lipids and lipoproteins. *Genetic Epidemiology, 2,* 227-254.

Napier, L. (1927). Caring for premature and underweight babies. *American Journal of Nursing, 27,* 1035-1037.

Natapoff, J. N. (1978). Children's views of health: A developmental study. *American Journal of Public Health, 68,* 995-1000.

Natapoff, J. N. (1990a). Introduction. In J. N. Natapoff & R. R. Wieczorek (Eds.), *Maternal-child health policy: A nursing perspective* (pp. 1-16). New York: Springer.

Natapoff, J. N. (1990b). Conclusions and recommendations: A policy agenda. In J. N. Natapoff & R. R. Wieczorek (Eds.), *Maternal-child health policy: A nursing perspective* (pp. 323-329). New York: Springer.

National Association of Children's Hospitals and Related Institutions. (1978). *Study to quantify the uniqueness of children's hospitals: Summary of major findings.* Alexandria, VA: Author.

National Association of Children's Hospitals and Related Institutions. (1996a). *Patient care FOCUS groups 1996: Executive summary.* Alexandria, VA: Author.

National Association of Children's Hospitals and Related Institutions. (1996b). *Pediatric excellence in health delivery systems.* Alexandria, VA: Author.

National Association of Children's Hospitals and Related Institutions. (1996c). *Points of FOCUS* [quarterly overview for participating hospitals]. Alexandria, VA: Author.

National Association of Children's Hospitals and Related Institutions. (1996d). *Managing clinical resources: "Out-of-the-box" collaborative solutions.* Alexandria, VA: Author.

National Association of Children's Hospitals and Related Institutions. (1997). *Overview of HEDIS 3.0.* Alexandria, VA: Author.

National Campaign to Prevent Teen Pregnancy. (1997). *Whatever happened to childhood: The problem of teen pregnancy in the United States.* Washington, DC: Author.

National Institute of Nursing Research. (1992). *Patient outcomes research: Examining the effectiveness of nursing practice* (NIH Publication No. 93-3411). Proceedings of the State of Science Conference, National Center for Nursing Research.

National Institute of Nursing Research. (1993). *Health promotion for older children and adolescents* (NIH Publication No. 93-2420). Bethesda, MD: National Institutes of Health & U.S. Department of Health and Human Services.

Naylor, M., Brooten, D., Jones, R., Lavizzo-Mourey, R., Mezey, M., & Pauly, M. (1994). Comprehensive dis-charge planning for hospitalized elderly: A randomized clinical trial. *Annals of Internal Medicine, 120,* 999-1006.

Neal, M. (1968). Vestibular stimulation and developmental behavior of the small premature infant. *Nursing Research, 17,* 568-569.

Neal, M., & Nauen, C. M. (1968). Ability of premature infant to maintain his own body temperature. *Nursing Research, 17,* 396-402.

Neff, E. J., & Beardslee, C. I. (1990). Body knowledge and concerns of children with cancer as compared with the knowledge and concerns of other children. *Journal of Pediatric Nursing, 5,* 179-189.

Nelms, B. C. (1989). Emotional behaviors in chronically ill children. *Journal of Abnormal Child Psychology, 17,* 657-668.

Newacheck, P., & Taylor, W. (1992). Childhood chronic illness: Prevalence, severity, and impact. *American Journal of Public Health, 82,* 364-371.

Newell, M. (1995). *Using nursing case management to improve health outcome: Recasting theory, tools and care delivery.* Gaithersburg, MD: Aspen.

Newhouse, J. P., Sloss, E. M., Manning, W. G., & Keeler, E. B. (1993). Risk adjustment for a children's capitation rate. *Health Care Financing Review, 15*(1), 39-54.

Newson, G., & Harvey, B. (1994). Assuring access to health care. In H. M. Wallace, R. P. Nelson, & P. J. Sweeney (Eds.), *Maternal and child health practices* (4th ed., pp. 11-17). Oakland, CA: Third Party Publishing Company.

Nightingale, F. (1858). *Notes on matters affecting the health, efficiency, in hospital administration of the British Army.* London: Harrison & Sons.

Nightingale, F. (1859). *Notes on hospitals.* London: Longman.

Nightingale, F. (1969). *Notes on nursing: What it is, and what it is not.* New York: Dover. (Original work published 1860)

Nolan, M., Keady, J., & Grant, G. (1995). Developing a typology of family care: Implications for nurses and other service providers. *Journal of Advanced Nursing, 21,* 256-265.

Norwood, S. L. (1996). The Social Support APGAR: Instrument development and testing. *Research in Nursing and Health, 19,* 143-152.

Nowacek, G. A., O'Malley, P. M., Anderson, R. A., & Richards, F. E. (1990). Testing a model of diabetes self-care management: A causal model analysis with LISREL. *Evaluation and the Health Professions, 13,* 298-314.

Nunnally, J. C. (1978). *Psychometric theory* (2nd ed.). New York: McGraw-Hill.

Nuttall, P., & Nicholls, P. (1992). Cystic fibrosis: Adolescent and maternal concerns about hospital and home care. *Issues in Comprehensive Pediatric Nursing, 15,* 199-213.

Nutting, P. L. (1987). *Community oriented primary care.* Washington, DC: U.S. Department of Health and Human Services.

Nyberg, D., Frink, B. B., Nolan, M., & Schauble, J. (1996, April). *Identification of key clinical indicators for patient response to conscious sedation.* Paper presented at the annual meeting of the Eastern Nursing Research Society, Pittsburgh, PA.

Oaks, J., Warren, B., & Harsha, D. (1987). Cardiovascular health knowledge of children and school personnel in Louisiana public schools. *Journal of School Health, 57,* 23-27.

Obrecht, J., Gallo, A., & Knafl, K. (1992). A case illustration of family management style in childhood end-stage renal disease. *American Nephrology Nurses Association Journal, 19,* 255-260.

Ogilvie, L. (1990). Hospitalization of children for surgery: The parents' view. *Children's Health Care, 19,* 49-56.

Olds, D. L., Henderson, C. R., & Kitzman, H. (1994). Does prenatal infancy home visitation have enduring effects on qualities of parental caregiving and child health at 25 to 50 months of life? *Pediatrics, 93,* 89-98.

Olds, D. L., Henderson, C., Kitzman, H., & Cole, R. (1995). Effects of prenatal and infancy nurse home visitation on surveillance of child maltreatment. *Pediatrics, 95,* 365-372.

Olds, D. L., Henderson, C. R., Tatelbaum, R., & Chamberlin, R. (1986). Improving the delivery of prenatal care and outcomes of pregnancy: A randomized trial of nurse home visitation. *Pediatrics, 77,* 16-28.

Olson, D. H., Portner, J., & Lavee, Y. (1985). *FACES III: Family Adaptability and Cohesion Evaluation Scales.* St. Paul: University of Minnesota, Family Social Science.

Olson, R. K, Heater, B. S., & Becker, A. M. (1990). A meta-analysis of the effects of nursing interventions on children and parents. *MCN: American Journal of Maternal Child Nursing, 15,* 104-108.

Orem, D. E. (1971). *Nursing: Concepts of practice.* New York: McGraw-Hill.

Orem, D. E. (1992). *Nursing: Concepts of practice* (2nd ed.). New York: McGraw-Hill.

Ory, M. G., & Kronenfeld, J. J. (1980). Living with juvenile diabetes mellitus. *Pediatric Nursing, 6,* 47-50.

Palfrey, J. S. (1994). *Community child health: An action plan for today.* Westport, CT: Praeger.

Palmer, M. (1922). The school nursing section. *Journal of Public Health Nursing, 7,* 512-513.

Patterson, J. (1995). Conceptualizing family adaptation to stress. In J. L. Tanner (Ed.), *Children, families and stress: Ross roundtable series* (pp. 11-21). Columbus, OH: Abbott Laboratories.

Patterson, J. M. (1990). Family and health research in the 1980's: A family scientist perspective. *Family Systems Medicine, 8,* 421-434.

Patterson, J. M., Jernell, J., Leonard, B. J., & Titus, J. C. (1994). Caring for medically fragile children at home: The parent-professional relationship. *Journal of Pediatric Nursing, 9,* 98-106.

Patterson, J. M., & McCubbin, H. I. (1991). Adolescent–Coping Orientation for Problem Experiences (ACOPE). In H. I. McCubbin & A. I. Thompson (Eds.), *Family assessment inventories for research and practice* (pp. 251-252). Madison, WI: Family Stress Coping and Health Project.

Patterson, J. M., McCubbin, H. I., & Grochowski, J. (1991). Young adult-coping orientation for problem experiences (YA-COPE). In H. I. McCubbin & A. I. Thompson (Eds.), *Family assessment inventories for research and practice* (pp. 263-264). Madison, WI: Family Stress Coping and Health Project.

Patton, A. C., Ventura, J. N., & Savedra, M. (1986). Stress and coping responses of adolescents with cystic fibrosis. *Children's Health Care, 14,* 153-156.

Pederson, C., & Harbaugh, B. L. (1995). Children's and adolescents' experiences while undergoing cardiac catheterization. *Maternal-Child Nursing Journal, 23,* 15-25.

Peebles, A. Y. (1933). Care of premature infants. *American Journal of Nursing, 33,* 866-869.

Pender, A. R. (1987). Economic incentives for prevention and health promotion. In N. Pender (Ed.), *Health promotion in nursing practice* (2nd ed., pp. 445-458). Norwalk, CT: Appleton & Lange.

Pender, N. J. (1982). *Health promotion in nursing practice.* Norwalk, CT: Appleton-Century-Crofts.

Pender, N. J. (1987). *Health promotion in nursing practice* (2nd ed.). Norwalk, CT: Appleton & Lange.

Pender, N. J. (1996). *Health promotion in nursing practice* (3rd ed.). Stamford, CT: Appleton & Lange.

Pender, N. J., Barkauskas, V. H., Hayman, L., Rice, V. H., & Anderson, E. T. (1992). Health promotion and disease prevention: Toward excellence in nursing practice and education. *Nursing Outlook, 40,* 106-112, 120.

Perkins, M. T. (1993). Parent-nurse collaboration: Using the caregiver identity emergence phases to assist parents of hospitalized children with disabilities. *Journal of Pediatric Nursing, 8,* 2-9.

Perlman, M., Claris, O., Hao, Y., Pandit, P., Whyte, H., Chipman, M., & Liu, P. (1995). Secular changes in the outcomes to eighteen to twenty-four months of age of extremely low birth weight infants, with adjustment for changes in risk factors and severity of illness. *Journal of Pediatrics, 126*(1), 75-87.

Perrin, E. C., & Gerrity, P. S. (1981). There's a demon in your belly: Children's understanding of illness. *Pediatrics, 67,* 841-849.

Perrin, E. C., Stein, R. E. K., & Drotar, D. (1991). Cautions in using the Child Behavior Checklist: Observations based on research about children with a chronic illness. *Journal of Pediatric Psychology, 16,* 411-421.

Perrin, J. (1985). Introduction. In N. Hobbs & J. Perrin (Eds.), *Issues in the care of children with chronic illness* (pp. 1-12). San Francisco: Jossey-Bass.

Perrin, J. M. (1994). Variations in pediatric hospitalization rates: Why do they occur? *Pediatric Annals, 23,* 676-677, 681-683.

Perrin, J. M., Greenspan, P., Bloom, S. R., Finkelstein, D., Yazdgerdi, S., Leventhal, J. M., Rodewald., L., Szilagyi, P., & Homer, C. J. (1996). Primary care involvement among hospitalized children. *Archives of Pediatric and Adolescent Medicine, 150,* 479-486.

Perrin, J., Shayne, M., & Bloom, S. (1993). *Home and community care for chronically ill children.* New York: Oxford University Press.

Perry, C., Baranowski, T., & Parcel, G. (1990). How individuals, environments, and health behavior interact: Social learning theory. In K. Glanz, F. M. Lewis, & B. K. Rimer (Eds.), *Health behavior and health education: Theory, research, and practice* (pp. 161-186). San Francisco: Jossey-Bass.

Perry, C., Luepker, R. V., Murray, D. M., Hearn, M. D., Halper, A., Dudovitz, B., Maile, M. C., & Smyth, M. (1989). Parent involvement with children's health promotion: A one-year follow-up of the Minnesota Home Team. *Health Education Quarterly, 16,* 171-180.

Peterson, L., & Brownlee-Duffeck, M. (1984). Prevention of anxiety and pain. In M. Roberst & L. Peterson (Eds.), *Prevention of problems in childhood* (pp. 266-309). New York: John Wiley.

Peto, R., Pike, M. C., & Armitage, P. (1976). Design and analysis of randomized clinical trials requiring prolonged observation of each patient. *British Journal of Cancer, 34,* 585-612.

Philichi, L. M. (1989). Family adaptation during a pediatric intensive care hospitalization. *Journal of Pediatric Nursing, 4,* 268-276.

Phillips, M. (1991). Chronic sorrow in mothers of chronically ill and disabled children. *Issues in Comprehensive Pediatric Nursing, 14,* 111-120.

Piaget, J. (1962). *Play, dreams, and imitation in childhood.* New York: Norton.

Piaget, J. (1969). *The theory of stages of cognitive development.* New York: McGraw-Hill.

Piaget, J., & Inhelder, B. (1969). *The psychology of the child* (H. Weaver, Trans.). New York: Basic Books.

Pianta, R. C., & Lothman, D. J. (1994). Predicting behavior problems in children with epilepsy: Child factors, disease factors, family stress, and child-mother interactions. *Child Development, 65,* 1415-1428.

Piers, E. V. (1984). *Piers-Harris Children's Self-Concept Scale: Revised manual.* Los Angeles: Western Psychological Services.

Pill, R. (1991). Issues in lifestyles and health: Lay meanings of health and health behavior. In B. Bandura & I. Kickbusch (Eds.), *Health promotion research: Towards a new social epidemiology* (WHO Regional Publications, European Series, No. 37, pp. 187-211). Copenhagen: World Health Organization.

Pine, M., Norusis, M., Jones, B., & Rosenthal, G. E. (1997). Predictions of hospital mortality rates: A comparison of data sources [see comments]. *Annals of Internal Medicine, 126*(5), 347-354.

Pinelli, J. (1981). A comparison of mothers' concerns regarding the care-taking of newborns with congenital heart disease before and after assuming their care. *Journal of Advanced Nursing, 6,* 261-270.

Pinyerd, B. J. (1983). Siblings of children with myelomeningocele: Examining their perceptions. *Maternal-Child Nursing Journal, 12,* 61-70.

Pless, I. B., Feeley, N., Gottlieb, L., Rowat, K., Dougherty, G., & Willard, B. (1994). A randomized trial of a nursing intervention to promote the adjustment of children with chronic physical disorders. *Pediatrics, 94,* 70-75.

Plomin, R. (1994). Behavioral genetic evidence for the importance of nonshared environment. In E. M. Hetherington, D. Reiss, & R. Plomin (Eds.), *Separate social worlds of siblings: The impact of nonshared environment on development* (pp. 1-32). Hillsdale, NJ: Lawrence Erlbaum.

Plomin, R. (1995). Genetics and children's experiences in the family. *Journal of Child Psychology and Psychiatry, 36,* 33-68.

Poets, C., & Southall, D. (1994). Noninvasive monitoring of oxygenization in infants and children: Practical considerations and areas of concern. *Pediatrics, 93,* 737-746.

Pollack, M. M., & Getson, P. R. (1988). *Reducing the nation's pediatric intensive care mortality.* Proposal to Bureau of Maternal Child Health, Washington, DC.

Pollack, M. M., Getson, P. R., Ruttimann, U. E., Steinhart, C. M., Kanter, R. K., Katz, R. W., Zucker, A. R., Glass, N. L., Spohn, W. A., Fuhrman, B. P., & Wilkinson, J. D. (1987). Efficiency of intensive care. A comparative analysis of eight pediatric intensive care units. *Journal of the American Medical Association, 258,* 1481-1486.

Pollack, M. M., Patel, K. M., & Ruttimann, U. E. (1996). PRISM III: An updated pediatric risk of mortality score. *Critical Care Medicine, 24,* 743-752.

Pollack, M. M., Patel, K. M., Ruttimann, U., & Cuerdon, T. (1996). Frequency of variable measurement in 16 pediatric intensive care units: Influence on accuracy and potential for bias in severity of illness assessment. *Critical Care Medicine, 24,* 74-77.

Pollack, M. M., Ruttimann, U. E., & Getson, P. R. (1988). Pediatric risk of mortality (PRISM) score. *Critical Care Medicine, 16,* 1110-1116.

Pollack, M. M., Ruttimann, U. E., Getson, P. R., & Members of the Multi-Institutional Study Group. (1987). Accurate prediction of the outcome of pediatric intensive care. *New England Journal of Medicine, 316,* 134-139.

Pollack, M. M., Ruttimann, U. E., Glass, N. L., & Yeh, T. S. (1985). Monitoring patients in pediatric intensive care. *Pediatrics, 76,* 719-724.

Pollack, M. M., Wilkinson, J. D., & Glass, N. L. (1987). Long-stay pediatric intensive care unit patients: Outcome and resource utilization. *Pediatrics, 80,* 855-860.

Pollack, M. M., Yeh, T. S., Ruttimann, U. E., Holbrook, P. R., & Fields, A. I. (1984). Evaluation of pediatric intensive care. *Critical Care Medicine, 12,* 376-383.

Pollitt, E. (1994). Poverty and child development: Relevance of research in developing countries to the United States. *Child Development, 65,* 283-295.

Pontius, S. L., Kennedy, A., Chung, K. L., Burroughs, T. E., Libby, L. J., & Vogel, D. W. (1994). Accuracy and reliability of temperature measurement in the emergency department by instrument and site in children. *Pediatric Nursing, 20,* 58-63.

Pontius, S. L., Kennedy, A. H., Shelley, S., & Mittrucker, C. (1994). Accuracy and reliability of temperature measurement by instrument and site. *Journal of Pediatric Nursing, 9,* 114-123.

Popenoe, D. (1993, April 14). Scholars should worry about the disintegration of the American family. *Chronicle of Higher Education,* p. A48.

Porter, C. (1994). As the twig is bent: Child rearing and working poor, older African-American mothers. *American Black Nursing Faculty Journal, 5*(3), 77-83.

Porter, C. P., Oakley, D., Ronis, D. L., & Neal, R. W. (1996). Pathways of influence on fifth and eighth graders' reports about having had sexual intercourse. *Research in Nursing and Health, 19,* 193-204.

Porter, J. E. (1995). The benchmarking effort for networking children's hospitals (BENCHmark). *Joint Commission Journal on Quality Improvement, 21*(8), 395-406.

Porter, L. S. (1972). The impact of physical-physiological activity on infants' growth and development. *Nursing Research, 21,* 210-219.

Price, J. H., Desmond, S. M., & Smith, D. (1991). A preliminary investigation of inner city adolescents' perceptions of guns. *Journal of School Health, 61,* 255-259.

Price, P. J. (1993). Parents' perceptions of the meaning of quality nursing care. *Advances in Nursing Science, 16*(1), 33-41.

Pridham, K. F. (1993). Anticipatory guidance of parents of new infants: Potential contribution of the internal working model construct. *Image: Journal of Nursing Scholarship, 25,* 49-56.

Pridham, K. F. (1995). *Support of mothers and family members in feeding an extremely low birth weight preterm infant at risk for chronic lung disease.* Grant Narrative No. MCJ-550806.

Pridham, K. F. (1997). Mothers' help-seeking as care initiated in a social context. *Image: Journal of Nursing Scholarship, 29,* 65-70.

Pridham, K. F., Broome, M., Woodring, B., & Baroni, M. (1996). Education for the nursing of children and their families: Standards and guidelines for prelicensure and early professional education. *Journal of Pediatric Nursing, 11*(5), 273-280.

Pridham, K. F., Limbo, R., Schroeder, M., Thoyre, S., & Van Riper, M. (in press). Guided participation and development of caregiving competencies for families of low birth-weight infants. *Journal of Advanced Nursing.*

Pridham, K. F., & Schutz, M. E. (1985). Rationale for naming problems from a nursing perspective. *Image: Journal of Nursing Scholarship, 17*(4), 122-126.

Prochaska, J. O., & DiClemente, C. C. (1983). Stages and processes of self-change of smoking: Toward an integrative model of change. *Journal of Consulting and Clinical Psychology, 51,* 390-395.

Proctor, D. L. (1987). Relationship between visitation policy in a pediatric intensive unit and parental anxiety. *Children's Health Care, 16,* 13-17.

Prugh, D. G., Staub, E., Sands, H. H., Kirschbaum, R. M., & Lenihan, E. A. (1953). A study of the emotional reactions of children and families to hospitalization and illness. *American Journal of Orthopsychiatry, 23,* 70-106.

Pulkininen, L. (1983). Youthful smoking and drinking in a longitudinal perspective. *Journal of Youth and Adolescence, 12,* 253-283.

Purcell, A. C., O'Brien, E., & Parks, P. L. (1996). Cholesterol levels in children: To screen or not to screen. *Journal of Pediatric Nursing, 11,* 40-44.

Radbill, S. X. (1955). A history of children's hospitals. *American Journal of Diseases of Children, 90,* 411-416.

Radbill, S. X. (1976). Reared in adversity: Institutional care of children in the 18th century. *American Journal of Diseases in Children, 130,* 751-761.

Radloff, L. S. (1977). The CES-D scale: A self-report depression scale for research in the general population. *Applied Psychological Measurement, 1,* 385-401.

Rafkin, H. S., & Hoyt, J. W. (1994). Objective data and quality assurance programs: Current and future trends. *Critical Care Clinics, 10,* 157-177.

Rausch, P. B. (1981). Effects of tactile and kinesthetic stimulation on premature infants. *Journal of Obstetric, Gynecologic, and Neonatal Nursing, 10,* 34-37.

Ray, L. D., & Ritchie, J. A. (1993). Caring for chronically ill children at home: Factors that influence parents' coping. *Journal of Pediatric Nursing, 8,* 217-225.

Report of the Executive Secretary. (1912). *Transactions of the American Association for the Study and Prevention of Infant Mortality, 1,* 19.

Research reporter. (1953). *Nursing Research, 2,* 41.

Reverby, S. M. (Ed.). (1987). *Ordered to care: The dilemma of American nursing, 1850-1945.* New York: Cambridge University Press.

Rew, L. (1987a). Children with asthma: The relationship between illness behaviors and health locus of control. *Western Journal of Nursing Research, 9,* 465-483.

Rew, L. (1987b). The relationship between self-care behaviors and selected psychosocial variables in children with asthma. *Journal of Pediatric Nursing, 2,* 333-341.

Rhiner, M., Ferrell, B. R., Shapiro, B., & Dierkes, M. (1994). The experience of pediatric cancer pain, Part II: Management of pain. *Journal of Pediatric Nursing, 9,* 380-387.

Rhodes, J., & Englund, S. (1993). School-based interventions for promoting social competence. In D. S. Glenwick & L. A. Jason (Eds.), *Promoting health and mental health in children, youth, and families* (pp. 17-31). New York: Springer.

Rice, R. (1977). Neurophysiological development in premature infants following stimulation. *Developmental Psychology, 13,* 69-76.

Richardson, D. K., Gray, J. E., McCormick, M. C., Workman, K., & Goldmann, D. A. (1993). Score for Neonatal Acute Physiology: A physiologic severity index for neonatal intensive care. *Pediatrics, 91,* 617-623.

Richardson, D. K., Phibbs, C. S., Gray, J. E., McCormick, M. C., Workman-Daniels, K., & Goldmann, D. A. (1993). Birth weight and illness severity: Independent predictors of neonatal mortality. *Pediatrics, 91,* 969-975.

Richardson, J. (1996, April 2). *Congressional Record service report for Congress.* Washington, DC: Congressional Record.

Richardson, L. A., Selby-Harrington, M., Krowchuk, H. V., Cross, A. W., & Quade, D. (1995). Health outcomes of children receiving EPSDT checkups: A pilot study. *Journal of Pediatric Health Care, 9,* 242-250.

Richmond, J. B. (1989). Early education. *Bulletin of the New York Academy of Medicine, 65,* 307-318.

Richmond, J. B. (1994). Foreword. In J. S. Palfrey, *Community child health: An action plan for today* (pp. xiii-xiv). Westport, CT: Praeger.

Richmond, J. B. (1995). The Hull House era: Vintage years for children. *American Journal of Orthopsychiatry, 65,* 10-20.

Richmond, J. B., & Fein, R. (1995). The health care mess: A bit of history. *Journal of the American Medical Association, 273,* 69-71.

Richmond, J. B., & Kotelchuck, M. L. (1983). Political influences: Rethinking national health policy. In C. H. McGuire, R. P. Foley, A. Gorr, R. W. Richards, & Associates (Eds.), *Handbook on health professions education* (pp. 386-404). San Francisco: Jossey-Bass.

Riddle, I. I., Hennessey, J., Eberly, T. W., Carter, M. C., & Miles, M. S. (1989). Stressors in the pediatric intensive care unit as perceived by mothers and fathers. *Maternal-Child Nursing Journal, 18,* 221-234.

Riesch, S. K. (1992). Nursing centers: An analysis of the anecdotal literature. *Journal of Professional Nursing, 8,* 16-25.

Riley-Lawless, K. (1995). *Family research in nursing: An integrative review.* Unpublished manuscript, University of Pennsylvania.

Riley-Lawless, K. (1996). *Health promotion during the adolescent transition: The role of the family.* Dissertation proposal in progress, University of Pennsylvania.

Ritchie, J. (1977). Children's adjustive and affective responses in the process of reformulating a body image following amputation. *Maternal-Child Nursing Journal, 6,* 25-35.

Roberts, C. S., & Feetham, S. L. (1982). Assessing family functioning across three areas of relationships. *Nursing Research, 31,* 231-236.

Roberts, M. X., Maieron, M. J., & Collier, J. (1988). *Directory of hospital psychosocial policies and programs.* Washington, DC: Association for the Care of Children's Health.

Robertson, J. (1958). *Young children in hospitals.* New York: Basic Books.

Robertson, J. (1993). Pediatric pain assessment: Validation of a multidimensional tool. *Pediatric Nursing, 19,* 209-213.

Robinson, C. (1996). Health care relationships revisited. *Journal of Family Nursing, 2,* 152-173.

Robinson, C. A. (1984). When hospitalization becomes an "everyday thing." *Issues in Comprehensive Pediatric Nursing, 7,* 363-370.

Robinson, C. A. (1985). Parents of hospitalized chronically ill children: Competency in question. *Nursing Papers, 17*(2), 59-68.

Robinson, C. A. (1987). Roadblocks to family centered care when a chronically ill child is hospitalized. *Maternal-Child Nursing Journal, 16,* 181-193.

Robinson, C. A. (1994). Nursing interventions with families: A demand or an invitation to change? *Journal of Advanced Nursing, 19,* 897-904.

Robinson, C. A. (1995a). Beyond dichotomies in the nursing of persons and families. *Image: Journal of Nursing Scholarship, 27,* 116-120.

Robinson, C. A. (1995b). Unifying distinctions for nursing research with persons and families. *Journal of Family Nursing, 1,* 8-29.

Rogers, J., Curley, M., Driscoll, J., Kerrigan, T., LeBlanc, G., Libman, M., & McCarty, K. (1991). Evaluation of tympanic membrane thermometer for use with pediatric patients. *Pediatric Nursing, 17,* 376-378.

Rogoff, B. (1990). *Apprenticeship in thinking: Cognitive development in social context.* New York: Oxford University Press.

Roper, W. L. (1994). Why the problem of leadership in public health? In D. M. Fox & W. L. Roper (Eds.), *Leadership in public health* (pp. 20-28). New York: Milbank Memorial Fund.

Rose, M. H. (1972). The effects of hospitalization on the coping behaviors of children. In M. V. Batey (Ed.), *Communicating nursing research.* Boulder, CO: Western Interstate Commission for Higher Education.

Rosenbaum, S. (1993). Providing primary health care to children: Integrating primary care services with health insurance principles. *The Future of Children, 3*(2), 60-76.

Rosenberg, C. E. (Ed.). (1987). *The care of strangers: The rise of America's hospital system.* New York: Basic Books.

Rosenstock, I. M. (1960). What research in motivation suggests for public health. *American Journal of Public Health, 50,* 295-301.

Rosenstock, I. M. (1966). Why people use health services. *Milbank Memorial Fund Quarterly, 44,* 94-124.

Rosenstock, I. M. (1990). The Health Belief Model: Explaining health behavior through expectancies. In K. Glanz, F. M. Lewis, & B. K. Rimer (Eds.), *Health behavior and health education: Theory, research, and practice* (pp. 39-62). San Francisco: Jossey-Bass.

Rosenstock, I. M., Strecher, V. J., & Becker, M. H. (1988). Social learning theory and the health belief model. *Health Education Quarterly, 15,* 175-183.

Rosenthal, C., Marshall, V., MacPherson, A., & French, S. (1980). *Nurses, patients, and families.* New York: Springer.

Rossi, P. H., & Freeman, H. E. (1989). *Evaluation: A systematic approach.* Newbury Park, CA: Sage.

Roy, C., & Roberts, S. L. (1981). *Theory construction in nursing: An adaptation model.* Englewood Cliffs, NJ: Prentice Hall.

Roy, M. C. (1967). Role cues and mothers of hospitalized children. *Nursing Research, 16,* 178-182.

Rozmus, C. L., & Edgil, A. E. (1993). Values, knowledge, and attitudes about Acquired Immunodeficiency Syndrome in rural adolescents. *Journal of Pediatric Health Care, 7,* 167-173.

Rudolph, R. (Ed.). (1991). *Aspects of child health: Rudolph's pediatrics.* Norwalk, CT: Appleton & Lange.

Russell, D., Peplau, H. E., & Cutrona, C. E. (1980). The revised UCLA Loneliness Scale: Concurrent and discriminant validity evidence. *Journal of Personality and Social Psychology, 39,* 472-480.

Russell, K., & Jewell, N. (1992). Cultural impact of health-care access: Challenges for improving the health of African Americans. *Journal of Community Health Nursing, 9,* 161-169.

Russell, K. M., & Champion, V. L. (1996). Health beliefs and social influence in home safety practices of mothers with preschool children. *Image: Journal of Nursing Scholarship, 28,* 59-64.

Ruttimann, U. E., Pollack, M. M., & Fiser, D. H. (1996). Prediction of three outcome states from pediatric intensive care. *Critical Care Medicine, 24,* 78-85.

Ryan, E. A., & Hayman, L. L. (1996). The role of the family coordinator in longitudinal research: Strategies to recruit and retain families. *Journal of Family Nursing, 2,* 325-335.

Ryan, N. M. (1989). Stress-coping strategies identified from school age children's perspective. *Research in Nursing and Health, 12,* 111-122.

Ryan-Wenger, N. M. (1990). Development and psychometric properties of the Schoolagers' Coping Strategies Inventory. *Nursing Research, 39,* 344-349.

Ryan-Wenger, N. M. (1996). Children, coping, and the stress of illness: A synthesis of the research. *Journal of the Society of Pediatric Nurses, 1*(3), 126-138.

Ryan-Wenger, N. M., & Copeland, S. G. (1994). Coping strategies used by Black school-age children from low-income families. *Journal of Pediatric Nursing, 9,* 33-40.

Ryan-Wenger, N. M., & Walsh, M. (1994). Children's perspectives on coping with asthma. *Pediatric Nursing, 20,* 224-298.

Saba, V. (1992). The classification of home healthcare nursing: Diagnoses and interventions. *Caring, 11*(3), 50-57.

Sachs, B. (1984). Contraceptive decision-making in urban, Black female adolescents: Its relationship to cognitive development. *International Journal of Nursing Studies, 22,* 117-126.

Sachs, B. (1986). Reproductive decisions in adolescence. *Image: Journal of Nursing Scholarship, 18,* 69-72.

Sallis, J. F., & Nader, P. R. (1988). Family determinants of health behavior. In D. S. Gochman (Ed.), *Health behavior: Emerging research perspectives* (pp. 107-124). New York: Plenum.

Sallis, J. F., & Owen, N. (1997). Ecological models. In K. Glanz, F. M. Lewis, & B. K. Rimer (Eds.), *Health behavior and health education: Theory, research, and practice* (2nd ed., 403-424). San Francisco: Jossey-Bass.

Sarvela, P. D., & Ford, T. D. (1992). Indicators of substance abuse among pregnant adolescents in the Mississippi Delta. *Journal of School Health, 62,* 175-179.

Saucier, C. P. (1984). Self-concept and self-care management in school-age children with diabetes. *Pediatric Nursing, 10,* 135-138.

Saucier, C. P., & Clark, L. M. (1994). The relationship between self-care and metabolic control in children with insulin dependent diabetes mellitus. *Diabetic Educator, 19,* 133-136.

Savedra, M., Gibbons, P. T., Tesler, M., Ward, J. A., & Wegner, C. (1982). How do children describe pain? A tentative assessment. *Pain, 14,* 95-104.

Savedra, M. C., Holzemer, W. L., Tesler, M. D., & Wilkie, D. J. (1993). Assessment of postoperative pain in children and adolescents using the adolescent pediatric pain tool. *Nursing Research, 42,* 5-9.

Savedra, M. C., & Tesler, M. D. (1981). Coping strategies of hospitalized school-age children. *Western Journal of Nursing Research, 3,* 371-384.

Savedra, M. C., Tesler, M. D., Holzemer, W. L., Wilkie, D. J., & Ward, J. A. (1989). Pain location: Validity and reliability of body outline markings by hospitalized children and adolescents. *Research in Nursing and Health, 12,* 307-314.

Sawin, K. J., & Harrigan, M. P. (1995). *Measures of family functioning for research and practice.* New York: Springer.

Sawyer, E. H. (1992). Family functioning when children have cystic fibrosis. *Journal of Pediatric Nursing, 7,* 304-311.

Scanlon, M. K. (1985). A chronically ill child's progress through the separation-individuation process. *Maternal-Child Nursing Journal, 14,* 91-102.

Scannell, S., Gillies, D. A., Biordi, D., & Child, D. A. (1993). Negotiating nurse-patient authority in pediatric home health care. *Journal of Pediatric Nursing, 8,* 70-78.

Scharer, K., & Dixon, D. (1989). Managing chronic illness: Parents with a ventilator-dependent child. *Journal of Pediatric Nursing, 4,* 236-247.

Schatzman, L. (1991). Dimensional analysis: Notes on an alternative approach to the grounding of theory in qualitative research. In D. R. Maines (Ed.), *Social organization and social process: Essays in honor of Anselm Strauss* (pp. 303-314). New York: Aldine de Gruyter.

Schepp, K. G. (1991). Factors influencing the coping effort of mothers of hospitalized children. *Nursing Research, 40,* 42-46.

Schepp, K. G. (1992). Correlates of mothers who prefer control over their hospitalized child's care. *Journal of Pediatric Nursing, 7,* 83-89.

Schlomann, P. (1988). Development gaps of children with a chronic condition and their impact on the family. *Journal of Pediatric Nursing, 3,* 180-187.

Schmeltz, K., & White, G. (1982). A survey of parent groups: Prehospital admission. *Maternal-Child Nursing Journal, 11,* 75-86.

Schmidt, F. L. (1992). What do data mean? Research findings, meta-analysis, and cumulative knowledge. *American Psychologist, 47,* 1173-1181.

Schmidt, F. L. (1995). The impact of data analysis methods on cumulative research knowledge. *Evaluation and the Health Professions, 18,* 407-427.

Schmidt, W. M., & Wallace, H. M. (1994). The development of health services for mothers and children in the United States. In H. M. Wallace, R. P. Nelson, & P. J. Sweeney (Eds.), *Maternal and child health practices* (4th ed., pp. 103-119). Oakland, CA: Third Party Publishing Company.

Schorr, L. B. (1988). *Within our reach: Breaking the cycle of disadvantage.* New York: Doubleday.

Schorr, L. B. (1991). *Successful programs and the bureaucratic dilemma: Current deliberations.* Washington, DC: National Center for Children in Poverty.

Schorr, L. B. (1997). *Common purpose: Strengthening families and neighborhoods to rebuild America.* New York: Anchor.

Schryer, N. M. (1993). Nursing case management for children undergoing craniofacial reconstruction. *Plastic Surgery Nursing, 13,* 17-26.

Schubiner, H., & Eggly, S. (1995). Strategies for health education for adolescent patients: A preliminary investigation. *Journal of Adolescent Health, 17,* 37-41.

Schultz, N. V. (1971). How children perceive pain. *Nursing Outlook, 19,* 670-673.

Schuman, A. J. (1990). Homeward bound: The explosion in pediatric home care [Special issue on technology]. *Contemporary Pediatrics, 7,* 26-54.

Schwarz, D., & O'Sullivan, A. (1993). *Health promotion with teenage mothers.* Grant Narrative No. RO1 NR 03565.

Schwirian, P. M. (1976). Effects of the presence of a hearing-impaired preschool child in the family on behavior patterns of older "normal" siblings. *American Annals of the Deaf, 121,* 373-380.

Scipien, G. M., & Chard, M. A. (1990). Nursing of children: The development of the specialty. In G. M. Scipien, M. A. Chard, J. Howe, & M. U. Barnard (Eds.), *Pediatric nursing care* (pp. 2-11). St. Louis: C. V. Mosby.

Scott, R. A., Aiken, L. H., Mechanic, D., & Moravcsik, J. (1995). Organizational aspects of caring. *Millbank Quarterly, 73,* 77-95.

Sears, P. S. (1964). Self-concept in the service of educational goals. *California Journal of Institutional Improvement, 7*(2), 3-17.

Sedlak, M., & Church, R. (1982). *A history of social services delivered to youth, 1880-1977* (Final report to the National Institute of Education). Washington, DC: National Institute of Education.

See, E. M. (1977). The ANA and research in nursing. *Nursing Research, 26,* 165-171.

Segall, M. E. (1972). Cardiac responsivity to auditory stimulation in premature infants. *Nursing Research, 21,* 15-19.

Seidl, F. W. (1969). Pediatric nursing personnel and parent participation: A study in attitudes. *Nursing Research, 18,* 40-44.

Seidl, F. W., & Pilletteri, A. (1967). Development of an attitude scale on parent participation. *Nursing Research, 16,* 71-73.

Select Panel for the Promotion of Child Health. (1981). *Better health for our children: A national strategy: Volume I. Major findings and recommendations.* Washington, DC: U.S. Public Health Service & U.S. Department of Health and Human Services.

Sellew, G. (1943). *Nursing of children* (5th ed.). Philadelphia: W. B. Saunders.

Shaftel, N. (1978). A history of the purification of milk in New York, or "How now brown cow." In J. Leavitt & R. Numbers (Eds.), *Sickness and health in America* (pp. 275-292). Madison: University of Wisconsin Press.

Shannon, B. M., Tershakovec, A. M., Martel, J. K., Achterberg, C. L., Cortner, J. A., Smicklas-Wright, H. S., Stallings, V. A., & Stolley, P. D. (1994). Reduction of elevated LDL-cholesterol levels of 4- to 10-year old children through home-based dietary education. *Pediatrics, 94,* 923-927.

Sharp, N. (1995). Community nursing centers coming of age. *Nursing Management, 23*(8), 18-29.

Sharrer, V. W., & Ryan-Wenger, N. M. (1995). A longitudinal study of age and gender differences of stressors and coping strategies in school-age children. *Journal of Pediatric Health Care, 9,* 123-130.

Shattuck, L. (1976). *Report to the committee of the city council appointed to obtain the census of Boston for the year 1845.* New York: Arno. (Original work published 1850)

Shea, S., Basch, C. E., Lantigua, R., & Wechsler, H. (1992). The Washington Heights-Inwood Healthy Heart Program: A third generation community-based cardiovascular disease prevention program in a disadvantaged urban setting. *Preventive Medicine, 21,* 203-217.

Shedler, J., & Block, J. (1990). Adolescent drug use and psychologic health, a longitudinal inquiry. *American Psychologist, 45,* 612-630.

Sigma Theta Tau. (1995). Nursing research improves patient care. *Reflections, 21,* 17-35.

Simeonsson, R. J. (1994). Promoting children's health, education, and well-being. In R. J. Simeonsson (Ed.), *Promoting the well-being of children* (pp. 3-12). Baltimore: Paul H. Brookes.

Simon, N. B., & Smith, D. (1992). Living with chronic pediatric liver disease: The parents' experience. *Pediatric Nursing, 18,* 453-458, 489.

Simons, C. J. R., Ritchie, S. K., & Mullett, M. D. (1992). Relationships between parental ratings of infant temperament, risk status, and delivery method. *Journal of Pediatric Health Care, 6,* 240-245.

Simons-Morton, D. G., Simons, B. G., Parcel, G. S., & Bunker, J. F. (1988). Influencing personal and environmental conditions for community health: A multilevel intervention model. *Family and Community Health, 11,* 25-35.

Sinai, N., & Anderson, O. (1948). *Emergency maternity and infant care.* Ann Arbor, MI: Bureau of Public Health Economic.

Skinner, B. F. (1953). *Science and human behavior.* New York: Macmillan.

Skinner, B. F. (1974). *About behaviorism.* New York: Knopf.

Skipper, J. K., Leonard, R. C., & Rhymes, J. (1968). Child hospitalization and social interaction: An experimental study of mothers' feelings of stress, adaptation, and satisfaction. *Medical Care, 6,* 496-506.

Smilkstein, G. (1978). The Family APGAR: A proposal for a family function test and its use by physicians. *Journal of Family Practice, 6,* 1231-1239.

Smillie, W. (1955). *Public health: Its promise for the future.* New York: Macmillan.

Smith, A. B., & Wilkinson-Faulk, D. (1994). Factors affecting the life span of peripheral intravenous lines in hospitalized infants. *Pediatric Nursing, 20,* 543-547.

Smith, E. A., & Udry, J. R. (1985). Coital and non-coital sexual behaviors of White and Black adolescents. *American Journal of Public Health, 75,* 1200-1203.

Smith, K., Schreiner, B.-J., Brouhard, B., & Travis, L. (1991). Impact of a camp experience on choice of coping strategies by adolescents with insulin-dependent diabetes mellitus. *Diabetes Educator, 17,* 49-53.

Smith, L. D. (1994). Continuity of care through nursing case management of the chronically ill child. *Clinical Nurse Specialists, 8*(2), 65-68.

Smith, M. C. (1990). Nursing's unique focus on health promotion. *Nursing Science Quarterly, 3*(3), 105-106.

Smith, M. D. (1911). Incubator babies. *American Journal of Nursing, 11,* 791-795.

SmithBattle, L. (1996). Teenage mothers' narratives of self: An examination of risking the future. *Advances in Nursing Science, 17,* 22-36.

Snowden, A. W., & Gottlieb, L. N. (1989). The maternal role in the pediatric intensive care unit and hospital ward. *Maternal-Child Nursing Journal, 18,* 97-115.

Sorenson, E. S. (1990). Children's coping responses. *Journal of Pediatric Nursing, 5,* 259-267.

Spicher, C. M., & Yund, C. (1989). Effects of preadmission preparation on compliance with home care instructions. *Journal of Pediatric Nursing, 4,* 255-262.

Spielberger, G. D. (1973). *Manual for the State-Trait Anxiety Inventory for children.* Palo Alto, CA: Mind Garden.

Spielberger, G. D., Gorusch, R. L., Lushene, R., Vagg, P. R., & Jacobs, G. A. (1983). *Manual for the State-Trait Anxiety Inventory.* Palo Alto, CA: Mind Garden.

Spinetta, J. J., McLaren, H. H., Fox, R. W., & Sparta, S. N. (1981). The kinetic family drawing in childhood cancer: A revised application of an age-independent measure. In J. J. Spinetta & P. Deasy-Spinetta (Eds.), *Living with childhood cancer* (pp. 86-120). St. Louis: C. V. Mosby.

Spitzer, A. (1992a). Children's knowledge of illness and treatment experiences in hemophilia. *Journal of Pediatric Nursing, 7,* 43-51.

Spitzer, A. (1992b). Coping processes of school-age children with hemophilia. *Western Journal of Nursing Research, 14,* 157-169.

Spitzer, A. (1992c). Illness and treatment appraisal processes of healthy and hemophiliac boys. *Research in Nursing and Health, 15,* 3-9.

Spitzer, A. (1993). The significance of pain in children's experiences of hemophilia. *Clinical Nursing Research, 2,* 5-18.

Spock, B. (1964). *Dr. Spock talks with mothers.* Greenwich, CT: Fawcett.

Stainton, C. (1974). Preschoolers' orientation to hospital. *The Canadian Nurse, 7*(9), 38-40.

Stanhope, M., & Lancaster, J. (Eds.). (1988). History of community health and community health nursing. In M. Stanhope & J. Lancaster (Eds.), *Community health nursing.* St. Louis: C. V. Mosby.

Stein, R. E., Gortmaker, S. L., Perrin, J., Pless, I. B., Walker, D. K., & Weitzman, M. (1987). Severity of illness: Concepts and measurements. *Lancet, 11*(pt. 2), 1506-1509.

Stein, R. E. K. (1992). Chronic physical disorders. *Pediatric Review, 13,* 224-229.

Stein, R. E. K., & Jessop, D. J. (1982). A noncategorical approach to chronic childhood illness. *Public Health Reports, 97,* 354-362.

Stein, R. E. K., & Riessman, C. K. (1980). The development of an impact-on-family scale: Preliminary findings. *Medical Care, 18,* 465-472.

Stein, R. E. K., & Tassi, A. (1997). Child health at a cross-roads: Choices for policymakers. In R. E. K. Stein (Ed.), *Health care for children: What's right, what's wrong, what's next* (pp. 369-383). New York: United Hospital Fund of New York.

Stember, M., Swanson-Kaufman, K., Goodwin, L., Rogers, S., & Mathews, S. (1984). *How often do you?* Denver: University of Colorado Health Sciences Center.

Stevens, M. (1986). Adolescents' perception of stressful events during hospitalization. *Journal of Pediatric Nursing, 1,* 303-313.

Stevens, M. (1994). Parents coping with infants requiring home cardiorespiratory monitoring. *Journal of Pediatric Nursing, 9,* 2-12.

Stevens, S. M., Richardson, D. K., Gray, J. E., Goldmann, D. A., & McCormick, M. C. (1994). Estimating neonatal mortality risk: an analysis of clinicians' judgments. *Pediatrics, 93,* 945-950.

Stewart, B. J., & Archbold, P. G. (1992). Nursing intervention studies require outcome measures that are sensitive to change: Part 1. *Research in Nursing and Health, 15,* 477-481.

Stewart, B. J., & Archbold, P. G. (1993). Nursing intervention studies require outcome measures that are sensitive to change: Part 2. *Research in Nursing and Health, 16,* 77-81.

Stewart, I. (1929). The science and art of nursing [editorial]. *Nursing Education Bulletin, 2*(1), 107-137.

Stewart, M. L. (1977). Measurement of clinical pain. In A. K. Jacox (Ed.), *Pain: A source book for nurses and other health professionals* (pp. 107-137). Boston: Little, Brown.

Stoeckle, J. D. (1995). The citadel cannot hold: Technologies go outside the hospital, patients and doctors too. *Millbank Quarterly, 73,* 3-17.

Stokols, D. (1992). Establishing and maintaining healthy environments: Toward a social ecology of health promotion. *American Psychologist, 47,* 6-22.

Stoll, C. (1969). Responses of three children to burn injuries and hospitalization. *Nursing Clinics of North America, 4,* 77-87.

Stone, E. J., McGraw, S. A., Osganian, S. K., & Elder, J. P. (1994). Process evaluation in the Multicenter Child and Adolescent Trial for Cardiovascular Health (CATCH). *Health Education Quarterly,* Suppl. 2, S1-S143.

Stone, E. J., Perry, C. L., & Luepker, R. V. (1989). Synthesis of cardiovascular behavioral research for youth health promotion. *Health Education Quarterly, 16,* 155-168.

Straus, L. (1917). *Disease in milk: The remedy pasteurization: The life work of Nathan Straus.* New York: E. P. Dutton.

Strobel, C. T., Byrne, W. J., Ament, M. E., & Euler, A. R. (1979). Correlation of esophageal lengths in children with height: Application to the Tuttle test without prior esophageal manometry. *Journal of Pediatrics, 94,* 81-84.

Struthers, L. (1917). *The school nurse.* New York: G. P. Putman.

Stuffelbeam, D. (1983). The CIPP for program evaluation. In G. Madaus, M. Scriven, & D. Stuffelbeam (Eds.), *Educational models* (pp. 117-141). Boston: Kluwer Nijhoff.

Stullenbarger, B., Norris, J., Edgil, A. E., & Prosser, M. J. (1987). Family adaptation to cystic fibrosis. *Pediatric Nursing, 13,* 29-31.

Suddaby, E. S., & Frink, B. B. (1991). PICU nursing resource consumption by heart transplant patients as compared to cardiovascular surgery patients [Abstract]. In *Proceedings of organ transplants in children.* Philadelphia: Temple University.

Suddaby, E. S., & Frink, B. B. (1993). PICU nursing resource consumption by pediatric heart transplant recipients. *Journal of Transplant Coordination, 3,* 2-6.

Swift, J. (1983). *Gulliver's travels.* New York: Penguin. (Original work published 1726)

Syme, S. L. (1986). Strategies for health promotion. *Preventive Medicine, 15,* 492-507.

Taquino, L., & Blackburn, S. (1994). The effects of containment during suctioning and heelstick on physiological and behavioral responses of preterm infants. *Journal of Neonatal Nursing, 13*(7), 55.

Taylor, S. C. (1980). The effects of chronic childhood illnesses upon well siblings. *Maternal-Child Nursing Journal, 9,* 109-116.

Teres, D., & Lemeshow, S. (1994). Why severity models should be used with caution. *Critical Care Clinics, 10,* 111-115.

Terhaar, M., & O'Keefe, S. (1995). A new advanced practice role focused on outcomes management in women's and children's health. *Journal of Perinatal and Neonatal Nursing, 9*(3), 10-21.

Tesler, M., & Savedra, M. (1981). Coping with hospitalization: A study of school-age children. *Pediatric Nursing, 7*(2), 35-38.

Tesler, M., Ward, J., Savedra, M., Wegner, C., & Gibbons, P. (1983). Developing an instrument for eliciting children's description of pain. *Perceptual and Motor Skills, 56,* 315-321.

Tesler, M. D., Savedra, M. C., Holzemer, W. L., Wilkie, D. J., Ward, J. A., & Paul, S. M. (1991). The word-graphic rating scale as a measure of children's and adolescents' pain intensity. *Research in Nursing and Health, 14,* 361-371.

Thompson, M. L. (Ed.). (1995). Evolution of child health care and pediatric nursing. In M. L. Thompson (Ed.), *Pediatric nursing* (pp. 1-7). Springhouse, PA: Springhouse Corporation.

Thompson, R. H. (1985). *Psychosocial research on pediatric hospitalization and health care: A review of the literature.* Springfield, IL: Charles C Thomas.

Thompson, R. J., & Gustafson, K. E. (1996). *Adaptation to chronic childhood illness.* Washington, DC: American Psychological Association.

Thorne, S. E. (1993). *Negotiating health care: The social context of chronic illness*. Newbury Park, CA: Sage.

Thorne, S. E., & Robinson, C. A. (1988a). Reciprocal trust in health care relationships. *Journal of Advanced Nursing, 13,* 782-789.

Thorne, S. E., & Robinson, C. A. (1988b). Health care relationships: The chronic illness perspective. *Research in Nursing and Health, 11,* 293-300.

Thorne, S. E., & Robinson, C. A. (1989). Guarded alliance: Health care relationships in chronic illness. *Image: Journal of Nursing Scholarship, 21,* 153-157.

Tiedeman, M. E., & Clatworthy, S. (1990). Anxiety responses of 5- to 11-year-old children during and after hospitalization. *Journal of Pediatric Nursing, 5,* 334-343.

Tinsley, B. J. (1992). Multiple influences on the acquisition and socialization of children's health attitudes and behavior: An integrative review. *Child Development, 63,* 1043-1069.

Tomlinson, P. S., Kirschbaum, M., Tomczyk, B., & Peterson, J. (1993). The relationship of child acuity, maternal responses, nurse attitudes and contextual factors in the bone marrow transplant unit. *American Journal of Critical Care, 2,* 246-252.

Tomlinson, P. S., & Mitchell, K. E. (1992). On the nature of social support for families of critically ill children. *Journal of Pediatric Nursing, 7,* 386-394.

Torrance, J. T. (1968a). Temperature readings of premature infants. *Nursing Research, 17,* 312-320.

Torrance, J. T. (1968b). *Children's reactions to intramuscular injections: A comparative study of needle and jet injections*. Unpublished doctoral dissertation, Case Western Reserve University, Cleveland, OH.

Trierweiler, K., Cotler, J., & McNally, J. (Eds.). (1996). *An introduction to home visitation*. Denver: Colorado Department of Public Health and Environment.

Tripp, S. L., & Stachowiak, B. (1992). Health maintenance, health promotion: Is there a difference? *Public Health Nursing, 9,* 155-161.

Tucker, S. K. (1990). Adolescent patterns of communication about the menstrual cycle, sex, and contraception. *Journal of Pediatric Nursing, 5,* 393-400.

Turner, M. A., Tomlinson, P. S., & Harbaugh, B. L. (1990). Parental uncertainty in critical care hospitalization of children. *Maternal-Child Nursing Journal, 19,* 45-62.

Turner-Henson, A. (1993). Mothers of chronically ill children and perceptions of environmental variables. *Issues in Comprehensive Pediatric Nursing, 16,* 63-76.

Turner-Henson, A., & Holaday, B. (1995). Daily life experiences for the chronically ill: A life-span perspective. *Family and Community Health, 17*(4), 1-11.

Turner-Henson, A., Holaday, B., Corser, N., Ogletree, G., & Swan, J. H. (1994). The experiences of discrimination: Challenges for chronically ill children. *Pediatric Nursing, 20,* 571-577.

Turner-Henson, A., Holaday, B., & O'Sullivan, P. (1992). Sampling rare pediatric populations. *Journal of Pediatric Nursing, 7,* 329-334.

U.S. Department of Health and Human Services. (1979). *Healthy people: Surgeon General's report on health promotion and disease prevention*. Washington, DC: U.S. Public Health Service.

U.S. Department of Health and Human Services. (1990). *Healthy people 2000: National health promotion and disease prevention objectives* (DHHS Publication No. PHS 91-50213). Washington, DC: Government Printing Office.

U.S. Department of Health and Human Services. (1995). Prevention and managed care: Opportunities for managed care organizations, purchasers of health care and public health agencies. Atlanta: Public Health Services, Centers for Disease Control.

U.S. Department of Health and Human Services. (Ed.). (1992). *Patient outcomes research: Examining the effectiveness of nursing practice* (NIH Publication No. 93-3411). Proceedings of a conference sponsored by the National Center for Nursing Research, September 1991. Rockville, MD: Author.

U.S. Department of Labor, Children's Bureau. (1923). *The promotion of the welfare and hygiene of maternity and infancy*. Washington, DC: Government Printing Office.

U.S. General Accounting Office. (1990). *Home visiting: A promising early intervention strategy for at-risk families*. Gaithersburg, MD: Author.

U.S. General Accounting Office. (1994). *School-based health centers can promote access to care* (GAO/HEHS Publication No. 95-35). Washington, DC: Author.

Umphenour, J. H. (1980). Bacterial colonization in neonates with sibling visitation. *Journal of Obstetric, Gynecologic, and Neonatal Nursing, 9,* 74-75.

Uphold, M., & Graham, C. (1993). Schools as centers for collaborative services for families: A vision for change. *Nursing Outlook, 41*(5), 204-211.

Uzark, K., LeRoy, S., Callow, L., Cameron, J., & Rosenthal, A. (1994). The pediatric nurse practitioner as a case manager in the delivery of services to children with heart disease. *Journal of Pediatric Health Care, 8*(2), 74-78.

Van Cleve, L. (1989). Parental coping response to their child's spina bifida. *Journal of Pediatric Nursing, 4,* 172-176.

Van Cleve, L. J., & Savedra, M. C. (1993). Pain location: Validity and reliability of body outline markings by 4 to 7-year-old children who are hospitalized. *Pediatric Nursing, 19,* 217-220.

Van Ingren, P. (1921). *A half century of public health*. New York: American Public Health Association.

Van Os, D. C., Clark, C. G., Turner, C. W., & Herbst, J. J. (1985). Life stress and cystic fibrosis. *Western Journal of Nursing Research, 7,* 301-315.

van Veen, A., Karstens, A., van der Hoek, A. C., Tibboel, D., Hahlen, K., & van der Voort, E. (1996). The prognosis of oncologic patients in the pediatric intensive care unit. *Intensive Care Medicine, 22,* 237-241.

Vardaro, J. A. (1978). Preadmission anxiety and mother-child relationships. *Journal of the Association of the Care of Children's Hospitals, 7*(2), 8-15.

Veit, C. T., & Ware, J. E. (1983). The structure of psychological distress and well-being in general populations. *Journal of Consulting and Clinical Psychology, 51,* 730-742.

Vernon, D., Foley, J., Sipowicz, R., & Schulman, J. (1965). *The psychological responses of children to hospitalization and illness.* Springfield, IL: Charles C Thomas.

Vernon, D. T. (1974). Modeling and birth order in responses to painful stimuli. *Journal of Personality and Social Psychology, 29,* 794-799.

Vernon, D. T. (1975). Use of modeling to modify children's responses to a natural, potentially stressful situation. *Journal of Applied Psychology, 58,* 351-356.

Verran, J. (1986). Testing a classification instrument for the ambulatory care setting. *Research in Nursing and Health, 9,* 279-287.

Vessey, J. A., Bogetz, M. S., Caserza, C. L., Liu, K. R., & Dunleavy, M. F. (1994). Parental upset associated with participation in induction of pediatric anaesthesia. *Canadian Journal of Anaesthesia, 41,* 276-280.

Vessey, J. A., & Carlson, K. L. (1996). Nonpharmacological intervention to use with children in pain. *Issues in Comprehensive Pediatric Nursing, 19,* 169-182.

Vessey, J. A., Carlson, K. L., & McGill, J. (1994). Use of distraction with children during an acute pain experience. *Nursing Research, 43,* 369-372.

Vessey, J. A., & Mahon, M. M. (1990). Therapeutic play and the hospitalized child. *Journal of Pediatric Nursing, 5,* 328-333.

Villarruel, A. (1995). Culturally competent nursing research: Are we there yet? *Capsules and Comments in Pediatric Nursing, 1*(4), 18-26.

Visintainer, M. A., & Wolfer, J. A. (1975). Psychological preparation for surgical pediatric patients: The effect of children's and parents' stress responses and adjustment. *Pediatrics, 56,* 187-202.

Vivier, P. M., Bernier, J. A., & Starfield, B. (1994). Current approaches to measuring health outcomes in pediatric research. *Current Opinion in Pediatrics, 6,* 530-537.

von Bertalanffy, L. (1968). *General systems theory.* New York: George Braziller.

Vredevoe, D. L., Kim, A. C., Dambacher, B. M., & Call, J. D. (1969). Aggressive post-operative play responses of hospitalized preschool children. *Nursing Research, 4,* 4-5.

Waechter, E. H. (1977). Bonding problems of infants with congenital anomalies. *Nursing Forum, 16,* 298-318.

Walker, L. O. (1992). *Parent-infant nursing science: Paradigms, phenomena, methods.* Philadelphia: F. A. Davis.

Walker, S. H. (1992). Teenagers' knowledge of Acquired Immunodeficiency Syndrome and associated behaviors. *Journal of Pediatric Nursing, 7,* 246-250.

Wallace, R. M. (1989). Temperament: A variable in children's pain management. *Pediatric Nursing, 15,* 118-121.

Wallander, J. (1993). Special section editorial: Current research on pediatric chronic illness. *Journal of Pediatric Psychology, 18,* 7-10.

Wallerstein, N. (1992). Powerlessness, empowerment, and health: Implications for health promotion programs. *American Journal of Health Promotion, 6,* 197-205.

Wallston, K. A., Wallston, B. S., & DeVillis, R. (1978). Development of the multidimensional health locus of control (MHLC) scales. *Health Education Monographs, 6,* 160-170.

Walsh, M., & Ryan-Wenger, N. M. (1992). Sources of stress in children with asthma. *Journal of School Health, 62,* 459-463.

Warady, B., Mudge, C., Wiser, B., Wiser, M., & Rader, B. (1996). Transplant allograft loss in the adolescent patient. *Advances in Renal Replacement Therapy, 3,* 154-165.

Warda, M. (1992). The family and chronic sorrow: Role theory approach. *Journal of Pediatric Nursing, 7,* 205-209.

Watson, A. (1972). A study of family attitudes to children with diabetes. *Community Health, 128,* 122-125.

Watt-Watson, J. H., Evernden, C., & Lawson, C. (1990). Parents' perceptions of their child's acute pain experience. *Journal of Pediatric Nursing, 5,* 344-349.

Weathersby, A. M., Lobo, M. L., & Williamson, D. (1995). Parent and student preferences for services in a school-based clinic. *Journal of School Health, 65,* 14-17.

Webb, C. J., Stergios, D. A., & Rodgers, B. M. (1989). Patient-controlled analgesia as postoperative pain treatment for children. *Journal of Pediatric Nursing, 4,* 162-171.

Wehr, E., & Jameson, E. J. (1994). Beyond benefits: The importance of a pediatric standard in private insurance contracts to ensuring health care access for children. *The Future of Children, 4*(3), 115-133.

Weichler, N. K. (1990). Information needs of mothers of children who have had liver transplants. *Journal of Pediatric Nursing, 5,* 88-96.

Weidman, W., Kwiterovich, P., Jesse, M. E., & Nugent, E. (1983). Diet in the healthy child: American Heart Association Nutrition Committee and the Cardiovascular Disease in the Young Council of the American Heart Association. *Circulation, 67,* 1411A-1414A.

Weissberg, R., & Elias, M. (1993). Enhancing young people's social competence and health behavior: An important challenge for educators, scientists, policy makers, and funders. *Applied and Preventive Psychology, 2,* 179-190.

Wells, M., Riera-Fanego, J. F., Luyt, D. K., Dance, M., & Lipman, J. (1996). Poor discriminatory performance of the pediatric risk of mortality (PRISM) score in a South African intensive care unit. *Critical Care Medicine, 24,* 1507-1513.

West, C. (1885). *The mother's manual of children's diseases.* New York: Appleton.

West, C. (1954). *How to nurse sick children.* London: Longman. (Original work published 1854)

Whalen, K. (1996). *Familial aggregation of health behaviors during the school-age adolescent transition.* Dissertation proposal in progress, University of Pennsylvania.

Whall, A., & Loveland-Cherry, C. (1993). Family unit research in nursing. In H. Werley & J. J. Fitzpatrick (Eds.), *Annual review of nursing research* (pp. 227-247). New York: Springer.

Whatley, J. H. (1991). Effects of health locus of control and social network on adolescent risk taking. *Pediatric Nursing, 17,* 145-148.

White, M. A., Williams, P. D., Alexander, D. J., Powell-Cope, G. M., & Conlon, M. (1990). Sleep onset latency and distress in hospitalized children. *Nursing Research, 39,* 134-139.

Whitehead, B. D. (1993). Dan Quayle was right. *Atlantic Monthly, 271,* 47-84.

Willard, J. C., & Schoenborn, C. A. (1995). Relationship between cigarette smoking and other unhealthy behaviors among our nation's youth: United States, 1992. *Advance Data, 263,* 1-12.

Williams, B. C., & Miller, C. A. (1992). Preventive health care for young children: Findings from a 10-country study and directions for United States policy. *Pediatrics, 89*(Suppl. 5), 983-998.

Williams, D. M. (1989). Political theory and individualistic health promotion. *Advances in Nursing Science, 12*(1), 14-25.

Williams, D. S., & Davis, C. E. (1994). Reporting of assignment methods in clinical trials. *Controlled Clinical Trials, 15,* 294-298.

Williams, J. K. (1995). Parenting a daughter with precocious puberty or Turner syndrome. *Journal of Pediatric Health Care, 9,* 109-114.

Williams, J. K., & Lessick, M. (1996). Genome research: Implications for children. *Pediatric Nursing, 22,* 40-46.

Williams, P. D., Lorenzo, F. D., & Borja, M. (1993). Pediatric chronic illness: Effects on siblings and mothers. *Maternal-Child Nursing Journal, 21,* 111-121.

Wills, J. M. (1983). Concerns and needs of mothers providing home care for children with tracheostomies. *Maternal-Child Nursing Journal, 12,* 89-108.

Wilson, C. C. (1991). The pet as an anxiolytic intervention. *Journal of Nervous and Mental Diseases, 179,* 482-489.

Wilson, C. J. (1987). Comparison of two methods of preparation for hospitalization. *Children's Health Care, 16,* 24-27.

Witter, D. M. (1996). Transforming paradigms for provider information systems. *Quality Management in Health Care, 4*(2), 7-13.

Wojner, A. (1996). Outcomes management: An interdisciplinary search for best practice. *American Association of Critical Care Nurses Clinical Issues, 7,* 135-145.

Wolfer, J. A., & Visintainer, M. A. (1975). Pediatric surgical patients' and parents' stress responses and adjustment as a function of psychological preparation and stress-point nursing care. *Nursing Research, 24,* 244-255.

Wolfer, J. A., & Visintainer, M. A. (1979). Prehospital psychological preparation for tonsillectomy patients: Effects on children's and parent's adjustment. *Pediatrics, 64,* 646-655.

Wood, M. (1992). The international classification in primary care: Health information for the future. In M. Stewart, F. Tudiver, M. J. Bass, E. V. Dunn, & P. G. Norton (Eds.), *Tools for primary care research* (pp. 36-49). Newbury Park, CA: Sage.

Woods, L. G. (1979). Dominant coping behaviors of a hospitalized four-year-old deaf boy. *Maternal-Child Nursing Journal, 8,* 181-193.

World Health Organization. (1984). *Health promotion: A discussion document on the concept and principles: Summary report of the working group on concept and principles of health promotion.* Copenhagen: Author.

Wright, L. M., & Leahey, M. (1990). Trends in nursing of families. *Journal of Advanced Nursing, 15,* 148-154.

Wright, L. M., & Leahey, M. (1994a). *Nurses and families: A guide to family assessment and intervention* (2nd ed.). Philadelphia: F. A. Davis.

Wright, L. M., & Leahey, M. (1994b). Calgary Family Intervention Model: One way to think about change. *Journal of Marital and Family Therapy, 20,* 381-395.

Wright, L. M., & Levac, A. M. (1992). The non-existence of non-compliant families: The influence of Humberto Maturana. *Journal of Advanced Nursing, 17,* 913-917.

Wright, L. M., Watson, W. L., & Bell, J. M. (1990). The family nursing unit: A unique integration of research, education and clinical practice. In J. M. Bell, W. L. Watson, & L. M. Wright (Eds.), *The cutting edge of family nursing* (pp. 95-112). Calgary, Alberta, Canada: Family Nursing Unit Publications.

Wuest, J. (1991). Harmonizing: A North American Indian approach to management of middle ear disease with transcultural nursing implications. *Journal of Transcultural Nursing, 3*(1), 5-14.

Wuest, J., & Stern, P. N. (1990a). Childhood otitis media: The family's endless quest for relief. *Issues in Comprehensive Pediatric Nursing, 13,* 25-39.

Wuest, J., & Stern, P. N. (1990b). The impact of fluctuating relationships with the Canadian health care system on family management of otitis media with effusion. *Journal of Advanced Nursing, 15,* 556-563.

Wuest, J., & Stern, P. N. (1991). Empowerment in primary health care: The challenge for nurses. *Qualitative Health Research, 1,* 80-99.

Yarcheski, A., Mahon, N. E., & Yarcheski, T. J. (1992). Validation of the PRQ85 social support measure for adolescents. *Nursing Research, 41,* 332-337.

Yeh, T. S., Pollack, M. M., Holbrook, P. R., Fields, A. I., & Ruttimann, U. (1982). Assessment of pediatric intensive care: Application of the therapeutic intervention scoring system. *Critical Care Medicine, 10,* 497-500.

Young, J. (1992). Changing attitudes towards families of hospitalized children from 1935 to 1975: A case study. *Journal of Advanced Nursing, 17,* 1422-1429.

Young, R. (1977). Chronic sorrow: Parents' responses to the birth of a child with a defect. *MCN: American Journal of Maternal-Child Nursing, 1,* 38-42.

Youngblut, J. M., Brennan, P. F., & Swegart, L. A. (1994). Families with medically fragile children: An exploratory study. *Pediatric Nursing, 20,* 463-468.

Youngblut, J. M., & Casper, G. R. (1993). Single-item indicators in nursing research. *Research in Nursing and Health, 16,* 459-465.

Youngblut, J. M., & Jay, S. S. (1991). Emergent admission to the pediatric intensive care unit: Parental concerns. *Clinical Issues in Critical Care Nursing, 2,* 329-337.

Youngblut, J. M., & Shiao, S.-Y. P. (1992). Characteristics of a child's critical illness and parents' reactions: Preliminary report of a pilot study. *American Journal of Critical Care, 1,* 80-84.

Youngblut, J. M., & Shiao, S.-Y. P. (1993). Child and family reactions during and after pediatric ICU hospitalization: A pilot study. *Heart and Lung, 22,* 46-54.

Youssef, M. M. S. (1981). Self-control behaviors of school-age children who are hospitalized for cardiac diagnostic procedures. *Maternal-Child Nursing Journal, 10,* 219-284.

Zadinsky, J. K., & Boettcher, J. H. (1992). Preventability of infant mortality in a rural community. *Nursing Research, 41,* 223-227.

Zelizer, V. (1985). *Pricing the priceless child: The changing social value of children.* New York: Basic Books.

Zhu, B. P., Lemeshow, S., Hosmer, D. W., Klar, J., Avrunin, J., & Teres, D. (1996). Factors affecting the performance of the models in the Mortality Probability Model II system and strategies of customizing: A simulation study. *Critical Care Medicine, 24,* 57-63.

Ziglio, E. (1991). Indicators of health promotion policy: Directions for research. In B. Bandura & I. Kickbusch (Eds.), *Health promotion research: Towards a new social epidemiology* (WHO Regional Publications, European Series, No. 37, pp. 55-83). Copenhagen: World Health Organization.

Zismer, D. K. (1994). *Integrated health systems.* Minneapolis: Partners Consulting Group.

NAME INDEX

Abbot, G., 10
Abbott, N. C., 105
Abrams, L., 105
Abramson, I. S., 74
Achenbach, T. M., 201, 202, 203, 216, 217, 239
Achterberg, C. L., 71
Ackerley, G., 4
Adamo, F., 136, 138
Adams, G., 201, 203
Aday, L. A., 281, 282
Agency for Health Care Policy and Research, 171, 274, 276, 284
Aiken, L. H., 272, 276
Ainsworth, M., 41
Airhihenbuwa, C. O., 85
Ajzen, I., 58, 61, 62
Alex, M. R., 133, 134, 135
Alexander, D. J., 152, 153
Alpert, J., 74
Alpha Center, 271, 272
Altimier, L., 134, 135
Altman, D., 159, 276
Ament, M. E., 136
American Academy of Pediatrics, 258, 259, 262
American Association of Critical Care Nurses, 170
American Heart Association, 69
American Nurses Association Commission on Nursing Research, 110
Anderson, E. T., 80, 81, 91
Anderson, G. C., 109, 194
Anderson, G. F., 285, 290
Anderson, J., 190
Anderson, J. M., 187, 190, 194, 245

Anderson, O., 253
Anderson, R. A., 85
Anderson, W. T., 205, 207
Andersson-Segesten, K., 187
Anglim, M. A., 222
Angst, D. B., 181, 185
Angulo, J., 40
Annie E. Casey Foundation, 275
Anthony, M. A., 251, 265, 266
Aradine, C., 186, 191, 192
Aradine, C. R., 107
Arbeit, M. L., 65, 66, 67, 78, 83, 85, 93
Archbold, P. G., 241, 288
Armitage, P., 159
Armstrong, G. D., 222, 255
Armstrong, M. A., 293
Asarnow, J. R., 80
Ashley, J., 264
Ashley, L. C., 107
Asprey, J. R., 134, 135
Atkins, C. J., 74
Atkinson, B. A., 100, 104
Austin, J. K., 182, 186, 189, 194, 197, 200, 202, 203, 204, 205, 207, 208, 216, 217, 218, 237, 239
Autio, L., 131, 132
Avrunin, J., 293
Ayres, L., 186, 190

Badger, G. J., 63
Bagarozzi, D. A., 207
Bailey, T. F., 105
Baker, C. D., 208
Baker, J. P., 9, 253, 256-257
Baker, S. J., 9, 10

Bakewell-Sachs, S., 223, 232, 260
Bales, S. N., 276, 277
Bandak, A. G., 125, 132
Bandura, A., 48, 58, 61, 63, 66, 68, 69, 72, 78, 83
Bane, M. J., 278
Bangdiwala, S. I., 69, 71, 77, 83
Bangdiwala, S. J., 69, 71
Baranowski, T., 63, 64
Barkauskas, V. H., 80, 81, 91
Barlow, J., 182
Barlow, R. S., 136, 137, 138
Barnard, K., 57
Barnard, K. E., 17, 23, 101, 109, 193, 222
Barnes, C. M., 108, 110, 125, 127, 130, 132
Barnsteiner, J., 170
Baroni, M., 91, 174
Bartlett, L., 273, 277
Barton, L., 128, 131, 204
Barton, W., 5
Basch, C. E., 84
Bates, J. E., 17
Batey, M. V., 193
Bauman, K. E., 17
Baumrind, D., 74
Bazron, B. J., 169
Beal, J., 193
Beal, J. A., 144, 169, 182, 194, 222, 234
Beardslee, C. I., 125, 132
Beardslee, C. J., 127, 128, 129, 132, 185
Beatrice, D., 276
Beaven, P. W., 114
Beaver, C. F., 84, 85
Beck, A. T., 201

Beck, C. T., 38, 39, 181, 182, 194
Beck, M., 186
Becker, A. M., 222, 234
Becker, M. H., 48, 53, 58
Beckett, L. A., 189, 202, 206, 208, 216
Beckstrand, J., 136, 137, 138
Bee, H. L., 109
Begley, C. E., 281, 282
Behar, L., 45
Behrman, R. E., 275
Bell, J., 194, 241, 242
Bell, J. M., 71, 244
Bell, M. A., 45, 46, 87
Bennett, D. S., 217
Bennion, L., 201, 203
Benoliel, J., 232
Benoliel, J. Q., 188
Berenson, G. S., 65, 66, 67, 78, 83, 85
Bergman, R. L., 265
Bernier, J. A., 283, 290
Bernier-Henn, M., 189
Bertram, D. A., 292
Best, J. A., 88
Betz, C. L., 144, 169, 182, 193, 194, 222, 234
Beuman, E., 205
Beyer, J. E., 107, 133
Beyers, M., 265
Bibace, R., 58, 63
Biordi, D., 192
Bixler, G. K., 100
Black, M., 225, 226, 229, 230, 231, 233, 241
Black, M. M., 75, 76
Blackburn, S., 109
Blain, M. D., 221, 223
Blake, F., 13
Blake, F. G., 179
Blehar, M., 41
Blendon, R. J., 276
Block, J., 74
Bloom, F., 277
Bloom, S., 236, 237
Bloom, S. R., 274, 290
Blumberg, M. S., 281, 282
Blumenthal, S. J., 57, 72
Bogetz, M. S., 104
Bolduan, C., 9
Bomar, P., 13
Bonner, M. J., 235, 243
Bonsel, G. J., 294
Bookbinder, M., 144, 145, 147
Borja, M., 188, 205, 209
Bossert, E., 126, 127, 130, 132, 184, 190

Both, D. R., 269, 270, 271, 274, 275
Bottorff, J. L., 85
Botvin, G. J., 83, 84
Bowditch, B., 188
Bowlby, J., 87, 88, 181
Boyce, W., 45
Bradbury, D., 10
Bradley, C. B., 69, 71
Bradley, R. H., 17
Brailer, D. J., 286, 292
Braithwaite, F. L., 93
Brandt, E. N., 81
Brandt, P., 222, 234
Brandt, P. A., 41, 225, 226, 228, 229, 231, 233, 241
Bransetter, E., 104
Brazelton, T. B., 17
Breitmayer, B., 188, 189, 190, 192, 193, 194, 197, 200, 202, 209, 210, 212, 213
Breitmayer, B. J., 184, 186, 197, 200, 202, 210, 213
Brennan, A., 222, 234
Brennan, P. F., 189
Brent, N., 260
Bretherton, I., 91
Brimmer, P. F., 112
Brittain, E., 159
Brodie, B., 4, 100, 111, 112, 113
Bronfenbrenner, U., 72, 75, 76, 78, 90, 191
Brook R., 282
Broome, M., 91, 168, 169, 170, 173, 174, 175, 184
Broome, M. E., 107, 132, 145, 146, 153, 160, 170, 184, 221
Brooten, D., 109, 223, 232, 260
Brostrom, M. B., 273, 277
Brouhard, B., 225, 227, 228, 231, 234
Brown, J. S., 102
Brown, L., 223, 232, 260
Brown, S. S., 272
Brownlee-Duffeck, M., 166
Bru, G., 144, 145, 147
Brubaker, B. H., 80
Bruhn, J. G., 53, 68, 69, 70, 71, 86
Bryant, G., 88
Buckwalter, K., 121
Budetti, P., 272, 273
Bulechek, G. M., 143, 160, 161, 167, 222, 234, 242, 243
Bullock, D. H., 87
Bunker, J. F., 63
Burch, S., 265, 266
Burdine, J. N., 92
Burke, M. L., 187

Burke, S. O., 122, 182, 183, 192, 193, 194, 221, 223
Burkhardt, P. V., 187, 211, 214
Burns, A. C., 58
Burns, C., 51, 52, 53
Burns, K., 168
Burroughs, T. E., 137
Bush, P. J., 58, 59, 60, 86
Butcher, A. H., 65, 66, 83, 85
Butts, P., 223, 232, 260
Butz, A. M., 261
Byers, M. L., 107
Byrne, W. J., 136

Caire, J. B., 145, 148, 153
Caldwell, B. M., 17
Call, J. D., 104
Call, T., 110
Callery, P., 192
Callow, L., 264
Cameron, J., 264
Cameron, M. E., 90, 126, 127, 129, 131, 132, 182, 183, 185, 200, 201, 202, 203, 204, 205, 206, 208
Camitta, B. M., 222
Camp, R. C., 294
Camp, T. L., 264
Campbell, L., 111
Canam, C., 187, 190
Caplan, G., 91
Capuzzi, C., 191
Carabott, J. A., 155, 158, 159
Carey, M. E., 183
Carey, T., 80
Carey, W. B., 17
Carlson, E., 91
Carlson, K., 170
Carlson, K. L., 45, 46, 93, 106, 107, 145, 156, 158
Carmody, S., 144, 145, 147
Carnegie Corporation of New York, 270, 275
Carnegie Council on Children, 269, 271, 276
Carnegie, M. E., 113
Carrieri, V. K., 183
Carter, M. C., 105, 108, 120, 121, 164
Carter, W., 276
Carter, W. B., 61, 62
Carty, R. M., 108
Caruso, J., 136, 138
Casanova, C., 289
Caserza, C. L., 104
Casper, G. R., 133

Cassetta, R. A., 93
Cassidy, J., 91
Castiglia, P., 23, 28, 87
Caty, S., 103, 105, 125, 126, 127,
    130, 132, 183
Cauble, E., 205, 208
Cavillari, K., 164
Cedargren, D., 189, 190
Center for Health Economics
    Research, 276
Center for Studying Health
    Systems Change, 275
Center for the Future of Children,
    271, 272, 275
Chafel, J. A., 273
Chamberlain, R. W., 93, 223
Chamorro, I., 109
Chang, W. S., 292
Chard, M. A., 257, 258
Charron-Prochownik, D., 182
Chiafery, M., 119, 120
Child, D. A., 192
Children's Defense Fund, 273
Childs, R. E., 191
Chiofalo, N., 225, 226, 227, 228,
    229, 231, 233, 234, 241
Chipman, M., 293
Chipman, S. S., 74
Christian, B. J., 187, 189
Chung, J., 190
Chung, K. L., 137
Church, R., 14
Clancy, C., 283
Clancy, G. M., 225, 226, 231, 233
Claris, O., 293
Clark, C. G., 187
Clark, L. M., 184
Clatworthy, S., 104, 126, 128, 129,
    131, 132, 144, 145
Clayton, S. L., 100
Clements, D. B., 186, 210, 211, 214
Clubb, R. L., 187
Coates, P. M., 72, 84, 87, 93
Cochran, S. W., 205, 207
Coffman, S., 37, 38, 40, 41, 87
Cohen, D. C., 74
Cohen, F., 187
Cohen, M. H., 186, 190, 211, 215
Cohen, S., 6
Cohens, N., 109, 260
Coie, J. D., 80
Cole, M., 111
Cole, R., 260
Collier, J., 103, 104
Comeau, J. K., 205, 208
Committee on Bioethics, 168
Condit, K., 273

Cone, T. E., Jr., 12, 100, 253, 257
Conlon, M., 152, 153
Connell, D. B., 231
Conway, A. E., 137, 138
Coontz, S., 237
Coopersmith, S., 201, 203
Copeland, L., 186, 189
Copeland, L. G., 186, 210, 211, 214
Copeland, S. G., 35, 40, 199
Corbo-Richert, B. H., 125, 127,
    130, 132
Corliss, L., 6
Cormier, P. P., 102, 103
Corser, N., 191
Cortner, J. A., 71
Costello, E. A., 122, 192
Cotler, J., 261
Coughlin, T. A., 273
Covotsos, L., 9, 10
Cowell, J., 51
Cowen, E. L., 93
Cowen, J. S., 293
Cox, C. L., 51
Coyne, J. C., 27
Crabtree, M. K., 171
Craft, M., 121
Craft, M. J., 194, 222, 225, 226,
    228, 231, 233, 234
Crain, W., 111
Crandall, E., 260
Crane, J., 171
Cranley, M. S., 41
Cravens, H., 8
Crockett, L. J., 85
Crooks, C. E., 93
Cross, T. L., 169
Crummette, B., 191, 192
Cruz-Collins, M., 61, 77, 89
Cuerdon, T., 293
Cunningham, P. J., 271, 273
Curley, M., 135
Currie, J., 254
Cutrona, C. E., 40
Cystic Fibrosis Foundation, 180
Czarnecki, M. T., 294, 296

Dabbs, J. M., 110
Dahlen, G., 72
Dahm, J., 109, 194
Dale, S., 184
Dambacher, B. M., 104
Damrosch, S. P., 187
Dance, M., 294
Danek, G. D., 154, 158
Danesco, E. R., 75, 76
D'Antonio, I., 191

Dashiff, C., 187, 190, 211, 214
D'Auria, J., 166
Davies, L. K., 188
Davies, R., 172
Davis, C. E., 159
Davis, H. W., 189
Davis, J. H., 104
Davis, K., 135
Davis, L. L., 222
Day, S. A., 100, 104
Deatrick, J., 183, 190, 193
Deatrick, J. A., 181, 185, 190, 193,
    194, 210, 212, 213, 218,
    231, 235, 242
Deeds, S. G., 68
DeFaire, U., 72
DeGood, D. E., 107
de LaPuente, J., 109
de la Sota, A., 225, 227, 228, 231,
    233, 234
Deliardo-Papadopoulos, M., 223,
    232, 260
DeMets, D. L., 159
Denehy, M. J., 91
Dennis, K., 169
Denyes, M., 133, 185
Denyes, M. J., 144, 185
DeVillis, R., 48
Dewis, M. E., 182, 183
Dick, M. J., 134, 135
DiClemente, C. C., 53
DiClemente, R. J., 23, 28
Dienneman, N., 170
Dierkes, M., 117, 122, 123, 124
Dihoff, R., 136, 138
Dillon, M. C., 122, 192
DiMarcello, K. J., 137, 139
Dittemore, I. L., 183, 184
Dixon, D., 164, 181, 187, 190, 193,
    240, 242
Dixon, D. M., 103
Dixon, P., 166
Dixon, S., 13
Doherty, W., 166
Donalson, G., 232
Donelan, K., 276
Donnelly, E., 189, 206, 207, 208
Donohue-Sword, B., 144, 145, 147
Dore, C. J., 159
Dougherty, G., 185, 225, 227, 228,
    229, 230, 231, 233, 234, 241
Driscoll, J., 135
Drotar, D., 217
Dryfoos, J., 262, 263
Dubovitz, B., 74
Duffy, J., 4, 11
Dunleavy, M. F., 104

Durand, B. A., 276, 286
Dusenbury, L., 83, 84, 88
Duvall, E. M., 124
Dye, J., 136, 137, 138

Eakes, G., 187
Eakes, G. G., 187
Earp, J. L., 81
Eberly, T. W., 120, 121, 164
Ebmeier, C., 131, 132
Eccles, J. S., 93
Edelbrock, C., 239
Edgil, A. E., 191
Edwards, J., 264
Edwards-Beckett, J., 189, 190
Egan, E., 168
Egeland, B., 91
Eggleston, P., 261
Eggly, S., 91
Eland, J. M., 105, 107
Elander, G., 134, 135
Elder, G. H., 93
Elder, J. P., 63, 64, 65, 71, 78, 79
Elfert, H., 187, 190
Elias, M., 263
Elizondo, A. P., 264
Elkind, D., 165
Ellerton, M., 105
Ellerton, M. L., 103, 125, 126, 130, 132, 183
Ellett, M., 136, 137, 138
Ellickson, P. L., 85
Ellis, J., 296
Ellis, M. K., 109, 194
Ellison, B. P., 278
Ellsworth, R. B., 201
Ellwood, D. T., 278
Ellwood, P., 281-282
Elston, R. C., 72
Endress, M., 105
Endress, M. P., 143
Endsley, R. C., 107, 145, 146, 153
Eng, B., 172
English, K., 285
Englund, S., 83
Epstein, L. H., 74
Erbaugh, J., 201
Erickson, R. S., 135
Erickson, S., 145, 148, 153
Erikson, E., 12, 111, 226
Escobar, G. J., 293
Esveldt-Dawson, K., 199
Ettinger, R. S., 225, 226, 228, 230, 231, 233, 234
Ettinger, S., 225, 226, 228, 230, 231, 233, 234
Euler, A. R., 136

Evans, K., 107
Evernden, C., 134, 135
Ewen, E., 9

Faber, H., 4
Fagan, C. L., 153, 154, 159
Fagin, C. M., 103
Faier-Routman, J., 182
Faulkner, M. S., 187
Faux, S. A., 183, 188, 191, 192, 193, 194, 218
Feather, N. T., 78
Federa, R. S., 264
Feeg, V., 170
Feeg, V. D., 290
Feetham, S., 68, 170, 222, 231, 235, 241, 286
Feetham, S. L., 71, 180, 188, 205, 207, 217, 276, 278, 285, 286
Fegley, B. J., 145, 148, 153
Fein, R., 278
Feinson, C., 272, 273
Feldman, H. A., 63, 71, 78
Ferguson, B. G., 105, 143
Ferguson, S., 254
Ferketich, S. L., 34, 40, 109
Ferrell, B. R., 117, 122, 123, 124
Feshbach, S., 201, 204
Field, M. J., 273
Fields, A. I., 293
Fine, G., 168
Fine, M., 205, 207
Fingerhut, L. A., 278
Fink, A., 173
Finkelstein, D., 274, 290
Finkler, S., 223, 232, 260
Finney, J. W., 235, 243
Fioravanti, I. D., 155, 158
Fischer, A., 293
Fiser, D. H., 294
Fishbein, M., 58, 61, 62
Fisher, K. W., 87
Fisher, M. D., 116, 117, 118, 122, 164
Fitzgerald, M., 101
Flaherty, M., 45
Flaskerud, J., 53
Fleming, J., 222, 234
Fleming, J. W., 128, 131, 204
Flexner, S., 100
Flint, S., 55
Flynn, B. S., 63
Foley, J., 163
Foley, M., 168
Folkman, S., 27, 183
Ford, M., 254
Ford, T. D., 16, 21, 87

Forrest, C. B., 283
Forsman, I., 84
Foster, M. S., 255, 256, 257
Foster, R., 133, 166
Fowler, E. J., 285, 290
Fox, H., 271
Fox, P. D., 263, 264
Fox, R. W., 201, 202
Fraley, A. M., 187
Frank, G. C., 65, 66, 83, 85
Frankish, C. J., 93
Frauman, A. C., 69, 71
Frauman, A. G., 69, 71, 77, 83
Fredrikzon, B., 145, 150, 153
Freeland, C. A. B., 17
Freeley, N., 185, 225, 227, 228, 229, 230, 231, 233, 234, 241
Freeman, H. E., 276, 277
Freire, P., 91
French, J. P., 136, 139
French, N. H., 199
French, S., 181
Freud, S., 12
Frey, M., 185
Friedman, L. M., 159
Frink, B. B., 170, 281, 283, 284, 285, 286, 288, 293, 294
Fuhrman, B. P., 293
Fullard, W., 17
Fuller, P. W., 109
Fulton, R. A. B., 184
Furberg, C. D., 159

Gaffney, K. F., 51, 52, 84
Gagliardi, B. A., 189, 190
Galanter, E., 87
Gallagher, J. J., 242
Gallagher, P. R., 72, 84, 87, 93
Gallo, A., 189, 190, 192, 193, 194, 210, 212
Gallo, A. M., 184, 186, 188, 190, 197, 200, 202, 209, 210, 213
Games, C., 136, 137, 138
Ganong, L. H., 194, 195, 240, 243
Gansky, S. A., 69, 71
Garcia Coll, C., 88
Garduque, L., 269, 270, 271, 274, 275
Garlinghouse, J., 184, 186
Gaut, D. A., 185
Gedaly-Duff, V., 107
Geeze, M. A., 264
Geis, D., 222
Geller, B. M., 63
Genet, M., 185
Gennaro, S., 109
Georgiadon, F., 232

Gerrity, P. S., 107
Gesell, A., 8
Getson, P. R., 117, 293
Gibbons, A., 223, 232, 260
Gibbons, C. L., 185
Gibbons, P., 107
Gibbons, P. T., 107
Gibson, C., 186, 187
Gibson, C. H., 187, 189
Gillies, D. A., 192
Gilliss, C. L., 71, 222
Gilliss, J. R., 237
Gillon, J. E., 191
Ginsburg, P. B., 273
Ginzberg, E., 88
Ginzburg, H., 111
Girouard, S., 276, 286, 289
Glass, N. L., 293
Glenister, A. M., 23, 28, 87
Glenville, C., 184
Glueck, C. J., 72
Gochman, D. S., 58
Godell, B., 232
Godfrey, A. E., 103
Goldman, L. R., 84
Goldmann, D. A., 293
Goldsmith, J. C., 265
Gonella, J. S., 293
Goodwin, L., 51
Goodwin, T., 40
Goon-Johnson, K., 225, 226, 228, 230, 231, 233, 234
Gordon, M., 51
Gortmaker, S., 181
Gortmaker, S. L., 196, 293
Gortner, S. R., 100, 101
Gorusch, R. L., 209
Gott, M., 91
Gottlieb, L., 185, 225, 227, 228, 229, 230, 231, 233, 234, 241
Gottlieb, L. N., 40, 122
Gottlieb, N. H., 92
Graeter, L. J., 289
Graham, C., 262
Graham, J., 291
Grant, G., 194
Grason, H. A., 273, 284
Gray, J. E., 293
Grebin, B., 297
Green, D., 109
Green, L. W., 68, 93
Green, M., 56, 58, 72, 74, 269, 270, 271, 274
Green, P., 72
Green, T., 65
Greenberg, L. G., 281, 282
Greenspan, P., 274, 290
Gremke, R. J., 294

Grey, M., 55, 90, 126, 127, 129, 131, 132, 182, 183, 185, 200, 201, 202, 203, 204, 205, 206, 208
Grey, M. J., 185
Grobe, S., 222
Grochowski, J., 204
Grodin, M. A., 113
Gröer, M. W., 40, 87
Gronseth, E., 222
Grotberg, E., 253, 261
Grotevant, H. D., 240
Guacci-Franco, N., 37, 38, 40, 41, 87
Gureno, M. A., 156, 158
Gustafson, K. E., 180
Gutierrez-Castrellon, P., 294
Guyer, B., 184, 273, 275, 284

Haase, J., 184, 275
Hader, D. F., 157, 158
Haggerty, J., 74
Haggerty, R. J., 277, 297
Hagopian, G. A., 194
Hahlen, K., 294
Hahn, B. A., 271, 273
Hainsworth, M. A., 187
Hainsworth, M. N., 187
Halfon, N., 284, 288, 290
Hall, C., 12
Hall, G. S., 8
Hall, J. H., 259
Halm, M., 121
Halper, A., 74
Halpern, S., 12
Hamburg, D. A., 269, 270, 273, 274, 275, 277
Hampshire, S., 87
Handley-Derry, M. H., 192
Hanrahan, K., 153, 154, 159
Hansen, P., 105
Hanson, J. L., 259
Hao, Y., 293
Harbaugh, B. L., 117, 184, 189
Harder, L., 188
Harkins, A., 185, 190
Harkins, J. A., 205, 208
Harlan, W. R., 57
Harless, L. S., 184
Harold, N., 262
Harper-Jacques, S., 245
Harrell, J., 78
Harrell, J. S., 69, 71, 77, 83
Harrigan, M. P., 200, 205, 207
Harris, D. M., 187
Harris, L. H., 205
Harrison, M. B., 223

Harsha, D., 65, 67, 70
Harsha, D. W., 65, 66, 67, 78, 83, 85
Hart, D., 126, 132, 184
Harter, S., 27, 201, 203
Harvey, B., 271, 273
Hasselmeyer, E. G., 109
Hatch, M. H., 74
Hatton, C., 225, 226, 229, 231, 241
Hatton, D., 187, 190
Hauck, M. R., 17, 24, 87
Haughey, B., 23, 28, 87
Hawkins, D., 80
Hawkins, J., 6
Hayduk, L. A., 85
Hayes, E., 6
Hayes, V. E., 192
Hayman, L., 80, 81, 91, 231
Hayman, L. L., 68, 72, 84, 87, 93
Hays, R. D., 85
Heamon, D. J., 185, 187
Hearn, M. D., 74
Heater, B. S., 222, 234
Heckel, R. N., 182, 188
Hedrick, G., 191
Heiney, S., 225, 226, 228, 230, 231, 233, 234
Heinrich, J., 288
Heller, D. A., 72
Hellier, A., 184
Hellier, A. P., 132, 184
Hellstrom, G., 134, 135
Henderson, C., 260
Henderson, C. R., 260
Hendricks, R., 255, 256, 257
Hennessey, J., 120, 121, 164
Hennessey, J. A., 103
Henrie, S., 136, 137, 138
Hepworth, J. T., 119, 120, 134, 135
Herbst, J. J., 187
Hess, J. H., 109
Hester, L., 171
Hester, N., 133, 166
Hester, N. K., 107
Hester, N. O., 51, 221
Heuch, I., 72
Heuer, L., 120, 121, 164
Hewitt, N., 61, 77, 89
Higgins, S. S., 193
Hill, C., 276
Hill, I. T., 273, 277
Hills, M. D., 91
Hills, R. G., 225, 226, 228, 230, 231, 233, 234
Hinds, P. S., 184
Hinshaw, A. S., 288
Hirose, T., 186
Hlusko, D. L., 285
Ho, V., 182

Hobbie, W. L., 84
Hobbs, N., 181, 182
Hobdell, E. F., 136, 138
Hochbaum, G. M., 58
Hodges, L. C., 186
Hoekelman, R. A., 275
Holaday, B., 23, 26, 180, 184, 185, 187, 190, 191, 194
Holbrook, P. R., 293
Holditch-Davis, D., 134, 135
Hollen, P. J., 84
Hollingsworth, A., 109, 260
Holman, E., 264
Holmes, S., 128, 131, 204
Holohan, J., 273
Holt, J. L., 104
Holt, L. E., 7-8, 13, 256, 257
Holzemer, W. L., 133, 134, 286
Homer, C. J., 274, 290
Horn, S. D., 292
Hornbrook, M. D., 293
Horsley, J., 171
Hosmer, D. W., 293
Hotaling, A. J., 260
Hougart, M. K., 285
Houtrouw, S. M., 45, 46, 93
Hovestadt, A. J., 205, 207
Hoyt, J. W., 292, 293
Huang, S. T. T., 189, 194
Hudson, W., 41
Hughes, A. M., 187, 190
Huh, K., 201, 203
Hunter, S. M., 65, 66, 67, 83, 85
Hurrelmann, K., 69, 83
Huss, K., 261
Huston, A. C., 88, 280
Hutchins, V., 252
Huth, M. M., 131, 132
Huttlinger, K., 171
Hymovich, D. P., 192, 194, 205, 208

Iannotti, R. J., 58, 59, 60, 86
Iezzoni, L. I., 281, 282, 292
Iffrig, S. M. C., 109
Iglehart, J. K., 272
Igoe, J. B., 78, 261, 262, 269, 273, 277, 296
Ilg, F., 8
Inhelder, B., 13, 58
Institute of Medicine, 281, 284
Ireys, H., 181, 182, 273, 284

Jackson, P. L., 187
Jacobi, Abraham, 7
Jacobs, G. A., 209
Jacobs, S., 292

Jaloweic, A., 204
James, S., 45
James, S. R., 267
Jameson, E. J., 273
Janson-Bjerklie, S., 183
Javaheri, Z., 155, 158, 159
Jean, S. L., 6-7
Jeans, P. C., 179
Jemmott, J. B., III, 61, 62, 77, 83, 87, 89
Jemmott, L. S., 61, 62, 77, 83, 87, 89
Jenson, E., 45
Jeppson, E., 163
Jeppson, E. S., 259
Jernell, J., 192
Jerrett, M. D., 107, 189, 190
Jesse, M. E., 65
Jessop, D. J., 180, 200, 201, 237
Jessop, S., 51
Jessor, R., 51
Jewell, N., 92, 93
John-Steiner, V., 111
Johnson, B., 163
Johnson, B. D., 134, 135
Johnson, B. H., 259
Johnson, C. C., 63, 65, 66, 67, 71, 78, 83, 85
Johnson, D. I., 288, 294
Johnson, J., 105
Johnson, J. E., 110, 143
Johnson, J. L., 85
Johnson, K., 286
Johnson, S. L., 121
Johnson, W. L., 112
Joint Commission for the Accreditation of Healthcare Organizations, 167, 281, 282
Jonas, S., 263
Jones, B., 293
Jones, D. C., 126, 127, 128, 131, 132
Jones, R., 232

Kachoyeanos, M., 136, 167
Kagan, B. M., 109
Kaiser Commission on the Future of Medicaid, 254
Kalberer, J. T., 57
Kalisch, B., 11
Kalisch, P., 11
Kanner, A. D., 27
Kanski, G., 23, 28, 87
Kanter, R. K., 293
Kaplan, E. B., 72
Kaplan, N., 91
Kaplan, S. C., 297

Karstens, A., 294
Katz, R. W., 293
Katz, V., 109
Katzman, E., 264
Kauffmann, E., 122, 192, 223
Kayser-Jones, J., 193
Kazdin, A. E., 199
Keady, J., 194
Keefe, M., 170
Keeler, E. B., 273
Keilty, K., 155, 158, 159
Keith, R. A., 218
Kelder, S. H., 63, 71, 78, 83
Keller, C., 184, 187, 203, 204, 208
Kelley, Florence, 9
Kelley, M. A., 293
Kelly, J., 286
Keniston, K., 269, 271, 276
Kennedy, A., 137
Kennedy, A. H., 18, 135
Kennedy, C. M., 149, 153
Kennedy-Malone, L., 173
Kenney, F. M., 110
Kerner, J. F., 88
Kerrigan, T., 135
Kersey, J., 222
Kessel, S. S., 278
Khampalikit, S., 191
Kiburz, J. A., 188
Kieckhefer, G. M., 182, 185
Kieckhefer, G., 183, 222, 234
Kikuchi, J. F., 191
Kim, A. C., 104
King, C., 252
Kirchhoff, K. T., 143
Kirchoff, K., 105
Kirschbaum, M., 118, 119, 123
Kirschbaum, M. S., 181, 193
Kirschbaum, R. M., 103
Kitzman, H., 260
Klar, J., 293
Kleiber, C., 121, 153, 154, 159, 165
Klerman, L., 262, 278
Klerman, L. V., 88, 93
Knafl, K. A., 103, 164, 169, 175, 181, 184, 186, 188, 189, 190, 192, 193, 194, 197, 200, 202, 209, 210, 212, 213, 218, 222, 235, 245
Knight, C., 225, 226, 229, 230, 231, 233, 241
Knox, J. E., 192
Knudtson, F., 109
Kogan, M. D., 278
Koizumi, S., 190
Kolbe, L. J., 53
Kollef, M. H., 293
Koontz, A. M., 278

Kosa, J., 74
Kotelchuck, M. L., 270, 274, 275, 278
Kovacs, M., 182, 201, 202, 217
Kozlowski, L. J., 137, 139
Kramer, M., 93, 109
Kremers, R., 293
Kreuter, M. W., 68
Kristensen, K., 133, 166
Kristjansdottir, G., 116, 122
Kronenfeld, J. J., 182
Kruger, S., 192
Krulik, T., 190
Ku, L., 273
Kueffner, M., 184
Kulwicki, A., 171
Kumar, S., 223, 232, 260
Kwiterovich, P., 65
Kyngas, H., 182

L'Abate, L., 207
LaBree, L., 74
Ladd-Taylor, M., 11
Laffrey, S. C., 80
La Greca, A. M., 217
Lai, M., 190
Lairson, D. R., 281, 282
Lakatos, I., 89, 91
Lakin, J. A., 225, 226, 231, 233
Lambert, S. A., 102
Lamberty, G., 57
Lammarino, N. K., 93
LaMontagne, L. L., 102, 103, 119, 120, 134, 135
Lancaster, J., 260
Lang, N. M., 288
Langley, P. A., 280
Lannon, C. M., 81
Lantigua, R., 84-85
Larner, M. B., 275
Larson, J., 11
Laskarzewski, P., 72
Latham, H. C., 182, 188
Lauer, M. E., 222
Lauffer, D., 264
Laughlin, J., 284
Lavee, Y., 205, 207
LaVigne, J., 182
Lavin, A. T., 27, 31, 83, 90
Lavizzo-Mourey, R., 232
Lawler, M. K., 185, 187, 200, 201, 202, 203, 204, 205, 206, 207
Lawless, S., 134, 135
Lawrence, M., 83
Lawson, C., 134, 135
Lazarus, R., 27, 183

Leahey, M., 41, 71, 180, 194, 222, 230, 231, 244, 245
Leake, B., 225, 226, 227, 228, 229, 231, 233, 234 241
LeBlanc, G., 135
Lederer, S. E., 113
Lee, B., 292
Lee, C. M., 221, 223
Leff, P., 236
Le Gall, J. R., 293
Leger, R. R., 137, 138
Leibowitz, A., 284, 288, 290
Leininger, L., 81
Lemeshow, S., 293
Lenart, J. C., 45, 46, 87
Lenihan, E. A., 103
Lenz, C., 264
Leonard, B. J., 192
Leonard, R. C., 105, 143
LeRoy, S., 264
Lessick, M., 84
Lessing, D., 259
Levac, A. M., 222
Leventhal, H., 110
Leventhal, J. M., 274, 290
Levine, A., 69, 71, 77, 83
Levitt, M. J., 37, 38, 40, 41, 87
Lewandowski, L. A., 108, 186
Lewin, D. J., 160
Lewis, C. E., 40, 58, 223, 241
Lewis, K., 105
Lewis, M. A., 40, 58, 223, 222, 225, 226, 227, 228, 229, 231, 233, 234, 241
Lewit, E. M., 273
Li, D. K., 293
Libby, L. J., 137
Libman, M., 135
Lightburn, A., 189
Lillis, P. P., 160
Limbo, R., 91
Linden, L., 285
Lindgren, C. L., 187
Lindgren, E. L., 187
Lindley, P., 85
Lindsay, E., 6, 91
Lipman, J., 294
Lipman, T. H., 90, 126, 127, 129, 131, 132, 182, 183, 185
Lipsey, M. W., 218
Lipshitz, M., 136, 137, 139
Little, S. D., 65, 66, 83, 85
Liu, K. R., 104
Liu, P., 293
LoBiondo-Wood, G., 189
Lockwood, N. L., 104, 144
Loehlin, J. C., 86
Loftus, L. G., 186, 210, 211, 214

Lohr, K., 282
Lohr, K. N., 281
Long, B., 80
Lord, S., 93
Lorenz, F. O., 217
Lorenzo, F. D., 188, 205, 209
Losty, M., 109
Lothman, D. J., 217
Lough, M. A., 131, 132
Louis, D. Z., 293
Lounsbury, M. L., 17
Loveland-Cherry, C., 71
Loveland-Cherry, C. J., 80
Luepker, R. V., 63, 67, 71, 74, 78
Luft, H. S., 287
Lum, M. R., 280
Lundeen, E., 109
Lundeen, E. C., 109
Luscher, M., 204
Lushene, R., 209
Lutkenhoff, M.L., 225, 226, 228, 230, 231, 233, 234
Luyt, D. K., 294
Lynch, M., 149, 153
Lynn, M. R., 103, 105
Lythcott, N., 93

Macbriar, B. R., 184
MacDonald, H., 187
MacDorman, M., 184, 275
MacInnis, H., 222
MacPherson, A., 181
Madden, M., 181, 185
Madgy, D. N., 260
Maglacas, A. M., 91
Magyary, D., 222, 234
Magyary, D. L., 225, 226, 228, 229, 231, 233, 241
Mahaffy, P. R., 102, 143
Mahon, M. M., 104
Maieron, M. J., 103, 104
Maile, M. C., 74
Maiman, L. A., 58
Main, M., 91
Maligalig, R., 165
Malm, K. C., 187
Malveaux, F., 261
Mandelblatt, J. S., 88
Manger, G., 155, 158, 159
Manning, W. G., 273
Mansson, M. E., 145, 150, 153
Mardiros, M., 186, 187
Marek, K. D., 288
Margolis, P. A., 80
Marino, B. L., 136, 137, 139
Marion, L., 51
Markman, H. J., 80

Marshall, V., 181
Martel, J. K., 71
Martin, J., 184
Martin, J. A., 184, 275
Martin, K., 222
Martinez-Natera, O., 294
Martinson, E., 222
Martinson, I., 191, 222
Martinson, I. M., 186
Mason, E., 231
Mason, J. O., 81, 82
Mathews, S., 51
Matthews, K., 57, 72
Matthews, K. A., 40
Maulen-Radovan, I., 294
McBride, A. B., 189, 194
McBride, M. R., 109, 194
McCaffery, M., 104
McCain, G. C., 103
McCarthy, S. M., 190, 210, 212
McCarty, K., 135
McClearn, G. E., 72
McCloskey, J. C., 143, 160, 161,
   167, 222, 234, 242, 243
McClowry, S. G., 102, 129, 131
McCorkle, R., 232
McCormick, M. C., 293
McCoy-Thompson, M., 277
McCubbin, H., 165, 166
McCubbin, H. I., 41, 71, 189, 195,
   204, 205, 206, 208
McCubbin, M., 165
McCubbin, M. A., 189, 194, 195,
   205, 208
McCurley, J., 74
McDermott, N., 189
McDevitt, S. C., 17
McGill, J., 145, 156, 158
McGillicuddy, M. C., 103
McGinnis, J. M., 81, 84
McGlynn, E. A., 284, 288, 290
McGrath, P. A., 107, 108
McGraw, S. A., 63, 64, 65, 78, 79
McIntosh, R., 4
McKeever, P. T., 186, 187
McKeon, T., 294
McKinlay, J. B., 84, 88
McKinlay, S. M., 63, 71, 78
McLaren, H. H., 201, 202
McLaughlin, J. S., 80, 84, 88
McLeroy, K. R., 92
McLoyd, V. C., 88
McManus, M., 271
McMullen, A., 155, 158
McMurray, R. G., 69, 71, 77, 83
McNally, J., 261
McNeeley, G., 13

McNelis, A. M., 189, 194, 200,
   202, 203, 204, 205, 207
Means, R., 7
Measel, C. P., 109
Mechanic, D., 276
Meckel, R., 5
Medoff-Cooper, B., 109
Meeropol, E., 137, 138
Megivern, K., 121
Meier, P., 109, 191
Meininger, J. C., 72, 84, 87, 93
Meister, S. B., 71, 273, 276, 277,
   278, 286
Melamed, B. C., 105
Melby, J. N., 217
Meleis, A. I., 81, 94
Melnyk, B. M., 145, 151, 153
Melvin, P. M., 5
Members of the Multi-Institutional
   Study Group, 293
Mendelson, M., 201
Mendelson, M. J., 40
Mendez, L., 40
Meng, A., 105
Mengel, M. B., 185, 200, 201, 202,
   203, 204, 205, 206, 207
Menke, E. M., 188
Mercer, R. T., 34, 40, 109, 191
Mezey, M., 232
Mickalide, A., 58, 63
Midence, K., 218
Miles, M., 78, 166
Miles, M. S., 105, 108, 120, 121,
   164
Miles, T., 100, 104, 111
Milio, N., 78, 85, 286
Miller, B. A., 87
Miller, B. C., 217
Miller, C. A., 94
Miller, E., 51
Miller, K. L., 184
Millstein, S. G., 57, 72, 84
Mitchell, K. E., 121
Mitchell, P. H., 288
Mittrucker, C., 18, 135
Mobley, C. E., 184
Mock, J., 201
Moinpour, C., 232
Monahan, G. H., 144, 149
Monroe, B. H., 109, 260
Monsen, R. B., 185
Montgomery, L., 165
Montgomery, L. A., 121
Moon, M., 273, 276
Moore, C., 190
Moore, C. M., 184, 193, 194, 218
Moore, J. B., 51, 52, 84, 185
Moos, B., 43, 45, 51

Moos, R., 43, 45, 51
Moos, R. H., 76
Moravcsik, J., 276
Moritz, P., 284
Morris, J. A., 74
Morris, N. M., 74, 205
Morrison, M., 109
Morrow, J. D., 183
Mortensen, M. E., 289
Mortiz, P., 288
Morton, L. I., 103
Moser Woo, T., 135
Mott, D. S., 65, 66, 67, 78, 83, 85
Mudge, C., 165
Mulhern, R. K., 222
Mulligan, J. E., 10
Mullins, J., 237
Munet-Vilaro, F., 185, 190
Murigande, C., 261
Murphy, K. M., 189, 190
Murphy, S. P., 204
Murray, D. M., 74

Nader, P. R., 63, 71, 72, 73, 74, 78
Nahm, H., 100, 101
Nair, P., 225, 226, 229, 230, 231,
   233, 241
Namboodiri, K. K., 72
Napier, L., 109
Natapoff, J., N., 58, 271, 273, 277
National Association of Children's
   Hospitals and Related
   Institutions, 168, 171, 172,
   285, 289, 294, 295, 297
National Campaign to Prevent Teen
   Pregnancy, 275, 276
National Institute of Nursing
   Research (NINR), 56, 61,
   69, 78, 94, 167, 172, 278
Nauen, C. M., 109
Naylor, M., 232
Neal, M., 109
Neal, M. V., 101, 193
Neff, E. J., 127, 128, 129, 132, 185
Nehring, W., 187
Nelms, B. C., 185, 200, 202, 203,
   204
Nesbit, M. E., 222
Neveling, E., 136, 138
Nevin, R. S., 205, 208
Newacheck, P., 180, 271
Newell, M., 264
Newhouse, J. P., 273
Newson, G., 271, 273
Nicholls, P., 184
Nicholls, R., 184, 187, 203, 204,
   208

Nichols, B. S., 285
Nicholson, A., 121
Nicklas, T. A., 65, 66, 67, 78, 83, 85
Nightingale, E. O., 84
Nightingale, F., 80, 86, 100, 260, 288
Nocera, M., 136, 139
Nolan, M., 194, 288
Noris, E. M., 154, 158
Norris, J., 191
Norusis, M., 293
Norwood, S., 134, 135
Nowacek, G. A., 85
Nugent, E., 65
Nunnally, J. C., 124
Nusbaum, J. G., 103
Nuttall, P., 184
Nutting, P. L., 23, 83
Nyamathi, A., 53
Nyberg, D., 288

Oaks, J., 70
Obrecht, J., 190
O'Brien, M., 91
Obrosky, D. S., 182
O'Connor-Von, S., 170
Ogilvie, L., 192
Ogletree, G., 191
O'Keefe, S., 297
Olds, D. L., 260
Oleson, R., 76
Olson, D. H., 205, 207
Olson, R. K., 222, 234
O'Malley, P. M., 85
Opper, S., 111
Oppliger, R. A., 225, 226, 231, 233
Orem, D. E., 51, 53, 111, 168
Orlofsky, I., 109
Ory, M. G., 182
Osbahr, B., 128, 131, 204
Osganian, S. K., 63, 64, 78, 79
O'Sullivan, A., 62
O'Sullivan, P., 194
Owen, N., 72, 75, 76, 84, 90

Padgett, D., 222, 234
Padrick, K. P., 102
Palfrey, J. S., 268, 269, 271, 272, 274, 275, 276, 277, 278
Palmer, I., 13
Palmer, M., 261
Pandit, P., 293
Parcel, G., 63, 64
Parcel, G. S., 53, 63, 68, 69, 70, 71, 78, 86
Parker, J., 186

Parker, J. B., 109
Partridge, K. B., 68
Patel, K. M., 293
Patterson, J., 168
Patterson, J. M., 192, 204, 205, 206, 240
Patterson, T. L., 74
Patteson, D., 109
Patton, A. C., 184
Paul, S. M., 133
Pauly, M., 232
Pawlak, R., 119, 120
Peacock, J., 45
Pedersen, N. L., 72
Pederson, C., 184
Peebles, A. Y., 109
Pender, A. R., 45, 48, 53, 57, 69, 71, 77, 85, 94
Pender, N. J., 45, 72, 77, 78, 80, 81, 91
Peplau, H. E., 40
Perkins, M., 231
Perkins, M. T., 122, 189, 192
Perlman, M., 293
Perrin, E. C., 107, 217
Perrin, J., 180, 181, 182, 236, 237, 285, 293
Perrin, J. M., 274, 290
Perry, C., 63, 64, 74
Perry, C. L., 63, 67, 71, 78, 83
Perry, L. A., 187
Petersen, A. C., 84, 85
Peterson, J., 118, 119, 123
Peterson, L., 166
Peto, R., 159
Phibbs, C. S., 293
Phifer, L. C., 137, 139
Philichi, L. M., 118, 123, 124
Phillips, M., 187, 211, 213
Piaget, J., 12-13, 58, 104, 111, 185
Pianta, R. C., 217
Picard, M., 221, 223
Piercy, F. P., 205, 207
Piers, E. V., 201, 203
Pike, M. C., 159
Pill, R., 88
Pilletteri, A., 192
Pine, M., 293
Pinelli, J., 191
Pinyerd, B. J., 188
Pless, B. P., 275
Pless, I. B., 185, 225, 227, 228, 229, 230, 231, 233, 234, 241, 277, 293
Plomin, R., 73, 74, 84
Plos, K., 187
Poets, C., 167
Pollack, M. M., 117, 293, 294

Pollack, V., 155, 158
Pollitt, E., 88
Pontius, S., 18, 135
Pontius, S. L., 137
Popenoe, D., 237
Porter, C., 43, 45, 87
Porter, J. E., 296
Porter, L. S., 109
Portner, J., 205, 207
Powell-Cope, G. M., 152, 153
Powers, M. J., 204
Price, P. J., 189
Pridham, K. F., 76, 80, 87, 88, 91, 174
Pridham, K. H., 87
Prochaska, J. O., 53
Proctor, D. L., 108
Prosser, M. J., 191
Prugh, D. G., 103
Pugh, E., 109
Pulkininen, L., 74

Qvarnstrom, B., 134, 135

Radbill, S. X., 100, 252, 255, 256
Rader, B., 165
Radloff, L. S., 41
Rafkin, H. S., 292, 293
Ramey, S. L., 80
Rancoli, M., 109, 260
Rand, C., 261
Rand, W., 179
Rao, D. C., 72
Rathbone, W., 260
Ratner, P. A., 85
Rausch, P. B., 109
Ray, L. D., 190, 192, 197, 201, 206, 208, 211, 213
Raya, P., 87
Redburn, L., 163
Rehwaldt, M., 168
Reilly, C. A., 286
Reinhart, J. B., 110
Reisinger, C. L., 156, 158
Research reporter, 101
Reverby, S. M., 256
Rew, L., 185
Rhiner, M., 117, 122, 123, 124
Rhodes, J., 83
Rhymes, J., 105, 143
Rice, R., 109
Rice, V. H., 80, 81, 91
Richards, F. E., 85
Richardson, D. K., 293
Richardson, J., 74, 254

Richmond, J. B., 81, 268, 270, 274, 277, 278
Riddle, I., 120, 121
Riddle, I. I., 120, 121, 149, 153, 164
Rideout, K., 155, 158
Riera-Fanego, J. F., 294
Riesch, S. K., 93
Riessman, C. K., 205, 207
Rifkind, B. M., 72
Riley-Lawless, K., 71, 73
Risinger, M. W., 189, 194, 200, 202, 203, 204, 205, 206, 207, 208, 216
Ritchie, J., 102
Ritchie, J. A., 103 105, 125, 126, 130, 132, 133, 134, 135, 183, 190, 192, 197, 201, 206, 208, 211, 213
Roberts, C. A., 182, 193, 194, 221
Roberts, C. S., 188, 205, 207
Roberts, M. X., 103, 104
Roberts, S. L., 27
Robertson, J., 13, 133, 181
Robinson, C., 242
Robinson, C. A., 190, 192, 194, 230, 231, 232, 241
Roby, P., 225, 226, 229, 230, 231, 233, 241
Rodewald, L., 274, 290
Rodgers, B. M., 155, 158
Rogers, J., 135
Rogers, S., 51
Roghmann, K. J., 277
Rogoff, B., 76, 86
Romano, P. S., 287
Roncoli, M., 136, 138
Roosevelt, T., 252
Roper, W. L., 274
Roppe, B. E., 74
Rosberg, B., 145, 150, 153
Rose, M. H., 102
Rosenbaum, S., 271, 273
Rosenberg, C. E., 252, 256, 257
Rosenstock, I. M., 58, 68
Rosenthal, A., 264
Rosenthal, C., 181
Rosenthal, G. E., 293
Rossi, P. H., 276, 277
Rotenberg, E. J., 87
Rowat, K., 185, 225, 227, 228, 229, 230, 231, 233, 234, 241
Roy, C., 27
Roy, M. C., 102
Rudolph, R., 252, 253, 254
Rupp, J. W., 74
Russell, D., 40
Russell, G. A., 107
Russell, K., 92, 93

Ruttimann, U., 293
Ruttimann, U. E., 117, 293, 294
Ryan, E. A., 68, 93
Ryan, N. M., 197, 198
Ryan-Wenger, N. M., 34, 35, 40, 103, 183, 197, 198, 199

Saba, V., 222
Sachs, B., 90
Salas, I., 225, 226, 227, 228, 229, 231, 233, 234, 241
Sallis, J. F., 72, 73, 74, 75, 76, 84, 90
Salmon, M. E., 272
Sanders, S. T., 136, 137, 139
Sands, H. H., 103
Sandstrom, K., 168
Sarvela, P. D., 16, 21, 87
Saucier, C. P., 184, 185, 201
Saucier, J., 58
Savedra, M., 102, 107, 184
Savedra, M. C., 102, 103, 133, 134, 135
Sawin, K. J., 200, 205, 207
Sawyer, E. H., 189, 207
Scanlon, M. K., 183
Scannell, S., 192
Schaefer, C., 27
Scharer, K., 190
Schatzman, L., 88
Schauble, J., 288
Scheck, A., 276
Scheet, N., 222
Schepp, K. G., 118, 120
Schesselman, J. J., 159
Schkade, J. K., 144, 149
Schlomann, P., 191
Schmeltz, K., 105
Schmidt, F. L., 160
Schmidt, W. M., 277
Schneider, S., 261
Schoenborn, C. A., 79
Schorr, L. B., 269, 271, 272, 273, 274, 275, 276, 277, 278
Schreiner, B.-J., 225, 227, 228, 231, 234
Schroeder, M., 76, 91
Schryer, N. M., 264
Schubiner, H., 91
Schuler, M., 225, 226, 229, 230, 231, 233, 241
Schulman, J., 163
Schultz, N. V., 107
Schuman, A. J., 260
Schuster, D. P., 293
Schutz, M. E., 80, 87
Schuurmann Baker, L., 273

Schwarz, D., 62
Schwirian, P. M., 188
Sciera, M., 155, 158
Scipien, G. M., 257, 258
Scott, R. A., 276
Scribner, S., 111
Sears, P. S., 201, 203
Seckler-Walker, R. H., 63
Sedlak, M., 14
See, E. M., 112
Segall, M. E., 109
Seidl, F. W., 192
Select Panel for the Promotion of Child Health, 270
Sellew, G., 192
Senn, K. L., 74
Serpas, D. C., 65, 66, 83, 85
Shafer, K., 109
Shaftel, N., 5
Shannon, B. M., 71
Shapiro, B., 117, 122, 123, 124
Shapiro, G. R., 27, 31, 83, 90
Shapiro, H. T., 273
Shapiro, V., 186, 192
Sharkey, P. D., 292
Sharp, L. J., 184, 186
Sharp, N., 254
Shattuck, L., 3, 14
Shayne, M., 236, 237
Shea, S., 84
Shedler, J., 74
Shelley, S., 18, 135
Shiao, S.-Y. P., 117, 118, 119, 123, 124
Shoffner, D., 40, 87
Shure, M. B., 80
Siegal, J. M., 40
Siegel, L. J., 105
Sigma Theta Tau, 111
Simeonsson, R. J., 80
Simon, N. B., 187
Simons, B. G., 63
Simons-Morton, D. G., 63
Simpson, L., 283
Sinai, N., 253
Sipowicz, R., 163
Skinner, B. F., 12, 72
Skipper, J. K., 105, 143
Slater, C. H., 281, 282
Sloss, E. M., 273
Smicklas-Wright, H. S., 71
Smilkstein, G., 197
Smillie, W., 4
Smith, A. B., 136, 138
Smith, D., 187
Smith, E. A., 23
Smith, K., 225, 227, 228, 231, 234
Smith, L., 192

Smith, L. D., 264
Smith, M. C., 80, 160
Smith, M. D., 109
Smith, M. S., 189, 194, 200, 202,
    203, 204, 205, 207
Smyth, M., 74
Snowden, A. W., 122
Snyder, C., 222
Snyder, M., 168
Sobol, A., 181
Sorensen, E. R., 157, 158
Soto-Torre, L. E., 278
Souberman, E., 111
Southall, D., 167
Souza, J., 183
Sparta, S. N., 201, 202
Spears, H., 61, 77, 89
Spence, J., 257-258
Spicher, C. M., 151, 153
Spielberger, G. D., 201, 209
Spietz, A., 222
Spinetta, J. J., 201, 202
Spitzer, A., 183, 185, 210, 214
Spock, B., 13
Spohn, W. A., 293
Sroufe, L. A., 91
St. Clair, P. A., 45, 46, 87
Stachowiak, B., 94
Stainton, C., 105
Stallings, V. A., 71
Stanhope, M., 260
Starfield, B., 283, 289, 290
Stashinko, E. E., 72, 84, 137, 139
Staub, E., 103
Stegman, M., 222
Steigall, C., 109
Stein, M., 13
Stein, R. E., 293
Stein, R. E. K., 180, 200, 201, 205,
    207, 217, 237, 274
Steinhart, C. M., 293
Stember, M., 51
Stergios, D. A., 155, 158
Stern, P. N., 189, 194
Stevens, M., 102, 184, 189
Stevens, S. M., 293
Stewart, B. J., 241, 288
Stewart, I., 99
Stewart, M. L., 107
Stoeckle, J. D., 272
Stokols, D., 76, 93
Stoll, C., 184
Stolley, P. D., 71
Stone, E. J., 63, 64, 65, 67, 71, 78,
    79
Strassner, L., 283
Straus, L., 5
Strecher, V. J., 58

Stringfield, S., 45
Strobel, C. T., 136
Strobino, D. M., 184, 275
Struthers, L., 6
Stuffelbeam, D., 173
Stullenbarger, B., 191
Suddaby, E. S., 285
Swan, J., 185
Swan, J. H., 23, 26, 187, 191, 194
Swanson-Kaufman, K., 51
Swegart, L. A., 189
Swift, J., 108
Syme, S. L., 84
Szilagyi, P., 274, 290

Tamborlane, W. V., 185
Tanner, C. A., 102
Taquino, L., 109
Tassi, A., 274
Tatman, M. A., 259
Taylor, S. C., 188
Taylor, W., 180
Temoshok, L., 23, 28
Teres, D., 293
Terhaar, M., 297
Terman, D. L., 275
Tershakovec, A. M., 71
Tesler, M., 102, 107
Tesler, M. D., 102, 103, 133, 134
Thomas, D., 254
Thomas, J., 259
Thomas, S. P., 40, 87
Thompson, A., 165
Thompson, A. I., 41, 71, 205, 208
Thompson, L., 261
Thompson, M. L., 258
Thompson, R. H., 104, 106, 163,
    164
Thompson, R. J., 180
Thorne, S., 187, 190
Thorne, S. E., 181, 192
Thoyre, S., 76, 91
Thurber, F. W., 90, 126, 127, 129,
    131, 132, 182, 183, 185,
    200, 201, 202, 203, 204,
    205, 206, 208
Tibboel, D., 294
Tiedeman, M. E., 126, 128, 129,
    131, 132
Tinker, T. L., 280
Tinsley, B. J., 59, 93
Titler, M., 121
Titus, J. C., 192
Tomczyk, B., 118, 119, 123
Tomlinson, P. S., 117, 118, 119,
    121, 123, 189
Torrance, J. T., 107, 109

Tortu, S., 83
Travis, L., 225, 227, 228, 231, 234
Trierweiler, K., 261
Tripp, S. L., 94
Turner, C. W., 187
Turner, M. A., 117, 189
Turner, R., 231
Turner-Henson, A., 23, 26, 180,
    185, 187, 190, 191, 194
Tweet, A. G., 294

U.S. Department of Health and
    Human Services, 56, 57,
    65, 77, 79, 82, 241, 261,
    263, 271
U.S. Department of Labor, 10, 11
U.S. General Accounting Office,
    223, 262, 263
Udry, J. R., 23, 205
Ueda, R., 186
Uman, H., 186, 192
Umphenour, J. H., 103
Unis, A. S., 199
Uphold, M., 262
Uzark, K., 264

Vagg, P. R., 209
Valoski, A., 74
Van Cleve, L., 187
Van Cleve, L. J., 133, 135
van der Hoek, A. C., 294
Vanderlinden, D. W., 225, 226, 231,
    233
van der Voort, E., 294
Van Ingren, P., 4
Vanneman, J., 277
Van Os, D. C., 187
Van Riper, M., 76, 91
van Veen, A., 294
Vardaro, J. A., 105
Vega, W. A., 74
Veit, C. T., 209
Ventura, J. N., 184
Ventura, S. J., 184, 275
Vernon, D., 163
Vernon, D. T., 105, 143
Verran, J., 222
Vessey, J., 170
Vessey, J. A., 104, 106, 107, 145,
    156, 158, 185, 187, 190
Vidyasagar, D., 109, 194
Villarruel, A., 133, 169, 225
Visintainer, M. A., 102, 105, 143,
    166, 167
Viviani, N., 185, 200, 201, 202,
    203, 204, 205, 206, 207

Vivier, P. M., 283, 290
Vogel, D. W., 137
Vogel, M. A., 57
Volk, R., 185, 200, 201, 202, 203, 204, 205, 206, 207
von Bertalanffy, L., 72
Vredevoe, D. L., 104
Vygotsky, L. S, 111

Wachtel, R., 225, 226, 229, 230, 231, 233, 241
Waechter, E. H., 191
Wald, L., 5, 6, 9, 261
Walizer, E., 236
Walker, D., 181
Walker, D. K., 293
Walker, L. O., 23, 80, 222, 230
Walker, S. N., 85
Wall, S., 41
Wallace, H., 109
Wallace, H. M., 277
Wallace, J. P., 74
Wallace, R. M., 134, 135
Wallander, J., 239
Wallerstein, N., 93
Wallskog, J. M., 222
Wallston, B. S., 48
Wallston, K. A., 48
Walsh, M., 183, 190, 199
Walsh, M. W., 58, 63
Wambsgans, K., 65
Warady, B., 165
Ward, C. H., 201
Ward, J., 107
Ward, J. A., 107, 133
Warda, M., 187
Ware, J. E., 209
Warren, B., 70
Waters, E., 41
Watson, A., 186
Watson, W. L., 244
Watt, N. F., 80
Watt-Watson, J. H., 134, 135
Wattigney, W., 65, 67
Webb, C. J., 155, 158
Webber, L. S., 63, 65, 66, 67, 71, 78, 83, 85
Wechsler, H., 85
Weeks, K., 261
Wegner, C., 107

Wehr, E., 273
Weichler, N. K., 116, 122
Weidman, W., 65
Weill, K. S., 27, 31, 83, 90
Weinberg, A. D., 93
Weinert, C., 41
Weiss, S. M., 57, 72
Weissberg, R., 263
Weitzman, M., 181, 293
Welch, J., 136, 137, 138
Wells, M., 294
Wenner, W. H., 109
Wesley, R., 171
West, C., 100, 102, 111
West, S. G., 80
Whalen, K., 72, 73
Whall, A., 71
White, G., 105
White, M., 171
White, M. A., 152, 153
Whitehead, B. D., 237
Whyte, H., 293
Wicks, L., 271
Wilkie, D. J., 133, 134
Wilkinson, J. D., 293
Wilkinson-Faulk, D., 136, 138
Willadsen, J. A., 194, 222, 228, 234
Willard, B., 185, 225, 227, 228, 229, 230, 231, 233, 234, 241
Willard, J. C., 79
Williams, B. C., 94
Williams, D. M., 93
Williams, D. S., 159
Williams, J. K., 84, 191
Williams, L., 189
Williams, P. D, 152, 153, 188, 205, 209
Wills, J. M., 186
Wilson, C. C., 104
Wilson, C. J., 105
Wilson, L. R., 205, 206
Wilson, T., 184
Windom, R. E., 81
Wing, R. R., 74
Winkler, S. J., 80
Wiser, B., 165
Wiser, M., 165
Wiskin, N., 183
Wiskin, N. M., 223
Witter, D. M., 286

Wolfer, J. A., 102, 105, 143, 166, 167
Wood, C. J., 104
Wood, D. J., 171
Wood, M., 53
Woodring, B., 91, 170, 174
Woods, L. G., 183
Worden, J. K., 63
Workman, K., 293
Workman-Daniels, K., 293
World Health Organization, 57
Wright, H., 13
Wright, L. M., 41, 71, 180, 194, 222, 230, 231, 244
Wu, M., 63, 71, 78
Wuest, J., 189, 190, 194

Yazgerdi, S., 274, 290
Yeaworth, R., 40
Yeh, T. S., 293
Yi-Hua, L., 191
York, J., 40
York, R., 109, 260
Young, D. A., 273
Young, J., 181, 257, 258
Young, R., 187
Youngblut, J. M., 117, 118, 119, 123, 124, 133, 189
Youssef, M. M. S., 102
Yund, C., 151, 153

Zablocki, H., 260
Zaldo-Rodriguez, R., 294
Zastowny, T., 105
Zelizer, V., 6
Zhu, B. P., 293
Ziglio, E., 93
Zismer, D. K., 265
Zittergruen, M. A., 153, 154, 159
Zoeller, L., 188, 189, 190, 192, 193, 194, 197, 200, 202, 209, 210, 212, 213
Zoeller, L. H., 184, 186, 197, 200, 202, 210, 213
Zorn, J., 23, 28
Zucker, A. R., 293

SUBJECT INDEX

Activity Scale, 126
Acutely ill children:
  behavioral responses, 125-133
  behavior/emotions, 131-132
  concerns/fears, 132
  medication effects, 136
  pain research, 133-135
  physiological interventions,
    153-158
  physiologic responses, 133-
    139
  psychosocial interventions,
    144-153
  stress/coping, 125, 130-131,
    141
  stressors, 163
  studying, 110-111
  temperature-measurement
    research, 135-136
Acutely ill children, families of:
  family system responses,
    123-124
  mother roles, 122-123
  parental needs, 116-117, 120
  parental role, 122-123
  parental stress/coping,
    120-122, 141
Acutely ill children and their
    families, models for
    intervention with, 166-167
  analysis strategies, 170
  designs/methods, 168
  future, 170-172
  measurement issues, 169
  patient outcomes, 172
  sampling strategies, 169-170
  theoretical adequacy, 167-168

Adolescent Coping Orientation for
    Problem Experiences
    (ACOPE), 204
Adolescent-Family Inventory of
    Life Events and Changes
    (AFILE), 205, 206
Adolescent Life Change Event
    Scale, 32, 40
Adolescent pregnancy, 23, 275
Advanced practice nurses (APNs),
    260
Agency for Health Care Policy and
    Research, 288
AIDS, 23, 27, 28, 30, 48, 51, 55,
    61, 87
  pediatric, 180, 249, 280
  See also HIV
AIDS Knowledge and Belief
    Survey, 50
AIDS Questionnaire, 53, 54
Aid to Families with Dependent
    Children (AFDC), 253
Almshouses, 255
  infant mortality, 100
American Academy of Nursing, 288
American Academy of Pediatrics
    (AAP), 258
  guidelines, 20
American Association of Critical
    Care Nurses (AACN), 112
  Thunder Project, 170
American Association of Public
    Health (AAPH):
    School Nursing Section, 261
American Home Economics
    Association, 7
American Hospital Association, 256

American Medical Association
    (AMA), 10, 253
American Nurses' Association
    (ANA), 112
  Maternal-Child Council, 112
American Pediatric Society, 256,
    257
American Public Health
    Association:
    Public Health Nursing, 7
American School Health
    Association, 261
American Social Hygiene
    Association, 7
APGAR, 133
Association for the Care of
    Children's Health (ACCH),
    113, 258
Association of Operating Room
    Nurses (AORN), 113
Association of Pediatric Oncology
    Nurses (APON), 112
Association of Women's Health,
    Obstetrical, and Neonatal
    Nursing (AWHONN), 112

Baby boom, post-WWII, 13
Bates Infant Temperament
    Questionnaire, 17, 24
Bayley Scale of Infant
    Development, 229
Beck Depression Inventory, 201
Behavioral Intention Theory (BIT),
    58
Behavioral theorists, 12
BENCHmark, 296
Benchmarking, 248, 294, 296

pediatric populations, 294-296
Bloomsday Cardiovascular Fitness
    Questionnaire, 16, 19
Bogalusa Heart Study, 65
Brazelton Neonatal Behavioral
    Assessment Scale
    (BNBAS), 17, 25
Bright Futures project, 270
Bureau of Child Hygiene, 9

Cardiovascular Health in Children
    (CHIC I), 69, 71
Caregiver uncertainty, 117
Carnegie Corporation task forces,
    270
Case management. *See* Nursing
    case management
Center for Epidemiologic
    Studies-Depression Scale
    (CES-D), 41, 42
Center for Population Option:
    School Board Health Clinics
    Model, 31
Center for the Study of Health
    Behaviors in Vulnerable
    Youth, 78
Child Abuse Potential Inventory,
    229
Child adjustment:
    instruments assessing, 201
Child and Adolescent Adjustment
    profile, 126, 201
Child and Adolescent Self-Care
    Practices Questionnaire, 185
Child Attitude Toward Illness Scale
    (CATIS), 198, 200, 204
Child behavioral response studies:
    instruments used, 126-129
Child Behavior Checklist (CBCL),
    201, 202, 203, 216, 217,
    229, 239
Child developmentalists, 3-4, 8
Child development field:
    beginnings, 7-8
    mid-20th century, 12-13
Child Drawing Hospital, 126
Child Evaluation Inventory,
    Revision of, 199
Child health care:
    creating integrated systems,
    263-266
Child Health Organization, 7
Child health services:
    beginnings, 8-9
    children in societal context,
    252-255, 266

community-based campaigns,
    278
core elements, 269
financing, 272-274
hospital care, 255
primary care model, 256-257
societal view of children,
    251-252, 266
tertiary-focused programs, 254
See also Children's hospitals;
    Hospitalization, children's
Child hygiene bureaus, 10
Child Medical Fears Scale, 126, 132
Child morbidity levels, 4, 100
Child mortality levels, 4, 100
Child Rating of Anxiety, 126
Childrearing Practice
    Questionnaire, 146
Children's Bureau, 9-11, 252, 277
    child care, 10
    child labor laws, 252
    infant mortality, 10
    information dissemination, 10
    prenatal care, 10
    purpose, 252
    rural health care, 10
Children's Coping Behaviors, 127
Children's Coping Strategies
    Checklist, 126, 130
    Intrusive Procedures, 126
Children's Depression Inventory
    (CDI), 127, 201, 202, 217
Children's Hospital of Eastern
    Ontario Pain Scale
    (CHEOPS), 156
Children's Hospital of
    Philadelphia, 100
Children's hospitals, 7, 100,
    255-256, 285
    first, 4, 255
Children's organizations, 7
    *See also specific children's
    organizations*
Children's Perceived
    Benefits/Barriers to
    Exercise Questionnaire, 47
Children's Self-Efficacy Survey, 47
Child's Health Self-Concept Scale,
    51, 52
Child's Pain Response Tool, 146
Chronically ill children:
    attributes, 200-205, 210-211
    characteristics/health, 200-201
    coping/social support, 203-204
    feelings, 204
    functioning/adaptation,
    184-185
    increase, 196

initial diagnosis, 182-183
    number, 180-181
    ongoing stress/coping, 183-184
    parenting, 191-192
    psychosocial adjustment,
    201-203
    self-care, 185-186
    social competence, 184
Chronically ill children, families of:
    attributes, 205-209, 211
    child-rearing
    concerns/practices, 191
    cultural/environmental
    influences, 190-191
    family functioning, 188-191,
    206-207
    family management style
    (FMS), 189-190, 210, 212,
    213
    family member
    involvement/adjustment,
    208-209
    family resources, 208
    family stress, 206
    fathers, 187
    health care provider
    relationship, 192-193
    mother-infant interactions, 191
    parental coping, 208
    parental functioning styles, 188
    parents' chronic sorrow, 187
    parents' ongoing stress/coping,
    186-187
    parents' reaction to initial
    diagnosis, 186
    siblings, 187-188
Chronically ill children and their
    families, research on:
    assessment data source, 217
    assessment data type, 217
    assessment themes/issues,
    238-240
    convenience samples, 194
    developmental issues, 218
    domains, 181-188
    focus, 216
    future, 195
    history, 181
    individual focus, 181-182
    instruments developed, 197-200
    interpretive methods, 193, 194
    knowledge development,
    218-219
    qualitative assessment,
    209-215, 239
    quantitative assessment,
    200-209, 239
    trends, 193-195

validity issues, 217-218
See also Chronically ill
children; Chronically ill
children, families of
Chronicity Impact and Coping
Instrument, 205, 208
CINHAL, 15, 57
CIPP model, 173
Clinical information management,
285-288
Clinician's Overall Burden Index
(COBI), 201
Clinics, nurse-managed, 264
Close Person Satisfaction Scale,
37, 40
Cognitive Development Theory
(CDT), 58
Communicable Disease Perceived
Vulnerability, 46
Community health centers, 14
Community health workers
(CHWs), 261
Community infrastructure:
as strategy, 269-274
effective, 269
frameworks/models, 269-271
improvement barriers, 274-277
improvement goals, 271-272
Competency-focused research,
83-84
Comprehensive Social-Competence
and Health Education
(C-SCAHE) programming,
263
Continuous quality improvement
(CQI), 295
Cooperation Scale, 127, 145, 148
Coping Health Inventory for
Children (CHIC), 198
Coping Health Inventory for
Parents (CHIP), 205, 208
Coping Orientation for Problem
Experiences, 127
Coping styles:
active, 102, 103, 130
comfort/help seeking, 130
control theory, 102
growth/independence, 130
inactive, 102, 130
information-seeking, 130
intrapsychic, 130
orienting, 102
Coronary Risk Profile, 19
Corporate Hospital Rating Project
(CHRP), 292
Critical Care Family Needs
Inventory-Modified
(CCFNI), 118

Cumulative Index to Nursing and
Allied Health Literature,
196
Current Health Status scale, 127

Data collection tool, 138
Department of Health and Human
Services, 11
Dependent Care Agent
questionnaire, 51, 52
Depression Scale, 26
Diabetes Self-Care Practice
Instrument, 185
Dietary Checklist, 20
Diet Habit Survey, 19
Disease prevention:
versus health promotion, 57
Dispensary for the Infant Poor, 255

Early and Periodic Screening,
Diagnosis, and Treatment
Program (EPSDT), 27, 30,
269
Emotion Triangulation Scale, 201,
202

FACES pain rating scale, 156
FACES III, 118
Family Adaptability and Cohesion
Evaluation (FACES), 205,
207
Family Adjustment and Adaptation
Response Model (FAAR),
168
Family APGAR, Revised, 197-198,
200, 205, 206-207
Family assessment instruments, 205
See also specific instruments
Family-centered care, 259
Family Environment Scale (FES),
43, 45, 51, 52
Family Hardiness Index (FHI),
205, 208
Family Health Promotion Program,
65
Family Inventory of Life Events
and Changes (FILE), 205,
206
Family Inventory of Resources for
Management (FIRM), 205,
208
Family of Origin Scale, 205, 207
Family Routines Inventory (FRI),
42, 45
Family system uncertainty, 117

Federal Emergency Maternal and
Infant Care Program
(EMIR), 253
Feel Bad Scale, 35, 40
Feetham Family Functioning
Survey (FFFS), 118,
188-189, 205, 207
Feshbach Aggression Measure, 201
Feshbach Audiovisual empathy
Measure, 204
Feshbach Emotional
Responsiveness Measure,
204
Floating Hospital, 100
Foundation for Accountability
(FACCT), 291
Functional Status Measure (FSM),
200

Gate theory, 137
General Systems Theory, 72
Global Mood Scale, 145, 149
Great Ormand Street Hospital for
Sick Children, 100, 104

Hall, G. Stanley, 8
stage theory of development, 8
study of adolescents, 8
Harter Self-Perception Profile for
Children, 27, 31, 129, 201,
203, 228, 233, 243
Hassles Scale, 27, 32, 37
Hazardous secrets, 122
Head Start, 14, 16, 249, 254, 269,
270-271, 277, 280
Health care delivery, 248
child health, 88
data/information systems, 248
Health care delivery systems, 280
Health Care Financing
Administration, 289
Health care systems:
emerging, 264-266
integrated, 265
Health maintenance organizations
(HMOs), 263
Healthnet, 143
Health Perceptions Questionnaire,
47
Health-promoting interventions, 57
Health promotion:
definition, 80
importance, 94
multidimensional activity, 92
multivariate phenomenon, 92
versus disease prevention, 57

Health promotion assessment
models:
community-oriented primary
care, 23, 27-31, 83
comprehensive assessment, 51
developmental, 17-26
family assessment/family
systems, 41, 45
family health promotion, 45-48
health belief, 48, 53
interaction model of client
health behavior, 51
maternal responsiveness,
38-39, 41
medical/physiologic, 16-22
problem-prone behavior, 51, 53
self-care, 51
social cognitive theory, 48, 50,
51, 83
stress-adaptation, 27, 32-37,
40-41, 82
Health promotion intervention
models:
children's health belief
(CHBM), 58-61, 85, 86
ecological models, 75-77, 84,
88, 90
health belief, 58-61
health promotion, 68-71,
77-78, 83, 85, 86
model of family influences on
health behavior, 71-74
social cognitive theory (SCT),
61, 63-68, 72, 74, 78, 83
social learning theory, 58,
63-64, 68-69
theory of planned behavior
(TPB), 61-63
theory of reasoned action
(TRA), 61-63
Health promotion movement, 94
beginnings, 3, 14
Health promotion practice:
future, 93-95
responsive, 92
sensitive, 92
Health promotion research:
agendas, 81-82, 89-90
assessment/intervention
models, 83-85, 89, 90
design/methods, 85-89
focus groups, 89
future, 89-91
programs, 89
questions, 82-83
See also Health promotion
studies
Health promotion studies:

community-oriented primary
care model, 28-31
comprehensive assessment
model, 52
developmental model, 24-26
family assessment/family
systems model, 42-44
family health promotion
model, 46-47
health belief model, 49-50
interaction model of client
health behavior, 52
maternal responsiveness
model, 38-39
medical/physiologic model,
18-22
problem-prone behavior
theory, 54
self-care model, 52
social cognitive theory, 50
stress-adaptation model, 32-37
See also Health promotion
assessment models
Health Self-Determination Index
for Children, 52
Health services research, 281-285
children and families, 282-284
definitions, 281-282
interdisciplinary, 281
NACHRI study, 285
purpose, 281
rationale for emphasis, 284
Health teaching, 90-91
anticipatory guidance, 91
guided participation, 91
Healthy Heart Program, 84
Healthy Kids, 277
Healthy Start, 277
Hearing screening, 12
Heart Smart Cardiovascular School
Health Promotion Program,
65, 66, 67-68, 70, 78, 83, 85
HEDIS, 289
Henry Street Settlement House, 9
Henry Street Visiting Nurses
Service, 5
HIV, 93, 113
pediatric cases, 180
See also AIDS
Holt, Luther Emmett, 7-8, 256, 257
child care manual, 7-8, 13
pediatric textbook, 8
Home care, 259-261
Home Environment Scale, 229
Home Observation for
Measurement of the
Environment (HOME), 17,
24

Hospital Coping Scale, 127
Hospitalism, 258
Hospitalization, children's:
early history, 255
family-centered care, 257-259
psychological preparation,
105-106, 143
Hospital-physician
organization/combined
provider organization
(HPO/CPO), 263
Hospital visitation, 257-258
intensive care units, 104
liberal, 259
management, 103-104
parental, 13, 103, 104
peer, 103
sibling, 103-104
Hull House, 277
Human Figure Drawings, 128
Human Genome Project, 84, 297

Illness prevention, 265
Illness uncertainty, 117
Immunizations, 11-12
Impact on Family Scale, 205, 207
Index of Body Knowledge, 127
Index of Parental Support During
Intrusive Procedures, 151
Index of Parenting Attitudes, 41, 42
Index of Parent
Participation/Hospitalized
Child, 151
Infant Feeding Behavior
Assessment Checklist
(CSIFBAC), 138
Infant Health Status Scale, 37
Infant hygiene development, 4
Infant morbidity:
decreasing, 11
Infant mortality, 256
decreasing, 11, 275
uneducated mothers, 5
See also Children's Bureau
Infectious diseases, 100
Institute for Family-Centered Care,
259
Institute of Medicine, 272
International Classification of
Primary Care, 53
International Health Board, 7
Intervention research:
emergent issues, 160-161
methodological challenges,
158-160
past, 222-224
programs, 159

randomization procedures, 159
replication studies, 159
sample size, 160
themes/issues, 240-243
See also Intervention studies
Interventions:
  levels, 222
  orientations, 242
Intervention studies, 234-235
  demographic data relevancy,
    230
  outcome of child-focused
    interventions, 228
  outcome of family-focused
    interventions, 228-229
  outcome of sibling-focused
    interventions, 228
  outcomes, 233
  results, 233-234
  scarcity, 240
  summary, 226-227
  treatment characteristics,
    230-233
  See also Intervention research
Intimate behaviors scale, Smith and
    Udry, 26
Intracranial pressure monitor, 138
Introspectiveness Scale for
    Adolescents, 32

Jaloweic Coping Scale (JCS), 204
Joint Commission on Accreditation
    of Healthcare Organizations
    (JCAHO), 106, 288, 291

Kinetic Family Drawing—Revised
    (KFD-R), 201, 202
Knowledge of Infant Development
    Inventory (KIDI), 26
Know Your Body Health Habits
    Survey, 70

Latex allergy, 137, 138
Life Event Scale, 206
Life Events Checklist, 33
Life Experiences Fetal Attachment
    Scale, 33, 34
Luscher Color Test, 128, 204

Managed care, 263, 265
Managed health care organizations
    (MCOs), 263
Manifest Anxiety Scale, 229

Manifest Upset Scale, 128, 145,
    148, 149
Maternal and Child Health Bureau,
    94
Maternal-Fetal Attachment Scale,
    38, 41
Maternal Vigilance, 118
Matthews Youth Test for Health
    (MYTH), 35, 40
McGill Model of Nursing, 227
Measurement issues:
  children versus adults, 288-291
Medicaid, 253-254, 262, 263, 269
  expansions, 271
  managed care, 254
Medicare, 263
MEDLINE, 15, 57, 196
Mental Health Inventory (MHI),
    209
Metropolitan Nursing Association
    of London, 260
Miller's Bother Scale, 25
Model of Health Promotion, 53
Multicenter Child and Adolescent
    Trial for Cardiovascular
    Health (CATCH), 63, 67,
    78, 79
  objectives, 64
  students, 64
Multidimensional Health Locus of
    Control Scale, 48, 50

National Ambulatory Medical
    Care Survey (NAMCS), 30
National Association for the Study
    of Epilepsy and Care of
    Epileptics, 7
National Association of Children's
    Hospitals and Related
    Institutions (NACHRI),
    265, 285
  Patient Care FOCUS Groups
    benchmarking initiative,
    294-296
National Association of Pediatric
    Nurse Associates and
    Practitioners (NAPNAP),
    112
National Association of School
    Nurses, 261
National Center for Health
    Statistics AIDS survey, 28
National Center for Nursing
    Research CORP, 110
National Child Welfare
    Association, 7

National Committee for Quality
    Assurance (NCQA), 289,
    291
National Congress of Parents and
    Teachers, 7
National Forum on the Future of
    Children and Families, 270
National Institute of Nursing
    Research (NINR), 113
National Institutes of Health (NIH),
    278
National League for Nursing, 112
National Organization for Public
    Health Nursing, 7
National School Health Services
    Program, 27, 30
Neonatal Abstinence Score Tool
    (NAST), 139
Neonatal care, 109
Neonatal intensive care unit
    (NICU), 136, 254
Neonatal Therapeutic Intervention
    Scoring System (NTISS),
    293
New Futures project, 275
Nightingale School, 100
Nurse-managed care, 264
Nurses:
  child advocates, 267
  children's welfare, 14, 56, 80
  health services program
    development, 14
  See also Advanced practice
    nurses (APNs); Pediatric
    nurse practitioners
Nursing, professional:
  health promotion, 80
  outcomes, 288
Nursing case management, 264
Nursing Child Assessment
    Teaching Scale (NCATS),
    17, 23, 26
Nursing education:
  critical curricula, 91
  dialogic approach, 93
  ethical issues, 91
  future, 173-174
  health promotion
    research/practice, 91-93
  learning experiences, 93
Nursing Interventions
    Classification (NIC)
    project, 161, 167, 242
Nursing organizations:
  nursing research agendas, 112
  pediatric, 112-113
Nursing research:
  barriers, 113-114

coping, 102-103
critique, 124-125
federal support, 113
history, 100-102
intensive care units, 108-109
journals, 143
neonatal care, 109
pain management, 106-108
play, 104
professional organizations,
  112-113
psychological preparation,
  105-106
psychosocial domain, 102-106
separation/visitation/rooming-in,
  103-104
  See also Intervention research
Nutrition, 12

Objective Measure of Ego Identity
  Status (EOMEIS), 201, 203
Office of Economic Opportunity,
  254
Oncology Nurses' Society (ONS),
  112
Oucher, 133
Outcomes movement, 281
Outpatient Experience
  Questionnaire, 151

PACU Parental Visitation Program
  Evaluation, 147
PACU Parent Observation
  Checklist, 147
Pain management, 106-108,
  133-135
  coping strategies, 134
  pharmacologic, 133
  undermedication, 134-135, 141
Parent Activities Questionnaire, 119
Parental Concerns Scale, 118
Parental Control Preference, 118
Parental Postdischarge Care
  Questionnaire, 151
Parental Satisfaction Scale, 119
Parental Stressor Scale, 119
Parent/family studies:
  instruments used, 118-119
Parenting Stress Index, 229
Parent Rating of Own Anxiety, 128
Parent Teacher Association, 7
Pediatric intensive care units
  (PICUs), 108-109, 117,
  120, 121, 123-124, 164, 293
Pediatric medicine, 7-8

Pediatric nurse practitioners, 14,
  51, 165
Pediatric nurse researchers:
  advanced education, 111-112
  clinical area studies, 113-114
  preparation, 111-112
Pediatric nurses, 114
  training schools, 100
Pediatric nursing, 100, 111
  play, 104
Pediatric Nursing Endocrinology
  Society, 113
Pediatric nursing intervention
  research:
  early, 143-144
  future, 174-175
  growth, 142
Pediatric Risk of Mortality
  (PRISM) severity
  instrument, 293-294
  scores, 117
Peer's Health Behavior Scale, 20
PEN3 model, 85
Pennsylvania Hospital, 255
Perceived Threats to Body
  Integrity, 128
Perception of Infant Scale, 43
Perinatal Extension (SNAPPE), 293
Personal Resource Questions
  (PRQ85) Social Support
  measure, 41
Physiological intervention studies,
  153-158
Piaget, Jean, 111
  child development theory,
  12-13
  cognitive theory, 185
Picture Test, 128
Play, therapeutic, 104, 144, 183
  Piagetian view, 104
Point of service plans (PPS), 263
Poker Chip Tool, 133
Posthospitalization Behavior
  Questionnaire, 129, 145,
  149, 151
Poverty, 268
  child health, 88
Predisposing, Reinforcing, and
  Enabling Courses in
  Educational Diagnosis and
  Evaluation (PRECEDE)
  community-planning
  model, 68
Preferred provider organization
  (PPO), 263
Preschool Behavioral Rating Scale,
  36, 40

Preschool Behavior Questionnaire
  (PBQ), 42, 45
Preschool Health Picture Interview,
  46
Preventive medicine
  advances, 11-12
Primary care, 265, 266
Primary care providers:
  gatekeepers, 263
Primary Health Care Needs
  Assessment (PHCNA), 199
Princess Margaret Hospital Pain
  Assessment Tool
  (PMHPAT), 133
Psychiatric nurse researchers, 111
Psychosocial interventions, 146-152
Public health departments,
  municipal, 11
Public health nursing, 272
Pulse oximetry, 137, 139

Readiness for Change Model, 53
Reagan administration:
  health policy changes, 254
Relationship Closeness Scale, 37,
  40
Resiliency Model of Family
  Adjustment and Adaptation,
  165, 189, 195
Revised Infant Temperament
  Questionnaire, 17, 24, 25
Risk analysis, 291-293
  illness severity exemplar,
  292-293
Role Model Scale, 20
Roy's Adaptation Theory, 137

Safe Sex Behavior Questionnaire
  (SSBQ), 50
Safety Institute of America, 7
"Save the Babies" campaign, 4-5
  milk depots, 5, 257
  prenatal stations, 5
  well-baby stations, 5, 257
Schoolagers' Coping Strategies
  Inventory (SCSI), 34, 35,
  40, 198-199
School-based clinics (SBCs), 262, 277
School health:
  CDC definition, 262
School Health Evaluation project, 231
School health promotion, 6-7
  free breakfasts/lunches, 6
  free medical/dental care, 6
  health education, 7
  "little mothers" clubs, 6

street safety classes, 6
See also School nurses
School nurses, 6, 261
  role, 261-262
Schools:
  full-service, 263
  health services, 261
Score for Neonatal Acute
    Physiology (SNAP), 293
Self-Assessment Faces Scale, 149
Self-Care Abilities Scale, 228
Self-Care Practice Instrument, 185
Self-Care Questionnaire (SCQ), 201
Self-care theory, 111
Self-Concept Inventory, 201
Self-Concept Scale, 201, 203
Self-Determinism Index for
    Children, 51
Self-efficacy studies, 83-84
Self-Esteem Inventory (SEI), 201, 203
Self-Report of Distress, 148
Sexual intercourse scale, Bauman
    and Udry, 26
Sheppard-Towner Act, 10-11,
    252-253, 257
  AMA opposition, 10, 11, 257
Sleep/Activity Record, 24
Sleep/Behavior inventory, 24
Sleep Onset Latency Behavior
    Catalog, 151
Smoking Behaviors Scale, 20
Social Competence Scale, 39

Social Support APGAR, 44, 45
Society for the Prevention of
    Cruelty to Children, 251
Society of Mental Health, 7
Society of Pediatric Nurses (SPN),
    113
Society of Pediatric Nursing
    (SPN), 170
Society of Research in Child
    Development (SRCD), 113
Sources of Family Annoyance
    (SOFA), 44, 45
Spock, Benjamin, 13
  books, 13
State-Trait Anxiety Inventory for
    Children, 129, 201
State-Trait Anxiety Inventory
    (STAI), 119, 129, 147, 151,
    209
Strength of Body Boundaries, 129
Stress theory, 124

Title V, Social Security Act (1935),
    11, 253, 269
Toddler Care Questionnaire (TCQ),
    26
Toddler Temperament Scale, 17,
    24, 26
Total quality management, 296
Tuberculosis testing, 12

U.S. Public Health Service, 58-61, 271
UCLA Loneliness Scale, 36, 40, 41
  Revised, 32, 50
University of Calgary, Family Nursing
    Unit (FNU), 244-245
University of Iowa researchers, 243

Value Survey, 50
Vision screening, 12
Visiting nurse society, first, 260
Visual Analog Scale, 150
Vitamins, 12

War on Poverty, 253
Ways of Coping Checklist, 27, 119
  Revised, 32, 33, 228
Wellness education, 265
White House Conference on
    Children, 252
WIC, 254, 269
Word graphic scale, 133

Young Adult Social Support
    Inventory, 204
Young Child Observation
    Checklist, 147
Youth Health Survey Physical
    Activity Checklist, 20
Youth Risk Behavior Survey, 53, 54

ABOUT THE CONTRIBUTORS

Joan K. Austin, DNS, RN, FAAN, is Professor of Nursing in the Department of Environments for Health at Indiana University School of Nursing in Indianapolis. She conducts research on child and family adaptation to childhood epilepsy and has been published in *Nursing Research, Epilepsia, Journal of Pediatric Psychology,* and *Journal of Pediatric Nursing.*

Doris J. Biester, PhD, RN, FAAN, is Executive Vice President and Chief Operating Officer at Children's Hospital in Denver, Colorado. She is a member of the Board of Directors for the National Perinatal Information Center. Formerly, she served as a member and chair of the Governing Board of the Maternal Child Health Section of the American Hospital Association and as president of the Society of Pediatric Nurses. Her research interests are the development and evaluation of systems and the impact on patient care outcomes.

Barbara Brodie, PhD, RN, is Professor and Director of the Center for Nursing Historical Inquiry at the University of Virginia School of Nursing in Charlottesville. The role of professional nurses in the development of medical and health services for children and their families has been the focus of her historical research.

Marion E. Broome, PhD, RN, FAAN, is a Professor at the University of Wisconsin–Milwaukee and the Research Chair in Nursing of Children at the Children's Hospital of Wisconsin. Studies in her program of research in pediatric pain interventions have been published in a variety of refereed journals in nursing, medicine, and other interdisciplinary journals as well as in several consumer publications and programs. Her specific area of expertise is the reduction of child distress during pain using relaxation, distraction, and simple imagery. She is a member of the Nursing Science Study Section at the National Institutes of Health (1997-2001) and serves on several professional organization governing boards, including the Midwest Nursing Research Society and the Association for Care of Children's Health.

Martha Craft-Rosenberg, RN, PhD, FAAN, is a Professor at the University of Iowa College of Nursing. Her research interests are siblings and nursing diagnoses, interventions, and outcomes for families. She is coeditor of *Nursing Interventions for Infants and Children* (1990) and is coediting *Nursing Interventions for Childbearing and Childrearing Families,* to be published in 1998 by Sage.

Janet A. Deatrick, PhD, RN, FAAN, is an Associate Professor in the School of Nursing at the University of Pennsylvania, where she is also Program Director of the Nursing of Children Graduate Program. Her work and interest in the family began as a staff nurse in pediatric nursing and was cultivated during her master's and doctoral studies. Special interests are the day-to-day management by families who have children with chronic conditions and the contribution of qualitative research to further the understanding of that phenomenon. She received the Christian and Mary Lindback Award for Distinguished Teaching at the University of Pennsylvania in 1995 and in 1997 won the Excellence in Nursing Research Award given by the Society of Pediatric Nurses.

Janice Denehy, RN, PhD, is an Assistant Professor at the University of Iowa College of Nursing. Her research interests are developing nursing interventions for children and families, parenting, and children's knowledge of their bodies, health, and illness. She is coeditor of *Nursing Interventions for Infants and Children* (1990) and is coediting *Nursing Interventions for Childbearing and Childrearing Families,* to be published in 1998 by Sage.

Sandra A. Faux, PhD, RN, is an Associate Professor and Practitioner-Teacher in the Department of Maternal Child Nursing, College of Nursing at Rush University. Her current research interests focus on families, particularly well siblings, across the life span dealing with and caring for a family member with physical and/or cognitive chronic illness. A recent study included families of adults with developmental disabilities/mental retardation. She coedited with Kathleen Knafl a special edition of *Journal of Family Nursing* (May 1996) that focused on family health care professional relationships.

Suzanne L. Feetham, PhD, RN, FAAN, is currently Professor, Harriet Werley Research Chair, College of Nursing, at the University of Illinois at Chicago. Formerly she was Chief Office of Planning, Analysis and Evaluation (1990-1996) and Deputy Director (1993-1996), National Institute of Nursing Research, National Institutes of Health. She also served part-time as a professor of the Associated Faculty of the University of Pennsylvania, School of Nursing. As Director of Education and Research for Nursing and Patient Services at Children's National Medical Center in Washington, D.C., she directed a study on nursing patient classification systems that was replicated in four other children's hospitals and the ambulatory services of the U.S. Navy. She has also conducted a program of research of families of children with health problems.

Barbara B. Frink, PhD, RN, FAAN, is Director of Nursing Systems and Research at the Johns Hopkins Hospital and holds a faculty appointment at The Johns Hopkins School of Nursing. She has administrative oversight for nursing performance improvement, education, clinical research, systems research, and nursing informatics at the John Hopkins Hospital. She was a Special expert in Nursing Systems at the National Institute of Nursing Research at the National Institute of Health in 1993-1994, and Director of Nursing Research and Development a the Children's Hospital National Medical Center in Washington, D.C. for several years. She received her PhD in Nursing Administration from the University of Pennsylvania. She has published in the areas of nursing administration; outcomes, evaluation and quality measurement; nursing informatics; and health care technology assessment. Her research interests focus on clinical and economic outcomes for patients and systems in rapidly changing environments.

Mary Jo Gagan, RNCS, FNP, PhD, is Assistant Professor of Nursing at the University of Arizona College of Nursing, where she coordinates the Nurse Practitioner Options. She is interested in nurse practitioner performance and domestic violence and is conducting research on roles of nurse practitioners in a low-income housing program. She is also a family nurse practitioner at a campus health clinic.

Margaret Grey, DrPH, FAAN, CPNP, is the Independence Foundation Professor of Nursing and Associate Dean for Research and Doctoral Studies at the Yale School of Nursing, where she has been since January 1995. Prior to her appointment at Yale, she was Associate Professor of Nursing and Director of the Primary Care Graduate Program at the University of Pennsylvania, where she was also Chairperson of the Family and Community Health Division at the School of Nursing. She is a graduate of the University of Pittsburgh and Yale University and holds a doctorate in public health from Columbia University. Her research has focused on primary care of young people and on the natural history of adaptation to chronic illness in childhood, with an emphasis on children with diabetes mellitus. She also maintains a clinical practice working with children with diabetes and has authored over 54 data-based and clinical publications.

Laura L. Hayman, PhD, RN, FAAN, is the Carl W. and Margaret Davis Walter Professor in the Frances Payne Bolton School of Nursing at Case Western Reserve University. She received her BSN, MSN, and PhD in interdisciplinary studies in human development from the University of Pennsylvania. Her program of research has focused on cardiovascular health promotion and risk reduction in childhood and adolescence. She recently conducted a longitudinal twin-family study, funded by the National Institute of Nursing Research, designed to examine the genetic and environmental influences on biobehavioral risk factors for cardiovascular disease (CVD) during the school-age years, adolescence, and the transition between these two developmental phases. The results of this study indicated the importance of a developmental, family-based, profile approach to CVD prevention and provided direction for her current work focused on the early childhood and family origins of CVD. Recent publications have appeared in *Nursing Research, Annals of Behavioral Medicine,* and *Journal of Pediatric Nursing.*

Kathleen A. Knafl, PhD, is a Professor in the Department of Maternal Child Nursing and Executive Associate Dean of the College of Nursing at the University of Illinois at Chicago. She serves as director of the college's graduate program and is responsible for its Office of Research Facilitation. Her research interests focus on family response to childhood illness and disability. She has been especially interested in developing the concept of normalization to understand how families adjust to the challenges of chronic illness.

Susan B. Meister, PhD, RN, FAAN, is a member of Harvard's Working Group on Early Life and Adolescent Health Policy. As Director of Health Services Research at Children's Hospital in San Diego, she was the first director of the California Association of Children's Hospitals' six-hospital project to quantify clinical resource consumption in children's hospitals. She was the principal investigator of a joint project of Children's Hospital in San Diego and Children's Memorial Hospital in Chicago; the project tested the impact of innovations in care for children with chronic illnesses. She has served on technical advisory panels for the Health Care Financing Administration. Her research focuses on child health policies.

Karen F. Pridham, PhD, RN, FAAN, is a Professor at the University of Wisconsin–Madison School of Nursing and Department of Family Medicine. Her research focuses on health promotion in the context of the feeding both of children who are healthy and born at term and of very-low-birth-weight children. She is specifically interested in guided participation as a socially structured form of helping mothers develop caregiving competencies, such as those in relating to the child, in technical aspects of caregiving, and in problem solving and communicating with family members and clinicians. Her interests in interdisciplinary practice and research began in community health and primary care settings. She is currently affiliated with the University of Wisconsin Pediatric Pulmonary Center Interdisciplinary Education Project.

Sharon L. Sims, RNCS, PhD, is Associate Professor of Nursing and Chair of the Department of Family Health at Indiana University School of Nursing. She conducts research on families caring for technology-dependent children at home and has been published in *Western Journal of Nursing Research, Image,* and *Journal of Advanced Nursing.*

Barbara Velsor-Friedrich, PhD, R.N., is Associate Professor in the Department of Maternal Child Health Nursing at the Niehoff School of Nursing, Loyola University Chicago. She conducts research on pediatric chronic illness. Her current funded research project is on promoting self-care in African-American chidren with asthma. She is the co-editor of the child health policy column in the *Journal of Pediatric Nursing.*

Judith Vessey, PhD, RN, FAAN, is a Professor in The Johns Hopkins Univerity School of Nursing. Her research focuses on developmental and behavioral issues of children with chronic conditions. She has published widely and serves as associate editor for *Nursing Research* and on the editorial boards of *Pediatric Nursing* and *The Journal of Pediatric Nursing.*

JoAnne M. Youngblut, PhD, RN, FAAN, is Associate Professor in the Frances Payne Bolton School of Nursing at Case Western Reserve University. Her NIH-funded studies include the effects of maternal employment on premature children and the family effects of a preschooler's head trauma. She has published extensively in prestigious journals and is the founding editor of *Journal of the Society of Pediatric Nurses.*